Hepatitis B and D Protocols
Volume 1

METHODS IN MOLECULAR MEDICINE™

John M. Walker, Series Editor

99. **Pain Research:** *Methods and Protocols,* edited by *David Z. Luo, 2004*
98. **Tumor Necrosis Factor:** *Methods and Protocols,* edited by *Angelo Corti and Pietro Ghezzi, 2004*
97. **Molecular Diagnosis of Cancer:** *Methods and Protocols, Second Edition,* edited by *Joseph E. Roulston and John M. S. Bartlett, 2004*
96. **Hepatitis B and D Protocols:** *Volume 2, Immunology, Model Systems, and Clinical Studies,* edited by *Robert K. Hamatake and Johnson Y. N. Lau, 2004*
95. **Hepatitis B and D Protocols:** *Volume 1, Detection, Genotypes, and Characterization,* edited by *Robert K. Hamatake and Johnson Y. N. Lau, 2004*
94. **Molecular Diagnosis of Infectious Diseases,** *Second Edition,* edited by *Jochen Decker and Udo Reischl, 2004*
93. **Anticoagulants, Antiplatelets, and Thrombolytics,** edited by *Shaker A. Mousa, 2004*
92. **Molecular Diagnosis of Genetic Diseases,** *Second Edition,* edited by *Rob Elles and Roger Mountford, 2004*
91. **Pediatric Hematology:** *Methods and Protocols,* edited by *Nicholas J. Goulden and Colin G. Steward, 2003*
90. **Suicide Gene Therapy:** *Methods and Reviews,* edited by *Caroline J. Springer, 2004*
89. **The Blood–Brain Barrier:** *Biology and Research Protocols,* edited by *Sukriti Nag, 2003*
88. **Cancer Cell Culture:** *Methods and Protocols,* edited by *Simon P. Langdon, 2003*
87. **Vaccine Protocols,** *Second Edition,* edited by *Andrew Robinson, Michael J. Hudson, and Martin P. Cranage, 2003*
86. **Renal Disease:** *Techniques and Protocols,* edited by *Michael S. Goligorsky, 2003*
85. **Novel Anticancer Drug Protocols,** edited by *John K. Buolamwini and Alex A. Adjei, 2003*
84. **Opioid Research:** *Methods and Protocols,* edited by *Zhizhong Z. Pan, 2003*
83. **Diabetes Mellitus:** *Methods and Protocols,* edited by *Sabire Özcan, 2003*
82. **Hemoglobin Disorders:** *Molecular Methods and Protocols,* edited by *Ronald L. Nagel, 2003*
81. **Prostate Cancer Methods and Protocols,** edited by *Pamela J. Russell, Paul Jackson, and Elizabeth A. Kingsley, 2003*
80. **Bone Research Protocols,** edited by *Miep H. Helfrich and Stuart H. Ralston, 2003*
79. **Drugs of Abuse:** *Neurological Reviews and Protocols,* edited by *John Q. Wang, 2003*
78. **Wound Healing:** *Methods and Protocols,* edited by *Luisa A. DiPietro and Aime L. Burns, 2003*
77. **Psychiatric Genetics:** *Methods and Reviews,* edited by *Marion Leboyer and Frank Bellivier, 2003*
76. **Viral Vectors for Gene Therapy:** *Methods and Protocols,* edited by *Curtis A. Machida, 2003*
75. **Lung Cancer:** *Volume 2, Diagnostic and Therapeutic Methods and Reviews,* edited by *Barbara Driscoll, 2003*
74. **Lung Cancer:** *Volume 1, Molecular Pathology Methods and Reviews,* edited by *Barbara Driscoll, 2003*
73. ***E. coli*:** *Shiga Toxin Methods and Protocols,* edited by *Dana Philpott and Frank Ebel, 2003*
72. **Malaria Methods and Protocols,** edited by *Denise L. Doolan,* 2002
71. ***Haemophilus influenzae* Protocols,** edited by *Mark A. Herbert, Derek Hood, and E. Richard Moxon,* 2002
70. **Cystic Fibrosis Methods and Protocols,** edited by *William R. Skach,* 2002
69. **Gene Therapy Protocols,** *Second Edition,* edited by *Jeffrey R. Morgan,* 2002
68. **Molecular Analysis of Cancer,** edited by *Jacqueline Boultwood and Carrie Fidler,* 2002

METHODS IN MOLECULAR MEDICINE™

Hepatitis B and D Protocols

Volume 1: Detection, Genotypes, and Characterization

Edited by

Robert K. Hamatake, PhD

Johnson Y. N. Lau, MD

Ribapharm Inc., Costa Mesa, CA

Forewords by

Timothy M. Block, PhD and Baruch S. Blumberg, MD, PhD

T. Jake Liang, MD

Humana Press Totowa, New Jersey

999 Riverview Drive, Suite 208
Totowa, New Jersey 07512

www.humanapress.com

This publication is printed on acid-free paper. ∞
ANSI Z39.48-1984 (American Standards Institute) Permanence of Paper for Printed Library Materials.

Cover design by Patricia F. Cleary.

Cover illustration: HBV genome. Artwork supplied by Robert Hamatake, PhD. Background: Figure 1, Chapter 13, K. Abid and F. Negro.

Printed in the United States of America. 10 9 8 7 6 5 4 3 2 1

ISSN 1543-1894

Library of Congress Cataloging in Publication Data
Hepatitis B and D protocols / edited by Robert K. Hamatake, Johnson Y. N. Lau
p. ; cm. —(methods in molecular medicine; 95-96)
Includes bibliographical references and indexes.
Contents: v. 1. Detection, genotypes, and characterization—v. 2. Immunology, model systems, and clinical studies.
ISBN 1-58829-105-7 (v. 1 : alk. paper) E-ISBN 1-59259-669-X (v. 1) — ISBN 1-58829-108-1 (v. 2 : alk. paper) E-ISBN 1-59259-670-3 (v. 2)
1. Hepatitis B—Laboratory manuals. 2. Hepatitis B virus—Laboratory manuals. 3. Delta -associated agent—Laboratory manuals. 4. Delta infection—Laboratory manuals. I. Hamatake, Robert Kiyoshi, 1953– . II. Lau, Johnson Y. N. (Johnson Yiu-Nam). III. Series
[DNLM: 1. Hepatitis B. 2. Hepatitis D. WC 536 H53335 2004]
QR201.H46H43 2004
616.3'623-1–dc21 2003011624

To our wives, April T.G. Hamatake and Jane W.S. Fang-Lau, for their unfailing support, and our children, Kyle Hamatake, David Hamatake, Grace (Ling-Ling) Lau, Gillian (Gi-Gi) Lau, and Gabrielle (Ching-Ching) Lau, for keeping us rejuvenated.

Foreword

Despite the availability of an effective vaccine, there are still 400 million people, worldwide who are chronically infected with hepatitis B virus (HBV). For them, the vaccine, as currently applied, has no value. Given the possible consequences of HBV infection, the number of those chronically infected with HBV presents an enormous public health challenge. For example, the major etiology of hepatocellular carcinoma (HCC) is chronic infection with HBV. Although fifth in cancer incidence, worldwide, HCC/liver cancer is the third leading cause of cancer death. The high mortality associated with HCC arises because the disease is often detected late and is unresponsive to treatment. The number of deaths caused by PHCC is expected to rise over the next 20 years. Those chronically infected with HBV have a life risk of death to HCC of between 10 and 25%. Even the limited efficacy of drugs for the treatment of chronic HBV helps underscore the point that this disease is responsive to therapy. Drugs that target the polymerase (e.g., hepsera and lamivudine) and interferon alpha represent two distinct strategies and show that both conventional antiviral and immunotherapeutic approaches can be used in management. However, the current inventory of therapeutics is inadequate. Interferon alpha is of limited value, only parenterally available, and fraught with adverse reactions. The polymerase inhibitors are undermined by either a high frequency of resistance or, in the case of hepsera, additional concerns about toxicity. Other areas of concern also remain. There is still no reliable means of predicting disease outcome for chronic carriers, making early detection of liver disease and decisions about drug efficacy, as well as who should be treated and for how long, difficult. Moreover, tests for HBV DNA levels (and other markers) are often of dubious quantitative value. Because HBV patients are becoming more sophisticated and more demanding about these markers and many follow their viremia (DNA) levels like investors follow the Dow Jones Industrial values, it is essential that meaningful lab values be provided. The current vaccines are effective, but they are expensive, and escape mutants may be a problem waiting to happen.

Thus, without a doubt, more work needs to be done in all of the key areas of the management of HBV.

The good news is that there have been important advances. A clearer picture about the kinds of drugs that can be effective, their pathogenesis, and the development of research tools should facilitate the discovery process.

It is the matter of research tools that these volumes address. In an almost encyclopedic fashion, Hamatake and Lau have assembled a comprehensive, "how to" guide for the study of HBV. It is worth noting that many of the methods described will have value in the study of other viruses and liver diseases in general, despite being highly focused upon HBV.

This is a very practical resource, in every respect. In more than 40 chapters, leaders in the field who have "been there" have contributed step-by-step "programmed" approaches, telling the readers how to reproduce their findings. It is something of a users guide for do-it-yourselfers.

It is not an overstatement to write that nearly every aspect of HBV research is covered, section by section, virus detection through vaccine and drug development. Thus, *Hepatitis B and D Protocols* is likely to become as essential a resource to those studying HBV as was the fabled Maniatis series (published by Cold Spring Harbor Press) for Molecular Biology. It is certainly going to get a great deal of attention in the Hepatitis B Foundation labs, and, because of its value, we hope it is used in labs throughout the world. The more it is used, the more likely HBV research will be advanced.

Timothy M. Block, PhD
Professor and Director of the Jefferson Center
and Hepatitis B Foundation Laboratory
Thomas Jefferson University
and President, Hepatitis B Foundation
Doylestown, PA

Baruch S. Blumberg, MD, PhD
Nobel Laureate, 1976
Senior Adviser to the President of Fox Chase Cancer Center
and Professor of Medicine and Anthropology
University of Pennsylvania
Philadelphia, PA

Foreword

The identification of the "Australian antigen" by Dr. Blumberg, which was subsequently recognized to be the hepatitis B virus surface antigen, marks the discovery of an important pathogen for liver diseases. The virus was the first hepatitis virus discovered almost four decades ago. Despite the magnitude of the infection and the significant efforts by the scientific community, hepatitis B continues to be a global health problem affecting more than 350 million people worldwide. Many scientific milestones in basic and clinical research on hepatitis B had profound impact on this viral infection in the history of medicine: hepatitis B virus vaccine was introduced two decades ago; interferon alpha was approved for the treatment of chronic hepatitis B and two other antiviral drugs have also been approved; liver transplantation under high dose hepatitis B immunoglobulin coverage can now be offered to patients with end-stage hepatitis B related liver disease. These advances have also introduced new paradigms in our understanding of the fundamental concepts of viral infection in general. Certainly, more work looms ahead of us in order to ultimately conquer this viral infection. To equip the basic and clinical investigators with all the available tools is of utmost importance in this quest. As illustrated in this book, the marriage between basic science and clinical medicine is critical.

In the last few decades, we have witnessed the groundbreaking progress and the introduction of new clinical paradigms in hepatitis B virus infection. The next decade must underscore further application of our knowledge to translational research, bridging basic science and clinical medicine, and to capitalize on our understandings to conquer this viral infection. Undoubtedly, with all the scientific efforts contributed by many dedicated scientists and with our willingness to share knowledge, the common goal of improving human health by eradicating this virus can be achieved in this millennium.

T. Jake Liang, MD
Chief, Liver Diseases Section
NIDDK National Institutes of Health
Bethesda, MD

Preface

The 36 years since the identification of hepatitis B virus (HBV) in 1967 has seen the establishment of HBV virology as a rich and extensive field of science and the recognition of HBV as one of the top 10 leading causes of death in the world. There are an estimated 400 million people chronically infected with HBV worldwide with 20–30% of these projected to die from complications of chronic liver disease, including cirrhosis and liver cancer. Hepatitis delta virus (HDV) was first identified in 1980 as a novel transmissible agent distinct from HBV that requires the HBV envelope protein for its infectivity. HDV co-infection in chronic HBV patients is associated with a more severe disease outcome than those not co-infected. HBV and HDV infections represent a significant health burden to the worldwide community.

Despite the lack of an inflectable cell culture system, an enormous amount of information has been obtained on the virology and immunology of HBV and HDV infections. Modern molecular biological techniques and research with related viruses have enabled much of the HBV and HDV life cycle to be elucidated, leading to a number of therapeutic approaches for treating chronically infected patients. Innovative detection methods based on these findings and techniques have led to diagnostic and clinical monitoring assays of increasing sensitivity. However, our understanding of the viral life cycle and virus–host interactions is incomplete and will require much more research for a complete comprehension of the pathogenesis of disease caused by viral infection. Hepatitis B and D Protocols contains a collection of research techniques, divided into two volumes, used in the study of HBV and HDV. The authors represent a number of scientific disciplines, but share in common their interest in hepatitis research and their expertise in their respective areas. Although most of these techniques have been described in peer-reviewed journals, these chapters provide far more detail and are written so that investigators can use them as manuals. A few reviews are included in some specialized areas such as antiviral testing and the design of clinical trials. We hope that this compilation of techniques used in the different areas of HBV and HDV research will prove useful to scientists and encourage multidisciplinary approaches to their research, so that clinical investigators will find it beneficial for their understanding of the current HBV and HDV research.

We would like to take this opportunity to extend our gratitude to our teachers and friends: Dr. Zhi Hong, Dr. Maria Seifer, Dr. David Standring, Professor P. C. Wu, Professor C. L. Lai, Dr. H. J. Lin, Professor Roger Williams, and Dr. Graeme J. M. Alexander. Without their guidance and support, we would not have the opportunity of presenting this highly practical manual to you today.

Robert K. Hamatake, PhD
Johnson Yiu-Nam Lau, MD

Contents

Contributors

KARIM ABID • *Division of Gastroenterology and Hepatology, University Hospital, Geneva, Switzerland*

ANNA AYRES • *Victorian Infectious Diseases Reference Laboratory, North Melbourne, Australia*

ANGELINE BARTHOLOMEUSZ • *Victorian Infectious Diseases Reference Laboratory, North Melbourne, Australia*

ASHRAF A. BASUNI • *West of Scotland Specialist Virology Centre, Gartnavel General Hospital, Glasgow, Scotland, UK*

JÜRGEN BECK • *Department of Internal Medicine II / Molecular Biology, University Hospital Freiburg, Freiburg, Germany*

SCOTT BOWDEN • *Victorian Infectious Diseases Reference Laboratory, North Melbourne, Australia*

VOLKER BRUSS • *Department of Virology, University of Goettingen, Göttingen, Germany*

W. F. CARMAN • *West of Scotland Specialist Virology Centre, Gartnavel General Hospital, Glasgow, Scotland, UK*

JINAH CHOI • *Department of Molecular Microbiology and Immunology, Keck School of Medicine, University of Southern California, Los Angeles, CA*

HAU TIM CHUNG • *5/25 Anderson St., Chatswood NSW 2067 Australia*

SIJA DE GENDT • *Hepatitis Diagnostics Program, Innogenetics N.V., Ghent, Belgium*

JANE W. S. FANG • *Research and Development, Ribapharm, Inc, Costa Mesa, CA*

MARK A. FEITELSON • *Department of Pathology, Anatomy and Cell Biology, Thomas Jefferson University, Philadelphia, PA*

WOLFRAM H. GERLICH • *Institute of Medical Virology, Justus Liebig University, Giessen, Germany*

DIETER GLEBE • *Institute of Medical Virology, Justus Liebig University, Giessen, Germany*

HANS JÖRG HACKER • *Department of Virus Host Interactions, Deutsches Krebsforschungszentrum, Heidelberg, Germany*

JIANMING HU • *Department of Microbiology, Boston University School of Medicine, Boston, MA*

KATHY JACKSON • *Victorian Infectious Diseases Reference Laboratory, North Melbourne, Australia*

JELENA JURAS • *Hepatitis Diagnostics Program, Innogenetics N.V., Ghent, Belgium*

MICHAEL KANN • *Institute of Medical Virology, Justus Liebig University, Giessen, Germany*

MICHAEL M.C. LAI • *Department of Molecular Microbiology and Immunology, Keck School of Medicine, University of Southern California, Los Angeles, CA*

VICKY C. H. LAI • *Research and Development, Ribapharm, Inc, Costa Mesa, CA*

ROBERT E. LANFORD • *Department of Virology and Immunology, Southwest Foundation for Biomedical Research, San Antonio, TX*

JOHNSON Y. N. LAU • *Former Chief Executive Officer, Ribapharm Inc., Costa Mesa, CA*
JIE LI • *Department of Molecular Microbiology and Immunology, Keck School of Medicine, University of Southern California, Los Angeles, CA*
HSIANG JU LIN • *Falls Church, VA*
MARGARET LITTLEJOHN • *Victorian Infectious Diseases Reference Laboratory, North Melbourne, Australia*
JIE LIU • *Department of Pathology, Anatomy and Cell Biology, Thomas Jefferson University, Philadelphia, PA*
STEPHEN LOCARNINI • *Victorian Infectious Diseases Reference Laboratory, North Melbourne, Australia*
LISA LOTT • *Department of Virology and Immunology, Southwest Foundation for Biomedical Research, San Antonio, TX*
GEERT MAERTENS • *Hepatitis Diagnostics Program, Innogenetics N.V., Ghent, Belgium*
THOMAS B. MACNAUGHTON • *Department of Molecular Microbiology and Immunology, Keck School of Medicine, University of Southern California, Los Angeles, CA*
MARIA MILDENBERGER • *Department of Virus Host Interactions, Deutsches Krebsforschungszentrum, Heidelberg, Germany*
MICHAEL NASSAL • *Department of Internal Medicine II / Molecular Biology, University Hospital Freiburg, Freiburg, Germany*
FRANCESCO NEGRO • *Division of Clinical Pathology, University Hospital, Geneva, Switzerland*
MARIA GRAZI NIRO • *Department of Gastroenterology, Casa Sollievo della Sofferenza, San Giovanni Rotondo, FG, Italy*
LENA NOTVALL • *Department of Virology and Immunology, Southwest Foundation for Biomedical Research, San Antonio, TX*
JING-HSIUNG OU • *Department of Molecular Microbiology and Immunology, Keck School of Medicine, University of Southern California, Los Angeles, CA*
ANNEKE K. RANEY • *Research and Development, Ribapharm, Inc, Costa Mesa, CA*
MARIO RIZZETTO • *Department of Gastroenterology, University of Torino and Azienda Ospedaliera S. Giovanni, Battista, Torino, Italy*
CHARLES E. ROGLER • *Marion Bessin Liver Research Center, Department of Medicine, Albert Einstein College of Medicine, Bronx, NY*
ERWIN SABLON • *Hepatitis Diagnostics Program, Innogenetics N.V., Ghent, Belgium*
CLAUS H. SCHRÖDER • *Department of Virus Host Interactions, Deutsches Krebsforschungszentrum, Heidelberg, Germany*
FRED SHAPIRO • *Department of Medical Affairs, Innogenetics N.V., Ghent, Belgium*
CHIAHO SHIH • *Departments of Pathology, and Microbiology & Immunology, WHO Collaborating Center for Tropical Diseases and Sealy Center for Vaccine Developments, University of Texas Medical Branch, Galveston, TX*
ANTONINA SMEDILE • *Department of Gastroenterology , University of Torino and Azienda Ospedaliera S. Giovanni, Battista, Torino, Italy*
QIN SU • *Department of Pathology, Tangdu Hospital, The Fourth Military Medical University, Xi'an, China*

PEI-CHING TAI • *Center for Tropical Diseases, Department of Pathology, University of Texas Medical Branch, Galveston, TX*

JOHN E. TAVIS • *Department of Molecular Microbiology and Immunology, St. Louis University School of Medicine, St. Louis, MO*

SHUPING TONG • *The Liver Research Center, Rhode Island Hospital and Brown University School of Medicine, Providence, RI*

CHRISTIAN TRÉPO • *INSERM U271, 151 Cours Albert Thomas, 69003, Lyon, France*

STEPHAN URBAN • *Department of Molecular Virology, University of Heidelberg, Heidelberg, Germany*

ELS VAN ASSCHE • *Hepatitis Diagnostics Program, Innogenetics N.V., Ghent, Belgium*

ULRIKE WEND • *Institute of Medical Virology, Justus Liebig University, Giessen, Germany*

ZHENMING XU • *Department of Molecular Microbiology and Immunology, Keck School of Medicine, University of Southern California, Los Angeles, CA*

ERMEI YAO • *Department of Molecular Microbiology and Immunology, St. Louis University School of Medicine, St. Louis, MO*

TA-TUNG THOMAS YUAN • *Departments of Pathology, and Microbiology & Immunology, WHO Collaborating Center for Tropical Diseases and Sealy Center for Vaccine Developments, University of Texas Medical Branch, Galveston, TX*

STEFAN ZEUZEM • *Professor of Medicine, Department of Internal Medicine II, University Hospital, Homburg/Saar, Germany*

WEI ZHANG • *Department of Virus Host Interactions, Deutsches Krebsforschungszentrum, Heidelberg, Germany*

YANYAN ZHENG • *Department of Molecular Microbiology and Immunology, University of Southern California, Keck School of Medicine, Los Angeles, CA*

FABIEN ZOULIM • *INSERM U271, 151 Cours Albert Thomas, 69003, Lyon, France*

Contents for Volume 2

I

Detection of Viral Markers

1

Overview of Commercial HBV Assay Systems

Stefan Zeuzem

1. Introduction

Measurement of viral nucleic acid in serum is often a valuable adjunct to the management of viral infections *(1)*. In hepatitis B, tests for hepatitis B virus (HBV) DNA have been used widely (**Table 1**), but their interpretation and significance have yet to be defined. HBV DNA assays are limited by lack of standardization and variable sensitivity. Because HBV may circulate in serum at high levels (as high as 10^{10} virions/mL), direct molecular hybridization assays are capable of detecting HBV DNA in a high proportion of patients, particularly those with active disease and both HBsAg (hepatitis B surface antigen) and HBeAg (hepatitis B e antigen) in serum. Commercial assays comprise the liquid hybridization assay (Genostics™, Abbott Laboratories, Chicago, IL), the hybridization capture assay (Digene, HC II), and branched DNA (bDNA) signal amplification assay (Versant, Bayer Diagnostics). Furthermore, a quantitative polymerase chain reaction (PCR) assay for HBV DNA has been developed (Amplicor Monitor HBV, Roche Diagnostics); it detects HBV DNA in a higher proportion of patients with chronic hepatitis B and often yields positive results, even in HBsAg carriers without apparent disease.

2. HBV DNA Quantification Assays

2.1. Liquid Hybridization Assay

The Genostics HBV DNA assay was a liquid-phase molecular hybridization assay (**Fig. 1A**) that involved the hybridization of HBV genomic DNA to single-stranded ^{125}I-DNA probes in solution *(2,3)*. A sepharose column was used to separate the base-paired HBV DNA from the excess single-stranded ^{125}I-DNA, and the radioactivity in the column eluate was measured in a gamma counter. The radioactivity in each specimen was compared with that of positive and negative control standards, and results were expressed as picograms per milliliter (pg/mL). The test required 100 μL of serum for a single deter-

From: *Methods in Molecular Medicine, vol. 95: Hepatitis B and D Protocols, volume 1*
Edited by: R. K. Hamatake and J. Y. N. Lau © Humana Press Inc., Totowa, NJ

Table 1
Different Principles of HBV DNA Quantification

Signal amplification assays
Liquid hybridization
DNA–RNA hybridization
Branched DNA technology, bDNA
Target amplification assays
Polymerase chain reaction (PCR)
Transcription-mediated amplification (TMA)
Nucleic acid based amplification (NASBA)
Ligase chain reaction (LCR)

mination. The positive control standard included in the assay consisted of M13 phage containing the 3.2 kb HBV DNA genome (-) strand, quantified by plaque assays and diluted into HBV-negative human serum to a final concentration of 103 ± 10 pg DNA/mL **(2,4)**. The assay was applied in many clinical trials. Sales, however, were discontinued in 1999.

2.2. Branched DNA Assay

As a solid-phase sandwich assay based on bDNA technology **(Fig. 1B)**, the Bayer Versant (previously Chiron Quantiplex) assay involves the specific capture of HBV genomic DNA to microwells by hybridization to complementary synthetic oligonucleotide target probes *(5,6)*. Detection of the captured HBV DNA is accomplished through subsequent hybridization of bDNA amplifier molecules containing repeated nucleotide sequences for the binding of numerous alkaline phosphatase-modified label probes. Upon addition of a dioxetane substrate, the alkaline phosphatase-catalyzed light emission is recorded as luminescent counts on a plate-reading luminometer. Light emission is proportional to the amount of HBV DNA present in each specimen, and results are expressed as milliequivalents per milliliter (Meq/mL).

The assay requires two 10-μL aliquots of serum for each determination. Serum specimens are measured in duplicate, and the quantity of HBV DNA is determined from a standard curve included on the same plate for each assay run. Four assay standards, prepared by dilution of HBV DNA-positive human serum into HBV DNA-negative human serum, which cover a 4 $\log_{10}$ range in concentration from approx 0.4 to 4000 HBV DNA meq/mL, are included. The assay standards are value-assigned against the primary HBV DNA standard representing the entire HBV genome, subtype adw2, which is purified from recombinant plasmid and quantified using different independent analytical methods *(5,7)*.

2.3. DNA–RNA Hybridization

This assay uses an HBV–RNA probe to capture sample HBV DNA that has been rendered single-stranded **(Fig. 1C)**. These hybrids are then bound onto a solid phase with an anti-RNA–DNA hybrid antibody. This bound hybrid is reacted with antihybrid antibody, which has been conjugated to alkaline phosphatase and reacts with a chemiluminescent substrate. The light emitted is measured on a luminometer, and the concentration of HBV DNA is determined from a standard curve *(8,9)*.

Recently, a second-generation (HBV Digene Hybrid Capture II) antibody capture solution hybridization assay was developed ***(10)***. In this test, 30 μL of serum samples, controls, and standards or calibrators are incubated with a denaturation reagent. No additional sample preparation step is required. After preparation of the probe mixture, an HBV RNA probe is added to each well and incubated for 1 h. To capture the DNA–RNA hybrids, an aliquot of the solution in the microplates is transferred to the corresponding well of the anti-RNA–DNA hybrid antibody-coated capture microplate. The hybrid is detected using an antihybrid antibody conjugated to alkaline phosphatase and detected with a chemiluminiscent substrate. To enable detection of HBV DNA levels of less than 1.42×10^5 copies/mL, the ultrasensitive format of the assay is used. Here, 1-mL serum samples and controls along with 50 μL of precipitation buffer are centrifuged at 33,000*g* for 110 min at 4°C. The supernatant is discarded, and the precipitated virus is dissolved. This procedure yields a 30-fold increase in sensitivity ***(10)***.

2.4. Polymerase Chain Reaction

HBV DNA is isolated from 50 μL of serum by polyethylene glycol precipitation followed by virion lysis and neutralization. A known amount of quantitation standard is added into each specimen and is carried through the specimen preparation, amplification, and detection steps subsequently used for quantification of HBV DNA in the specimen **(Fig. 1D)**.

In the Amplicor Monitor HBV test a 104-bp segment of the highly conserved precore–core region is amplified by PCR by using one biotinylated primer and one nonbiotinylated primer ***(11,12)***. The quantitation standard is amplified with the same primers as target HBV. After 30 PCR cycles, HBV and quantitation standard are chemically denatured to form single-stranded DNA. The biotinylated amplicon is then captured on streptavidin-coated microwells and hybridized with HBV and internal standard-specific dinitrophenyl (DNP)-labeled oligonucleotide probes. Following an incubation with alkaline-phosphatase-conjugated anti-DNP antibodies and a colorimetric substrate, the amount of HBV DNA in each specimen is calculated from the ratio of the optical density for the HBV-specific well to the optical density for the quantitation-standard-specific well. The number of HBV DNA copies is calculated from a standard curve prepared from each amplification run. If the result exceeds 4.0×10^7 HBV DNA copies/mL, serum is diluted and retested.

The quantitative analysis of HBV DNA can be automated using the Cobas Amplicor Monitor HBV test. In this system, viral DNA is still manually extracted. Quantitative results of the Cobas Amplicor Monitor HBV test are interchangeable with measurements by the manual microwell plate version of Amplicor ***(13)***. Future systems will also automate extraction (e.g., Ampliprep), and fully automated analyzers will finally become available.

2.5. Other HBV DNA Quantification Assays

Other HBV DNA quantification systems comprise the transcription-mediated amplification (TMA)–based assay ***(14)***, the ligase-chain-reaction (LCR) assay ***(15)***,

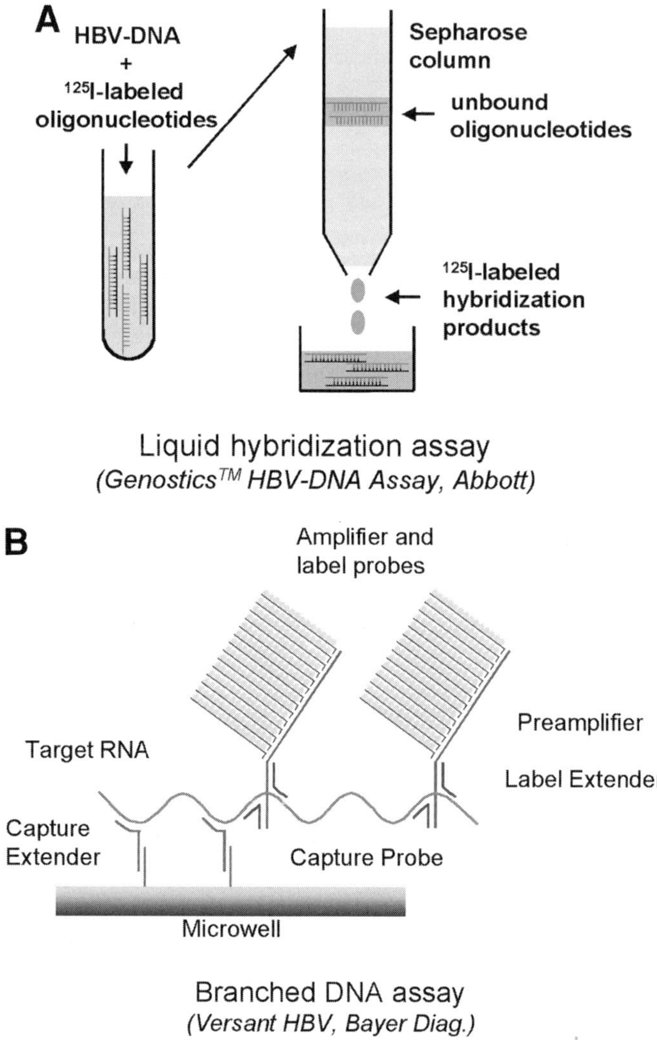

Fig. 1. Test principles of **(A)** Liquid hybridization assay (Genostics™ HBV-DNA Assay, Abbott Laboratories), **(B)** Branched DNA assay (Versant HBV, Bayer Diagnostics), **(C)** Hybrid Capture II Technology (Hybrid Capture™ II System, Digene), and **(D)** Polymerase chain reaction (Amplicor Monitor HBV, Roche Diagnostics).

the nucleic acid–based amplification (NASBA) assay ***(16)***, and various variations of the mentioned technologies ***(17–22)***. TMA-, LCR-, and NASBA-based assays for HBV DNA quantification are currently not commercially available in Europe or the United States.

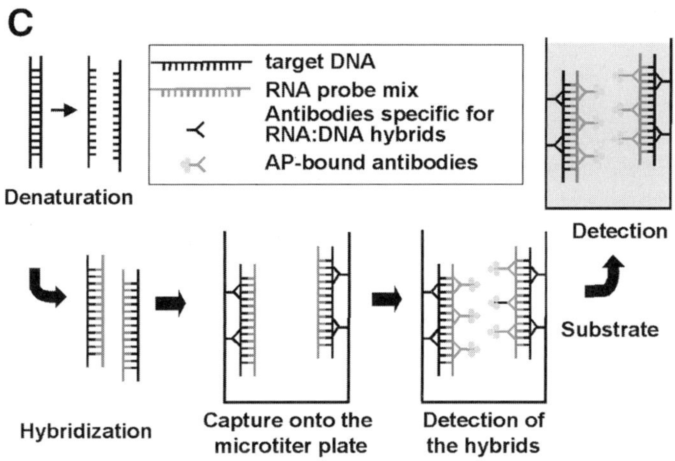

Hybrid Capture II Technology
(Hybrid Capture™ II System, Digene)

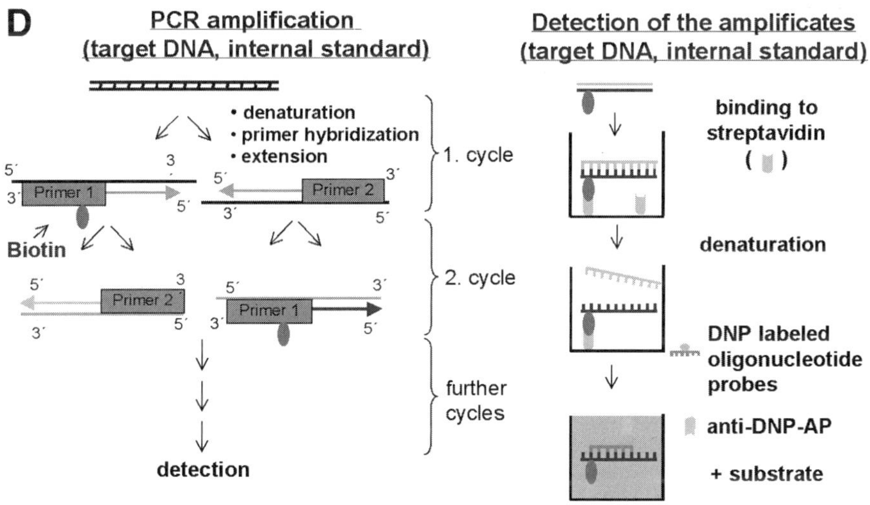

Polymerase chain reaction
(Amplicor Monitor HBV, Roche Diag.)

3. Sensitivity and Dynamic Range

Specimens tested with the liquid hybridization assay were considered positive for HBV DNA at 1.5% of the positive control standard quantification value, or approx 1.6 pg/mL *(3)*. The clinical quantification limit of the bDNA assay has been set at 0.7 HBV

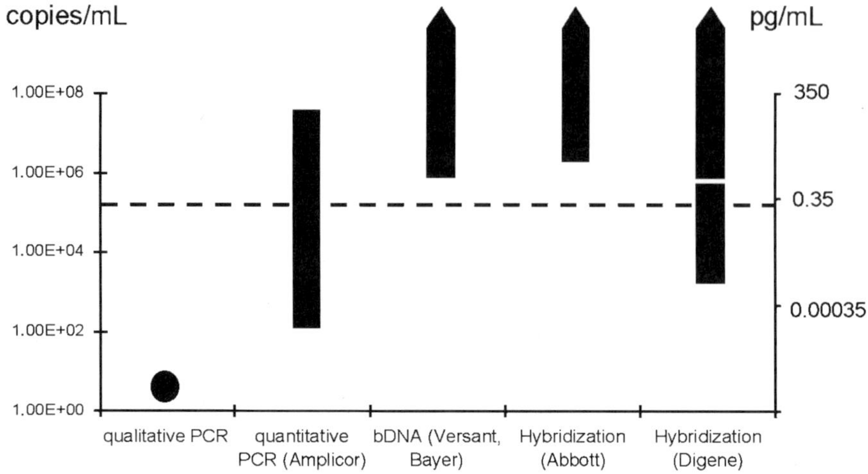

Fig. 2. Sensitivity and range of detection of different HBV DNA assays.

DNA meq/mL *(5)*. Similar to the HIV (Human Immunodeficiency Virus) or HCV (hepatitis C virus) RNA bDNA tests, sensitivity will be considerably improved in the next version of the assay. The lower detection limit of the HBV DNA–RNA hybridization capture assay in its ultrasensitive format is around 5000 copies/mL ***(10)***. The highest sensitivity of HBV DNA quantification assays, however, is achieved by the PCR-based assay (400 copies/mL) ***(13)*** **(Fig. 2)**. A limitation of this PCR assay is the relatively narrow linear range, requiring predilution of high-titer samples ***(13)***. These problems can be solved by real-time PCR detection assays based on TaqMan technology ***(21–23)***. All assay characteristics are summarized in **Table 2**.

4. Interassay Correlation Between HBV DNA Quantification Assays

The HBV DNA quantification values generated by the liquid hybridization assay are expressed as pg/mL. Values of the branched DNA assay are expressed as MEq/mL, and those of the DNA–RNA hybridization assay and the quantitative PCR are expressed as copies/mL.

For evaluation of the theoretical relationship between pg and MEq/copies, the following assumptions are required ***(24)***:

- HBV DNA comprises 3200 base pairs
- The molecular weight of a base pair is 666 g/mole
- Avogadro's number = 6.023×10^{23} molecules or copies mole.

According to the following calculations:

- 3200 base pairs × 666 g/mole = 2.13×10^{6} g/mole
- (6.023×10^{23} copies/mole)÷ (2.13×10^{6} g/mole) = 2.83×10^{17} copies/g

Table 2
Comparison of the Characteristics of Different HBV DNA Quantification Assays

	Liquid hybridization assay (Abbott Lab.)	Branched DNA assay (Bayer Diag.)	DNA-RNA hybridization assay (Digene II)	Polymerase chain reaction assay (Roche Molec. Systems)
Volume	100 μL	2 × 10 μL	30 μL/1 mL	50 μL
Sensitivity				
pg/mL	1.6	2.1	0.5 / 0.02	0.001
copies/mL	4.5×10^5	7×10^5	1.4×10^5 / 5×10^3	4×10^2
Linearity (copies/mL)	5×10^5–approx 10^{10}	7×10^5–5×10^9	2×10^5–1×10^9 5×10^3–3×10^6	4×10^2–1×10^7 *Cobas*: 10^6 *TaqMan*: 10^{10}
Genotype independence	D>A	A,B,C,D,E,F	A,B,C,D	(A),B,C,D,E
Coefficient of variation	12–22%	6–15%	10–15%	14–44%

- $(2.83 \times 10^{17}$ copies/g$) \div (1 \times 10^{12}$ g/pg$) = 2.83 \times 10^5$ copies/pg

The theoretical conversion equation is calculated as 1 pg/mL = 2.83×10^5 copies/mL = 0.283 meq/mL.

Several direct comparisons among different assays have been performed *(8,9,23–31)*. Conversion factors are summarized in **Fig. 3**. Large discrepancies were observed between the liquid hybridization assay and the other signal and target amplification systems. A good concordance exists between the DNA–RNA hybridization assay (Hybrid Capture II) System and the quantitative PCR detection assay (Amplicor Monitor HBV).

5. Standardization of HBV DNA Assays

Different extraction procedures of HBV DNA from serum generate different results in hybridization assays when compared with cloned DNA *(32)*. Because HBV contains viral polymerase covalently bound to genomic DNA, extraction procedures that remove protein from DNA extract the HBV DNA together with the polymerase. Proteinase K digestions of serum or plasma are often incomplete, and, thus, losses of HBV DNA occur during the subsequent phenol extraction. In contrast, lysis procedures without proteases do not remove a large amount of plasma protein, which may interfere with the assay. Cloned HBV DNA without covalently bound polymerase binds less efficiently to filters than does the virion-derived HBV polymerase/DNA complex in the presence of large amounts of plasma proteins. Thus, cloned HBV DNA cannot directly be used as a reference sample for virion-derived HBV DNA unless the polymerase and plasma protein have been carefully removed from the sample. Purity and quantity of cloned HBV DNA have to be assessed accurately.

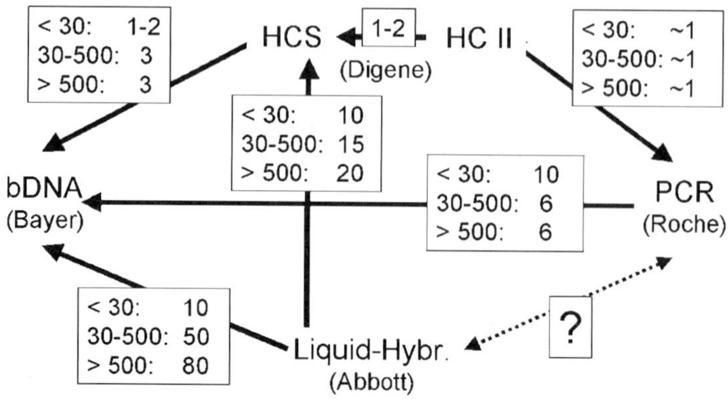

Fig. 3. Correlation between HBV DNA assays. Concentration ranges (< 30; 30–500; > 500) are given in pg/mL.

In view of these problems, the Eurohep Pathobiology Group decided to generate two reference plasma samples for HBV DNA. Plasma donations from two single, highly viremic carriers of HBV genotype A (HBV surface antigen subtype adw2) and genotype D (awy2/3), respectively, were collected, and the accurate number of HBV DNA molecules was determined (2.7×10^9 and 2.6×10^9 HBV DNA molecules/mL, respectively) ***(33)***. Genotypes A and D are predominant in Europe and North America. Pooling of donations from different HBV carriers was avoided because many infected patients carry antibodies against epitopes of heterologous HBV genotypes. This could cause aggregation of HBV and difficulties in testing of dilutions made from the reference samples. The two Eurohep reference plasma samples have already been used for the standardization of test kits ***(25)*** and in quality control trials ***(34)***, and the plasma from the carrier of genotype A will be the basis of a World Health Organization (WHO) reference sample.

6. Clinical Impact of HBV DNA Quantification

Quantitative detection of HBV DNA allows identification of patients with highly replicative hepatitis B who are HBeAg-negative ***(35)***. Furthermore, HBV DNA quantification in serum or plasma provides a means of measuring the viral load in patients before, during, and after antiviral therapy. There appears to be a level of HBV DNA below which hepatitis B is inactive and nonprogressive; this level may vary within the patient population and depending on the assay may be as high as 10^6 to as low as 10^4 copies mL ***(1,35)***. Nevertheless, cases with suppressed HBV activity, despite the very low levels of viremia, maintain a relatively high amount of intrahepatic viral genomes ***(36)***. The generation of treatment-resistant HBV mutants can be suspected when serum HBV DNA increases in patients during therapy. Furthermore, the level of HBV DNA makes it possible to estimate the potential infectivity of HBV-infected patients. Highly sensitive tests for HBV DNA are useful for detection of blood donors who express no serological markers and for detection of HBV in therapeutic plasma protein preparations *(37)*.

7. Conclusions

HBV DNA quantification assays suffer limitations in standardization. The liquid hybridization assay produced HBV DNA levels that are 10- to 80-fold lower than results reported from the bDNA assay and 10–20 times lower than the Digene Hybrid Capture assay. Different assays also have different linear ranges of accuracy. The introduction of the WHO HBV DNA standard will facilitate standardized quantification. In the future, a panel of standards for all HBV genotypes may be necessary to achieve genotype-independent HBV DNA quantification.

In view of the limitations surrounding viral assays, it is currently still difficult to assess the clinical significance of different levels of HBV DNA. Empirally, it appears that patients with an inactive carrier state generally have viral load of less than 10^5–10^6 copies/mL, whereas patients with an active carrier state exhibit HBV DNA levels above 10^5–10^6 copies/mL. High-sensitivity quantification of HBV DNA may particularly be clinically useful in the diagnosis of HBeAg-negative patients and for monitoring response to therapy. Careful assessment of the clinical implications of different viral levels using standardized reagents is much needed. In addition to HBV DNA quantification, clinical evaluation of HBV genotyping assays and molecular tests for specific mutations (pre-core, core promotor, surface, and polymerase) are required *(38)*.

References

1. Lok, A.S., Heathcote, E.J., Hoofnagle, J.H. (2001) Management of hepatitis B: 2000—summary of a workshop. *Gastroenterology* **120**, 1828–1853.
2. Kuhns, M.C., McNamara, A.L., Cabal, C.M., et al. (1988) A new assay for the quantitative detection of hepatitis B viral DNA in human serum. In: Zuckerman, A.J. (ed.) *Viral Hepatitis and Liver Disease*, Alan Liss, New York, 258–262.
3. Kuhns, M.C., McNamara, A.L., Perrillo, R.P., Cabal, C.M., and Campbel, C.R. (1989) Quantitation of hepatitis B viral DNA by solution hybridization: comparison with DNA polymerase and hepatitis B e antigen during antiviral therapy. *J. Med. Virol.* **27,** 274–281.
4. Kuhns, M., Thiers, V., Courouce, A., Scotto, J., Tiollais, P., and Bréchot, C. (1984) Quantitative detection of HBV DNA in human serum. In: Vyas, G., Dienstag, J., Hoofnagle, J. (eds.) *Viral Hepatitis and Liver Disease*, Grune and Stratton, Orlando, FL, 665–670.
5. Hendricks, D.A., Stowe, B.J., Hoo, B.S., et al. (1995) Quantitation of HBV DNA in human serum using a branched DNA (bDNA) signal amplification assay. *Am. J. Clin. Pathol.* **104,** 537–546.
6. Chen, C.H., Wang, J.T., Lee, C.Z., Sheu, J.C., Wang, T.H., and Chen, D.S. (1995) Quantitative detection of hepatitis B virus DNA in human sera by branched-DNA signal amplification. *J. Virol. Methods* **53,** 131–137.
7. Urdea, M.S. (1992) Theoretical aspects of nucleic acid standardization for HBV DNA detection. Report on the Sixth Eurohep Workshop, 3.1.2c.
8. Butterworth, L.-A., Prior, S.L., Buda, P.J., Faoagali, J.L., and Cooksley, G.E. (1996) Comparison of four methods for quantitative measurement of hepatitis B viral DNA. *J. Hepatol.* **24,** 686–691.

9. Pawlotsky, J.M., Bastie, A., Lonjon, I., et al. (1997) What technique should be used for routine detection and quantification of HBV DNA in clinical samples? *J. Virol. Methods* **65,** 245–253.
10. Niesters, H.G., Krajden, M., Cork, L., et al. (2000) A multicenter study evaluation of the digene hybrid capture II signal amplification technique for detection of hepatitis B virus DNA in serum samples and testing of EUROHEP standards. *J. Clin. Microbiol.* **38,** 2150–2155.
11. Kessler, H.H., Pierer, K., Dragon, E., et al. (1998) Evaluation of a new assay for HBV DNA quantitation in patients with chronic hepatitis B. *Clin. Diagn. Virol.* **9,** 37–43.
12. Gerken, G., Gomes, J., Lampertico, P., et al. (1998) Clinical evaluation and applications of the Amplicor HBV Monitor test, a quantitative HBV DNA PCR assay. *J. Virol. Methods* **74,** 155–165.
13. Noborg, U., Gusdal, A., Pisa, E.K., Hedrum, A., and Lindh, M. (1999) Automated quantitative analysis of hepatitis B virus DNA by using the Cobas Amplicor HBV Monitor test. *J.Clin. Microbiol.* **37,** 2793–2797.
14. Ide, T., Kumashiro, R., Hino, T., et al. (2001) Transcription-mediated amplification is more useful in the follow-up of patients with chronic hepatitis B treated with lamivudine. *Hepatol. Res.* **21,** 76–84.
15. Trippler, M., Hampl, H., Goergen, B., et al. (1996) Ligase chain reaction (LCR) assay for semi-quantitative detection of HBV DNA in mononuclear leukocytes if patients with chronic hepatitis B. *J. Viral Hepatitis* **3,** 267–272.
16. Yates, S., Penning, M., Goudsmit, J., et al. (2001) Quantitative detection of hepatitis B virus DNA by real-time nucleic acid sequence-based amplification with molecular beacon detection. *J. Clin. Microbiol.* **39,** 3656–3665.
17. Erhardt, A., Schaefer, S., Athanassiou, N., Kann, M., and Gerlich, W.H. (1996) Quantitative assay of PCR-amplified hepatitis B virus DNA using a peroxidase-labelled DNA probe and enhanced chemiluminescence. *J. Clin. Microbiol.* **34,** 1885–1891.
18. Lai, V.C., Guan, R., Wood, M.L., Lo, S.K., Yuen, M.F., and Lai, C.L. (1999) Nucleic acid-based cross-linking assay for detection and quantification of hepatitis B virus DNA. *J.Clin. Microbiol.* **37,** 161–164.
19. Cane, P.A., Cook, P., Ratcliffe, D., Mutimer, D., and Pillay, D. (1999) Use of real-time PCR and fluorimetry to detect lamivudine resistance-associated mutations in hepatitis B virus. *Antimicrob. Agents Chemother.* **43,** 1600–1608.
20. Defoort, J.P., Martin, M., Casano, B., Prato, S., Camilla, C., and Fert, V. (2000) Simultaneous detection of multiplex-amplified human immunodeficiency virus type 1 RNA, hepatitis C virus RNA, and hepatitis B virus DNA using a flow cytometer microsphere-based hybridization assay. *J. Clin. Microbiol.* **38,** 1066–1071.
21. Loeb, K.R., Jerome, K.R., Goddard, J., Huang, M., Cent, A., and Corey, L. (2000) High-throughput quantitative analysis of hepatitis B virus DNA in serum using the TaqMan fluorogenic detection system. *Hepatology* **32,** 626–629.
22. Chen, R.W., Piiparinen, H., Seppanen, M., Koskela, P., Sarna, S., and Lappalainen, M. (2001) Real-time PCR for detection and quantitation of hepatitis B virus DNA. *J. Med. Virol.* **65,** 250–256.
23. Pas, S.D., Fries, E., de Man, R.A., Osterhaus, A.D.M.E., and Niesters, H.G.M. (2000) Development of a quantitative real-time detection assay for hepatitis B virus DNA and comparison with two commercial assays. *J. Clin. Microbiol.* **38,** 2897–2901.
24. Kapke, G.E., Watson, G., Sheffler, S., Hunt, D., and Frederick, C. (1997) Comparison of the Chiron Quantiplex branched DNA (bDNA) assay and the Abbott Genostics solution hybridization assay for quantification of hepatitis B viral DNA. *J. Viral Hepat.* **4,** 67–75.

25. Zaaijer, H.L., ter Borg, F., Cuypers, H.T., Hermus, M.C., and Lelie, P.N. (1994) Comparison of methods for detection of hepatitis B virus DNA. *J. Clin. Microbiol.* **32,** 2088–2091.
26. Khakoo, S.I., Soni, P.N., and Dusheiko, G.M. (1996) A clinical evaluation of a new method for HBV DNA quantitation in patients with chronic hepatitis B. *J. Med. Virol.* **50,** 112–116.
27. Hwang, S.J., Lee, S.D., Lu, R.H., et al. (1996) Comparison of three different hybridization assays in the quantitative measurement of serum hepatitis B virus DNA. *J. Virol. Methods* **62,** 123–129.
28. Krajden, M., Minor, J., Cork, L., and Comanor, L. (1998) Multi-measurement method comparison of three commercial hepatitis B virus DNA quantification assays. *J. Viral Hepat.* **5,** 415–422.
29. Ho, S.K.N., Chan, T.M., Cheng, I.K.P., and Lai, K.N. (1999) Comparison of the second-generation Digene hybrid capture assay with the branched DNA assay for measurement of hepatitis B virus DNA in serum. *J. Clin. Microbiol.* **37,** 2461–2465.
30. Pawlotsky, J.M., Bastie, A., Hezode, C., et al. (2000) Routine detection and quantification of hepatitis B virus DNA in clinical laboratories: performance of three commercial assays. *J. Virol. Methods* **85,** 11–21.
31. Chan, H.L., Leung, N.W., Lau, T.C., Wong, M.L., and Sung, J.J. (2000) Comparison of three different sensitive assays for hepatitis B virus DNA in monitoring of responses to antiviral therapy. *J. Clin. Microbiol.* **38,** 3205–3208.
32. Gerlich, W.H., Heermann, K.-H., Thomssen, R., and the Eurohep Group (1995) Quantitative assays for hepatitis B virus DNA: standardization and quality control. *Viral Hep. Rev.* **1,** 53–57.
33. Heermann, K.-H., Gerlich, W.H., Chudy, M., Schaefer, S., Thomssen, R., and the Eurohep Pathobiology Group (1999) Quantitative detection of hepatitis B virus DNA in two international reference plasma preparations. *J. Clin. Microbiol.* **37,** 68–73.
34. Quint, W.G., Heijtink, R.A., Schirm, J., Gerlich, W.H., and Niesters, H.G. (1995) Reliability of methods for hepatitis B virus DNA detection. *J. Clin. Microbiol.* **33,** 225–228.
35. Lindh, M., Horal, P., Dhillon, A.P., and Norkrans, G. (2000) Hepatitis B virus DNA levels, precore mutations, genotypes and histological activity in chronic hepatitis B. *J. Viral Hepat.* **7,** 258–267.
36. Cacciola, I., Pollicino, T., Squadrito, G., et al. (2000) Quantification of intrahepatic hepatitis B virus (HBV) DNA in patients with chronic HBV infection. *Hepatology* **31,** 507–512.
37. Otake, K., and Nishioka, K. (2000) Nucleic acid amplification testing of hepatitis B virus. *Lancet* **355,** 1460.
38. Hunt, C.M., McGill, J.M., Allen, M.I., and Condreay, L.D. (2000) Clinical relevance of hepatitis B viral mutations. *Hepatology* **31,** 1037–1044.

2

Detection of HBV DNA in Serum Using a PCR-Based Assay

Hau Tim Chung

1. Introduction

Detection of minute amounts of hepatitis B virus (HBV) DNA in the serum using polymerase chain reaction (PCR)–based assay involves extracting the viral DNA from the viral particle in the serum, removing inhibitors of PCR, performing the PCR, and detecting the PCR product. PCR is an extremely sensitive assay, and preventing cross contamination is an important part of the assay.

1.1. HBV DNA Extraction from Viral Particles and Removal of Inhibitor of PCR

HBV DNA in viral particles in serum is covered by a coat of hepatitis B core antigen (HBcAg) particles and a lipid coat with hepatitis B surface antigen (HBsAg) in it. Removal of the HBcAg and the HBsAg with the lipid coat can be easily accomplished by treatment with a detergent or alkali. However, there are many inhibitors of the PCR reaction in the serum. Deproteinization removes most of these inhibitors and it forms the basis of the procedure being described and used by the author. Alternatively, PCR can also be performed from DNA extracted directly from serum.

1.1.1. Proteinase K/Phenol/Phenol Chloroform/Ethanol Precipitation

Extraction of HBV DNA from serum is a tedious procedure, and its yield is variable, which directly affects the sensitivity or detection limit of the assay. Moreover, each step in the procedure creates a risk for cross contamination. However, it will also serve as a concentration method. The sensitivity of the assay can be improved by simply increasing the amount of serum used for the extraction. The volume limit of the actual PCR, which is a result of the need to change the temperature at a rapid pace, does not count here. The negative strand of the HBV DNA molecule is covalently bound to a small piece of protein, and thus the whole molecule may stay in the interface if the proteinase K digestion is not performed well. This is one of the many problems that affect the yield

From: *Methods in Molecular Medicine, vol. 95: Hepatitis B and D Protocols, volume 1*
Edited by: R. K. Hamatake and J. Y. N. Lau © Humana Press Inc., Totowa, NJ

in HBV DNA extraction using proteinase K/phenol/phenol chloroform/ethanol precipitation. In a well-digested specimen, the interface between the aqueous and phenol phase should be almost nonexistent. The presence of any significant amount of interface will drastically reduce the yield and thus affects the detection limit of the assay.

1.1.2. Alkali Denaturization

PCR can also be performed using neat deproteinized serum that has been treated with a denaturing agent to release the nucleic acid from the lipid and protein coat. Proteinase K digestion is one of the methods for removing protein, but this process can also be achieved by alkali treatment of the serum and heat denaturing of the protein. PCR can be performed in the same tube with the denatured protein spun down. This method reduces dramatically the number of steps needed in the procedure and saves time, labor, and cost. More important, fewer steps and tube changes also reduce the risk of cross contamination.

1.2. Performing PCR and Detection of Its Products

PCR can be performed in the standard way using the deproteinized neat serum. When two sequential PCR steps of 30 cycles each are used with two sets of nested primers, the level of DNA can be amplified from as low as one molecule to a level that can easily be detected using ethidium bromide staining of a polyacrylamide gel. This method is much easier and less expensive than using a more sensitive detection method, such as Southern blotting, to detect a smaller amount of product from a single round of 30-cycle PCR. The turnaround time of the protocol described below is within one working day, compared with at least five for PCR-Southern blotting. It also removes the need to work with radioisotopes.

1.2.1. Choice of Primers

All published sequences of the hepatitis B virus ***(1–10)*** were aligned using a computer program. The HBV sequences have a reasonably conserved sequence among various isolates. There are only a few regions with significant variations: 851–999, 1977–2203, 2513–2815, and 2852–57 (HBV DNA sequence numbering system is according to Galibert et al. **[1]**). Regions of fewer than 300 base pairs in length of highly conserved regions were deemed suitable to be amplified using PCR and will achieve a high yield. This region has to be framed by two pairs of perfectly conserved short sequences, each about 20 nucleotides long, to be used as pairs of nested primers. One set of nested pairs of primers was chosen from the surface-antigen-coding region and another from the core-coding region. Running two PCR's for each specimen using two different sets of nested primers reduces the theoretical risk of variant viruses failing to be detected if one of the primers does not match the target sequence. It may also pick up cases of false-positive results caused by inadvertent cross contamination by PCR products from previous reactions.

1.2.2. Sequence of the Chosen Primers

Nested primer sets for surface-antigen-coding region:

Primer set for first PCR:

Primer 1: CCTGCTGGTGGCTCGAGTTC (58–77)
Primer 2: CAAACGGGCAACATACCTTG (486–467)

Primer set for the second PCR:
Primer 3: ACATCAGGATTCCTAGGACC (169–188)
Primer 4: CGCAGACACATCCAGCGATA (389–370)

These sets of primers used in a nested PCR will give a product of 221 base pairs in length.

Nested primer sets for the core-antigen-coding region:
Primer set for the first PCR:
Primer 5: GGAGTGGGATTCGCACTCC (2269–2288)
Primer 6: ATACTAACATTGAGATTCCC (2457–2438)

Primer set for the second PCR:
Primer 7: AGACCACCAAATGCCCCTAT (2299–2318)
Primer 8: GATCTTCTGCGACGCGGCGA (2429–2410)

These sets of primers used in a nested PCR will give a product of 131 or 137 base pairs in length, depending on the subtype of the HBV target.

1.3. Prevention of Cross Contamination

Cross contamination can be caused by HBV DNA present in the laboratory environment, on bench tops, on utensils, and as aerosol within the piston mechanism of pipetting instruments left from previous experiments performed in the same laboratory. More important, PCR products are short DNA sequences that can survive in the environment for a long period and are potential target sequences that will give a positive result in an assay. The number of copies of these PCR products totals millions- to trillions-fold that of HBV DNA handled in a clinical specimen and thus has a much higher risk of cross contamination. The following steps are used to reduce the chance of cross contamination:

1. Most instruments should be used only once when collecting a blood specimen from the subject. They include needles, needle holders, specimen tubes, and syringes. Gloves should be changed in between subjects, and extra care should be taken to avoid soiling of the tourniquet by blood.
2. Care should be taken to avoid contamination of the laboratory environment or cross contamination when centrifuging blood and separating serum from the specimen. Serum should be sucked out using a single-use Pasteur pipet with bulbs attached. Reusable bulbs cannot be used.
3. Consideration in avoiding cross contamination should be observed in storing specimens for future analyses, when thawing the specimen, and when aliquoting specimens for assay. Serum should not be stored in Eppendorf tubes with flip-open lids. Tiny amounts of serum always get into the lid when it is inverted for mixing after thawing and contaminate the glove

used to open it. Serum should be stored in screw-top tubes designed in such a way that serum will not get onto the glove when it is handled, inverted for mixing, or opened.

4. Procedures before PCR should be physically isolated from those after PCR. Ideally, they should be performed on different benches using different sets of instruments, in particular, pipettors. Gloves should be changed in between handling samples in the steps before and after PCR.
5. All solutions should be prepared using single-use utensils. They are prepared in large lots, aliquoted to portions sufficient for a single run, and stored in a refrigerator or freezer until used. Unused portions are discarded. The only exception to this rule is the *Taq* polymerase enzyme. It is added into the PCR mix just before it is dispensed into the reaction tube.
6. All pipetting should be performed using either a positive displacement pipet (Microman, Gilson, France) or an ordinary pipettor with filtered pipet tips (United States Biochemical Corps., Cleveland, OH, USA). This approach was found to be the single most important step in preventing cross contamination, with the vast majority of cases containing aerosol contaminations.
7. All PCR products should be disposed of carefully to avoid contaminating the laboratory environment. The protocol described in the following paragraphs used a minimum number of steps, a minimum number of pipettings, and a minimum number of tubes. Pipet tips, Eppendorf tubes, electrophoresis apparatus, the polyacrylamide gel, and the ultraviolet (UV) light box used to view the gel are potential sources of PCR products that could cause cross contamination. Eppendorf tubes are disposed of with lids closed, and pipet tips and gel are disposed of carefully, making sure the bench top and environment are not contaminated. Electrophoresis solutions are discarded carefully into the sink and flushed with ample amounts of water. The electrophoresis apparatus is washed with plenty of water. The UV light box can be wiped with 1 *N* HCl and neutralized with 1 *M* Tris-HCl pH 7 5 minutes later. Gloves are changed after handling these steps.

2. Materials

1. 1 *N* NaOH.
2. Tris-HCl/HCl: mixture of equal volume of 2 *M* Tris HCl, pH 8.3 and 2 *N* HCl.
3. PCR mix 1–2: 12.5 m*M* Tris-HCl, pH 8.3, 62.5 m*M* KCl, 1.875 m*M* $MgCl_2$, 250 μ*M* each of the four deoxyribonucleotides (dATP, dTTP, dCTP, and dGTP), 1.25 μM each of primer 1 and primer 2.
4. PCR mix 3–4: same as PCR mix 1–2, but use primer 3 and primer 4 instead of primer 1 and primer 2.
5. PCR mix 5–6: same as PCR mix 1–2, but use primer 5 and primer 6 instead of primer 1 and primer 2.
6. PCR mix 7–8: same as PCR mix 1–2, but use primer 7 and primer 8 instead of primer 1 and primer 2.
7. *Taq* polymerase enzyme.
8. 6X loading buffer: 15% Ficoll 400/0.15% bromphenol blue.

3. Methods

The following protocol utilizing alkali denaturization was used regularly by the author and will work, except if the specimen is heavily hemolyzed before separation ***(11–14)***.

1. Serum has to be separated from the blood specimen in a timely fashion to avoid hemolysis.
2. Put 10 μL of serum into a 500-μL Eppendorf tube.

3. Add 1 μL of 1 *N* NaOH solution.
4. Cover with 10 μL of mineral oil.
5. Heat to 37°C for 1 hour.
6. Add 1 μL of Tris-HCl/HCl. Care has to be taken that the solution is added into the aqueous phase of the tube and is not floating on the top of the mineral oil layer as a result of surface tension.
7. Heat to 98°C for 5 min, Protein will be denatured and come out of the solution as a yellowish precipitate.
8. Centrifuge in a microcentrifuge for 5 min. The denatured protein precipitate will stay in the bottom of the tube and will not interfere with the subsequent reaction.
9. Add *Taq* polymerase enzyme into a volume of PCR mix 1–2 just enough for the total number of tubes in the run. The final amount of enzyme should be 2.5 U per 40 μL of PCR mix.
10. Add 40 μL of solution from step 9 into the aqueous phase of specimen in step 8. There is no need for mixing, and care has to be taken not to disturb the protein precipitate at the bottom of the tube.
11. Put the Eppendorf tube into a PCR machine.
12. Run 30 cycles of PCR, each consisting of 54 seconds at 94°C, 1 minute at 50°C, and 1 minute at 72°C.
13. When PCR in step 12 is about to finish, add *Taq* polymerase enzyme into a volume of PCR mix 3–4 just enough for the total number of tubes in the run. The final amount of enzyme should be 2.5 U per 40 μL of PCR mix.
14. Set up the same number of Eppendorf tubes as the number of specimens run in step 2. Fill each of them with 40 μL of solution from step 13 and cover with 10 μL of mineral oil.
15. Pipet 10 μL of the PCR product from step 12 into each of the tubes from step 14.
16. Run 30 cycles of PCR, each consisting of 54 seconds at 94°C, 1 minute at 50°C, and 1 minute at 72°C.
17. Add 10 μL 6X loading buffer into each tube. Mix by pipetting and load 10 μL into a 5% polyacrylamide gel using the same pipet tip. Run electrophoresis and stain with ethidium bromide. Lanes with staining at 221 base pairs are positive.
18. Each run should include negative and positive controls. The positive control is made by diluting a positive serum with a known amount of hepatitis B virus (determined using dot blot hybridization) using a negative serum. The concentration of the positive control should be about 1–2 molecules of HBV DNA (the author used the equivalent of about 5×10^{18} g HBV DNA) per 10 μL.
19. The above steps are also run using the core protein-coding region primers by substituting PCR mix 1–2 in step 9 with PCR mix 5–6 and PCR mix 3–4 in step 13 with PCR mix 7–8. In step 17, lanes with staining at 131 or 137 base pairs are positive.
20. One way of controlling for the absence of PCR inhibitors in each specimen is to run a positive control for each specimen by spiking it with a known positive serum.

References

1. Galibert, F., Mandart, E., Fitoussi, F., Tiollais, P., and Charnay, P. (1979) Nucleotide sequence of the hepatitis B virus genome (subtype ayw) cloned in *E. coli. Nature* **281**, 646–650.
2. Pasek, M., Goto, T., Gilbert, W., et. al. (1979) Hepatitis B virus genes and their expression in *E. coli. Nature* **282**, 575–579.
3. Valenzuela, P., Gray, P., Quiroga, M., Zaldivar, J., Goodman, H. M., and Rutter, W. J. (1979) Nucleotide sequence of the gene coding for the major protein of hepatitis B virus surface antigen. *Nature* **280**, 815–819.

4. Valenzuela, P., Quiroga, M., Zalvidar, J., Gray, P., Rutter, W. J. (1980) The nucleotide sequence of the hepatitis B viral genome and the identification of the major viral genes. In: Fields, B.N., Jaenisch, R. (eds.) *Animal Virus Genetics*, 57–70.
5. Ono, Y., Onda, H., Sasada, R., Igarashi, K., Sugino, Y., and Nishioka, K. (1983) The complete nucleotide sequences of the cloned hepatitis B virus DNA: subtype adr and adw. *Nucleic Acids Res.* **11**, 1747–1757.
6. Fujiyama, A., Miyanohara, A., Nozaki, C., Yoneyama, T., Ohtomo, N., and Matsubara, K. (1983) Cloning and structural analyses of hepatitis B virus DNAs, subtype adr. *Nucleic Acids Res.* **11**, 4601–4610.
7. Pumpen, P. P., Kozlovskaya, T. M., Borisova, G. L., et al. (1984) Synthesis of the surface antigen of hepatitis B virus in *Escherichia coli. Dokl. Biochem. Sect.* **271**, 246–249.
8. Kobayashi, M., and Koike, K. (1984) Complete nucleotide sequence of hepatitis B virus DNA of subtype adr and its conserved gene organization. *Gene* **30**, 227–232.
9. Bichko, V., Dreilina, D., Pushko, P., Pumpen, P., and Gren, E. (1985) Subtype ayw variant of hepatitis B virus. *FEBS Lett.* **185**, 208–212.
10. Lo, S. J., Chen, M.-L., Chien, M.-L., and Lee, Y.-H.W. (1986) Characteristics of pre-S2 region of hepatitis B virus. *Biochem. Biophys. Res. Commun.* **135**, 382–388.
11. Chung, H.T., Lai, C.L., and Lok, A.S.F. (1989) Hepatitis B virus has an etiological role in the pathogenesis of cirrhosis in patients positive for anti-HBs or anti-HBc. *Hepatology* **10**, 577.
12. Chung, H.T., Lok, A.S.F., and Lai, C.L. (1993) Re-evaluation of alpha-interferon treatment of chronic hepatitis B using polymerase chain reaction. *J. Hepatol.* **17**, 208–214.
13. Chung, H.T., Lee, J.S.K, and Lok, A.S.F. (1993) Prevention of post-transfusion hepatitis B and C by screening for antibody to hepatitis C virus and antibody to hepatitis B core antigen. *Hepatology* **18**, 1045–1049.
14. Chung, H.T., Lai, C.L., and Lok, A.S.F. (1995) Pathogenic role of hepatitis B virus in hepatitis B surface antigen negative cirrhosis. *Hepatology* **22**, 25–29.

3

Detection of HBV DNA by Oligonucleotide Probing

Hsiang Ju Lin

1. Introduction

Hepatitis B virus (HBV) DNA is present in the blood of patients with acute or chronic HBV infection at concentrations representing up to hundreds of millions of virions per milliliter of plasma. Detection of HBV DNA was feasible, if not particularly sensitive, even before development of methods based on the polymerase chain reaction (PCR).

The procedure described in this chapter was published in 1987 *(1)*. It makes use of a specific oligonucleotide labeled with ^{32}P. Detection is carried out by means of radioautography. This method is useful for detection of hepatitis B viremia in studies where quantification of the viral load is not critical. It is particularly suited for screening large numbers of samples for the presence of HBV DNA. The methodology can be adapted for other applications. For example, some HBV variants could be detected using similar methodology with other HBV-specific primers *(2)*.

The chief advantage of employing the oligonucleotide probe is that it is simpler to prepare, compared with HBV DNA probes. The oligonucleotide probe was as sensitive as nick-translated HBV DNA for the detection of HBV DNA in serum **(Fig. 1)**. Furthermore, hybridization time could be reduced because short oligonucleotide probes anneal more rapidly to their targets than do DNA probes. Hybridization of the oligonucleotide probe to patient samples could be as short as 2 h, compared with 16 h for the DNA probe *(1)*.

The principle of the method is simple. With appropriate choices of temperature and medium for different steps in membrane processing, an HBV-specific oligonucleotide will hybridize specifically to HBV DNA in the sample. Under the correct conditions, other nucleic acids that may be present in the sample, such as human DNA or nucleic acids from other viruses, do not hybridize to the sample because they do not possess sites complementary to the probe sequence.

From: *Methods in Molecular Medicine, vol. 95: Hepatitis B and D Protocols, volume 1*
Edited by: R. K. Hamatake and J. Y. N. Lau © Humana Press Inc., Totowa, NJ

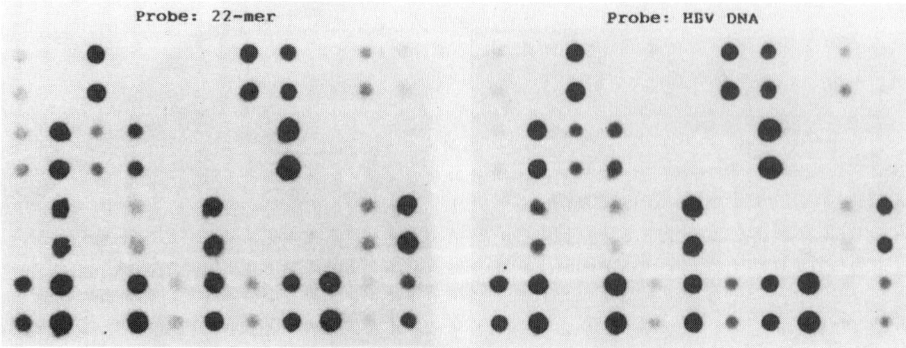

Fig. 1. Similarity of radioautograms obtained with oligonucleotide and HBV DNA probes. A set of 48 serum samples was applied in duplicate to two nylon membranes that were tested with the different probes. The concentrations per mL were: 10^7 dpm, about 10 ng (1.4 pmol) of oligonucleotide probe, and 5×10^6 dpm, 2.5 ng (1.25 fmol) HBV DNA. Hybridization and exposure times were 16 and 22 hours, respectively, for both probes. Reprinted from Lin, H. J., Wu, P. C., and Lai, C. L. (1987). An oligonucleotide probe for the detection of hepatitis B virus DNA in serum. *J. Virol. Method.* **15,** 139–149. Copyright (1987) with permission from Elsevier Science.

However, several conditions must be met. The choice of oligonucleotide is paramount. Ideally, it must be conserved across all HBV sequences. It is not difficult to locate conserved sequences in the HBV genome; they can be found predominantly in the S, pre-core, and core genes. Originally, the choice of oligonucleotide was based on analysis of only five complete HBV genomes representing the serotypes *adr*, *adw*, and *ayw* ***(1)***. A 21-nucleotide sequence homologous to the S-strand sequence in positions 1584–1604 (*Eco*RI site, ***1***) was conserved across these genomes. The choice proved to be sound, even with the inclusion of nine more genomes, including serotype *ayr* ***(3)***.

A recent search of complete human HBV genomes recorded in GenBank showed conservation of the selected 21-nucleotide sequence across 168 of the latest 173 entries, comprising genotypes A through G ***(4)***. Overall, the oligonucleotide was 97% conserved among 187 complete genomes. Point mutations (G → C, C → T, and T → C) were present in three isolates ***(5–7)***, and the sequence was absent from two HBV variants bearing 76- and 338-bp deletions in the X gene ***(8)***.

A BLAST search through current databases showed the probe sequence to be in some duck hepatitis B viruses and in orangutan hepadnavirus but not in woolly monkey hepatitis B virus ***(9)***. The search failed to reveal the presence of the 21-nucleotide sequence in human DNA, with two exceptions: It was present in human liver specimens where the HBV DNA was integrated into the human genome ***(9,10)***.

Aside from the high degree of conservation associated with the sequence, its location on the HBV genome was noteworthy. The HBV genome consists of two linear DNA strands of unequal length that form a partially doubled-stranded circle with a single-stranded gap. The selected oligonucleotide was complementary to the L-strand region that typically is found in the single-stranded form. Thus, the probe would hybridize to HBV DNA in the sample, even if denaturation (separation of the long and short strands) were incomplete.

The pitfalls in this procedure are common to many techniques that are based on hybridization of a probe to membrane-bound samples. Molecules of the oligonucleotide probe can and probably would interact with the membrane if they were allowed to, producing a useless autoradiogram that was the image of the membrane. Several steps in the procedure are performed to reduce nonspecific binding, i.e., the use of specific reagents for treating the membrane, hybridization, and washing.

Figure 2 illustrates the necessity of using the correct temperature and medium for washing the probed membrane. The figure brings up a second point. Trapping of nucleic acids on the membrane depended on the presence of the serum matrix. Purified DNA (from HBV or salmon) did not adhere to the membrane unless it was first mixed with serum. In summary, the interactions of nucleic acids or oligonucleotides with the membrane are highly dependent on the choice of temperature and on the presence of salts and macromolecules.

2. Materials

2.1. Specimen Handling (see Note 1)

Serum samples should be promptly separated and stored at –70°C. They may be subjected to several freeze–thaw cycles.

2.2. Membrane Filters

Nitrocellulose and nylon membranes have been used for this technique. Nylon membranes are strongly recommended because they are tougher. They also can be stripped and reused several times (see **Subheadings 2.8.** and **3.5.**). Nitrocellulose membranes are brittle and cannot be stripped and reprobed.

2.3. Oligonucleotide Probe (see Note 2)

The probe is 5'-d(CTTCGCTTCACCTCTGCACGT), a 21-mer labeled at the 3' end with [^{32}P]ddAMP. The 21-mer can be synthesized in-house or custom synthesized commercially. After the ^{32}P-labeled residue is added by means of 3' end labeling, the 21- and 22-mers are separated from unincorporated [^{32}P]ddATP (*see* **Subheading 3.2.**) and used as the probe.

2.4. Preparation of Membranes (see Note 3)

1. Lysis reagent: 5% Nonidet P-40, 1.5% 2-mercaptoethanol, and 0.002% bromophenol blue. Stored at 4°C.
2. Denaturing reagent: 0.667 *M* NaCl and 0.667 *M* NaOH.
3. 1X SSC (standard saline citrate): SSC is 0.15 *M* NaCl, 0.015 *M* Na citrate, pH 7.5. Stored at 20–25°C.
4. Denhardt's solution: 6X SSC containing 0.2% each of bovine serum albumin (BSA), Ficoll, and polyvinylpyrrolidone (PVP). For 2 L of reagent, mix 4 g each of BSA, Ficoll, and PVP with 6X SSC. Stir overnight at 20–25°C and store at 4°C.

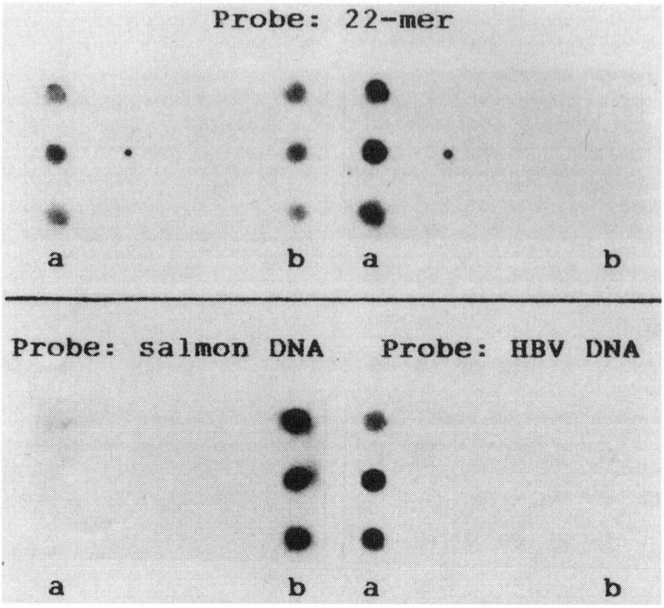

Fig. 2. Effect of washing conditions on the specificity of binding to the oligonucleotide probe. Dot samples were HBsAg-negative serum spiked with (a) HBV DNA or (b) salmon DNA. (**Top**): Membranes that were probed with the oligonucleotide and washed with 6X SSC at 4°C (**Left**) or with NEPS at 45°C (**Right**). See text (**Subheadings 2.4.** and **2.6.**) for composition of reagents. (**Bottom**): Hybridization of the dots to homologous DNA under the prescribed procedure. Reprinted from Lin, H. J., Wu, P. C., and Lai, C. L. (1987) An oligonucleotide probe for the detection of hepatitis B virus DNA in serum. *J. Virol. Method.* **15,** 139–149. Copyright (1987) with permission from Elsevier Science.

2.5. Hybridization

1. NETFAP: 2.7 *M* NaCl, 0.018 *M* ethylenediaminetetraacetic acid (EDTA), 0.54 *M* Tris-HCl (pH 7.8), and 0.3% each of Ficoll, BSA, and PVP. Stored at 20–25°C.
2. 20% PEG: Dissolve 6 g polyethylene glycol (PEG) in water and bring the total volume to 30 mL with water. Stored at 4°C.
3. Denatured salmon DNA (200 μg/mL): Dissolve 4 mg of salmon DNA in 20 mL water. Autoclave the solution for 5 min. Distribute the solution in 5-mL portions and store them in the freezer (–20°C).
4. Heparin solution: 50 mg heparin per mL, dissolved in 0.1 *M* NaCl, 0.0004 *M* EDTA, 0.006 *M* Tris-HCl, pH 7.4. Stored at 4°C.
5. 10% Na pyrophosphate: For 200-mL reagent, dissolve 20 g tetrasodium pyrophosphate. Add HCl solution to pH 7. Stored at 4°C.
6. 10% SDS: 100 g of sodium lauryl (dodecyl) sulfate (SDS) per L. Stored at 20–25°C.
7. [^{32}P]Oligonucleotide probe: The probe is stored at 4°C. It is essential to warm the preparation in a water bath for 5 min and to mix it gently before adding it to the other components of the hybridization mix (*see* **Note 4**).

8. Hybridization mix: Four milliliters of the mix was employed for each membrane (15 × 10 cm). Each milliliter contained 10^7 dpm oligonucleotide probe, 333 μL NETFAP, 300 μL 20% PEG, 100 μL denatured salmon DNA (200 μg/mL), 10 μL heparin solution, 10 μL 10% Na pyrophosphate, and 30 μL 10% SDS. (*see* **Note 4**)

2.6. Washing Probed Membranes (see Note 5)

1. NEPS: 1 *M* NaCl, 0.01 *M* EDTA, 0.05 *M* disodium phosphate, and 0.5% SDS, pH 7. Stored at 20–25°C.
2. Low salt wash: 0.2X SSC containing 0.1% SDS. Stored at 20–25°C.

2.7. Sephadex Column

1. Sephadex solution: 0.15 *M* NaCl containing 0.1% SDS and 0.5 *M* Tris-HCl, pH 7.5. Stored at 20–25°C.
2. Sephadex beads suspension: Put Sephadex G-25–150 beads in a jar, leaving it two-thirds empty. Fill the jar about two-thirds full with Sephadex solution. Let stand at 20–25°C before use.

2.8. Reagents for Stripping Membranes

1. Stripping solution: 0.4 *M* NaOH.
2. Neutralizing reagent: 0.2 *M* Tris-HCl (pH 7.5), 0.1% SDS, and 0.1X SSC.

3. Methods

3.1. Preparation of Membranes

1. Clamp the nylon membrane (Hybond, Amersham Pharmacia Biotech, Piscataway, NJ) in a plastic manifold.
2. Mix 25 μL serum with 20 μL lysis reagent. After 10 min, add 135 μL of denaturing reagent and mix.
3. Apply 170 μL to the membrane.
4. After filtration, soak the membrane in 200 mL of 6X SSC for 20 min and air-dry it.
5. Subject the membrane to ultraviolet irradiation for 20 min and then place it in Denhardt's solution for 16 h at 63°C.
6. Blot the membrane with filter paper and store it in a plastic bag at 4°C.

3.2. Preparation of Oligonucleotide Probe (see Note 6)

1. 3'-End labeling was carried out using per 100 μL: 48 pmol 21-mer, 320 μCi ddATP (dideoxyadenosine 5'-[α-^{32}P]triphosphate, specific activity about 5000 Ci/mmol) and 20 units terminal deoxynucleotidyl transferase (2 h, 37°C).
2. To separate the probe from ddATP, prepare a 20-cm column (diameter, 0.8–1.0 cm) of Sephadex G-25-150.
3. Develop the column with Sephadex solution, collecting fractions of approx 1 mL.
4. The oligonucleotides appear in the exclusion volume. Locate them precisely with the aid of Cerenkov counting: mix 10-μL samples with 5–10 mL water for scintillation counting.
5. Pool the appropriate fractions and store them at 4°C. The specific activity of the probe was about 10^9dpm/μg (7 × 10^6 dpm/pmol).

3.3. Hybridization and Washing of Membranes (see Note 7)

1. Transfer the membrane to a fresh plastic bag and pour in the hybridization mix.
2. Gently wet the membrane, avoiding bubble formation. Exclude air as much as possible before heat-sealing the bag.

3. Sandwich the bag between two glass plates and place 800 g of weights on top of the sandwich.
4. The assembly is placed at 63°C for 2 to16 h.
5. Over a period of 20 h, wash the membrane at 63°C with five portions of NEPS. Then place it in the low salt wash, with shaking, for 10 min at 20–25°C.
6. For each step, use 100 mL of fluid per membrane.
7. Blot the membrane between sheets of filter paper and air dry it.

3.4. Autoradiography

1. Place the membrane between polypropylene sheets.
2. Expose it to X-ray film with intensifying screens for 22–46 h at–70°C.

3.5. Stripping Membranes for Reuse (see Note 8)

1. Immerse the membrane in 100-mL portion stripping solution (45°C, 30 min).
2. Repeat this step.
3. Transfer it to the neutralizing reagent (45°C, 30 min).
4. Check for the complete removal of the probe by means of autoradiography.

4. Notes

1. Quantitative studies showed daily decreases in HBV DNA concentrations in serum samples stored at 45°C *(12)*. No significant decreases were observed in specimens subjected to eight freeze–thaw cycles *(13)*.
2. The 21-mer could be labeled at either end. 5'-End labeling was rejected because it was more expensive, with a fivefold excess of radioactive adenosine triphosphate (ATP) over oligonucleotide needed.
3. The serum sample volume may vary from 1 to 50 µL. The reagents are based on published procedures *(14, 15)*. HBV DNA is released by the actions of Nonidet P-40 (a nonionic detergent), the reducing agent 2-mercaptoethanol, and the alkali in the denaturing reagent. The latter also serves to separate the DNA strands. The purpose of the bromophenol blue in the lysis reagent is to make the sample visible to the naked eye. Treatment of membranes with Denhardt's solution reduces background.
4. The individual components of the hybridization medium were warmed to 37°C before being mixed, and the mixture was held at the hybridization temperature (63°C) for 10 min before application to the membrane. Failure to prewarm the oligonucleotide probe before its addition to the hybridization mix resulted in totally black autoradiograms.

   Several components of the hybridization medium were added for the purpose of producing light backgrounds: heparin and pyrophosphate *(16)*, polyethylene glycol *(17)*, and the Ficoll, BSA, and PVP specified by Denhardt *(15)*.
5. As shown by **Fig. 2**, use of NEPS resulted in appearance of HBV-specific signals and the absence of false-positive signals. The low salt wash was essential for a clean background *(18)*.
6. The use of a 3'-end labeling kit is recommended. In the presence of terminal transferase, oligonucleotides are labeled at the 3' end, with any deoxyribonucleoside-5' triphosphate labeled in the α position. Use of dideoxynucleoside triphosphate ensures that the oligonucleotide is extended by only one residue. With the given procedure, over 60% of the 21-mers were labeled, enabling use of the resulting preparation without separation of the 22-mer from the 21-mer. It is important to achieve the high specific activities because the 21-mer competed with the radioactive 22-mer. Addition of a sevenfold excess of the 21-mer to the hybridization mix completely suppressed the signal *(1)*.

7. For most patient samples, the signals obtained after 16 h hybridization were marginally stronger than those obtained with 2 h hybridization. But as expected, some samples produced positive signals only with the longer hybridization time ***(1)***.

   Several membranes may be washed in the same box. Stacking of membranes could be avoided by the use of spacers cut from plastic flyswatters.
8. There is gradual loss of the samples with repeated cycles of stripping and reprobing. Generally, up to five such cycles can be performed on the same membrane ***(19)***.

References

1. Lin, H. J., Wu, P. C., and Lai, C. L. (1987) An oligonucleotide probe for the detection of hepatitis B virus DNA in serum. *J. Virol. Methods* **15**, 139–149.
2. Lin, H. J., Lai, C.L., Lau, J. Y. N., Chung, H. T., Lauder, I. J., and Fong, M. W. (1990). Evidence for intrafamilial transmission of hepatitis B virus from sequence analysis of mutant HBV DNAs in two Chinese families. *Lancet* **336**, 208–212.
3. Lauder, I. J., Lin, H. J., Lau, J. Y. N., Siu, T. S., and Lai, C. L. (1993) The variability of the hepatitis B virus genome: statistical analysis and biological implications. *Mol. Biol. Evol.* **10**, 457–470.
4. Benson, D. A., Boguski, M. S., Lipman, D. J., Ouellete, B. F., Rapp, B. A., and Wheeler, D. L. (1999) GenBank. *Nucleic Acids Res* **27**, 12–17.
5. Renbao, G., Meijin, C., Lueping, S., Suwen, Q., and Zaiping, L. (1987) The complete nucleotide sequence of the cloned DNA of hepatitis B virus subtype adr in pADR-1. *Sci. Sin.* **30**, 507–521.
6. Mulaide, M., Kumazawa, T., Hoshi, A., Kawaguchi R., and Hikiji, K. (1992) The complete nucleotide sequence of hepatitis B virus, subtype adr (SRADR) and phylogenetic analysis. *Nucleic Acids Res.* **20**, 6105.
7. Imamichi, T., Murphy, M. A., Falloon, J., Brust, D. G., and Lane, H. C. Unpublished (GenBank accession number, AY034878).
8. Pult, I, Chouard, T., Wieland, S., Klemenz, R., Yaniv, M., and Blum, H. E. (1997) A hepatitis B virus mutant with a new hepatocyte nuclear factor 1 binding site emerging in transplant-transmitted fulminant hepatitis B. *Hepatology* **25**, 1507–1515.
9. Altschul, S. F., Madden, T. L., Schaffer, A. A., et al. (1997) Gapped BLAST and PSI-BLAST: a new generation of protein database search programs. *Nucleic Acids Res.* **25**, 3389–3402.
10. Quade, K., Saldanha, J., Thomas, H., and Monjardino, J. (1992) Integration of hepatitis B virus DNA through a mutational hotspot within the cohesive region in a case of hepatocellular carcinoma. *J. Gen. Virol.* **73 (Pt 1)**, 179–182.
11. Tsuei, D. J., Chen, P. J., Lai, M. Y., et al. (1994) Inverse polymerase chain reaction for cloning cellular sequences adjacent to integrated hepatitis B virus DNA in hepatocellular carcinomas. *J. Virol. Methods* ***49***, 269–284.
12. Krajden, M., Comanor, L., Rifkin, O., Grigoriew, A., Minor, J. M., and Kapke, G. (1998) Assessment of hepatitis B virus DNA stability in serum by the Chiron Quantiplex branched-DNA assay. *J. Clin. Microbiol.* **36,** 382–386.
13. Krajden, M., Minor J. M., Rifkin, R., and Comanor, L. (1999) Effect of multiple freeze-thaw cycles on hepatitis B virus DNA and hepatitis virus C RNA quantification as measured with branched-DNA technology. *J. Clin. Microbiol.* **37**, 1683–1686.
14. Harrison, T. J., Bal, V., Wheeler, E. G., et al. (1985) Hepatitis B virus DNA and e antigen in serum from blood donors in the United Kingdom positive for hepatitis B surface antigen. BMJ. **290**, 663–664.

15. Denhardt, D. T. (1966). A membrane-filter technique for the detection of complementary DNA. *Biochem. Biophys. Res. Commun.* ***23***, 641.
16. Singh, L. and Jones, K. W. (1984). The use of heparin as a simple cost-effective means of controlling background in nucleic acid hybridization mixture. *Nucleic Acids Res.* ***12***, 5627–5638.
17. Renz, M., and Kurz, C. (1984) A colorimetric method for DNA hybridization. *Nucleic Acids Res.* **12**, 3435–3444.
18. Berninger, M., Hammer, M., Hoyer, B., and Gerin, J. L. (1982) An assay for the detection of the DNA genome of hepatitis B virus in serum. *J. Med. Virol.* ***9***, 57–68.
19. Lin, H. J., Wu, P. C., Lai, C. L., and Leong, S. (1986) Molecular hybridization study of plasma hepatitis B virus DNA from different carriers. *J. Infect. Dis.* ***154***, 983–989.

4

Detection of HBV RNA in Serum of Patients

**Wei Zhang, Hans Jörg Hacker,
Maria Mildenberger, Qin Su, and Claus H. Schröder**

1. Introduction

Cell-free RNA of a different origin is known to circulate in the blood *(1–3)*. This finding has also been reported for RNA specified by viruses with a DNA genome, such as the hepatitis B virus (HBV)*(4)*. In the infected cell, genomic and subgenomic HBV–RNA molecules are synthesized from episomal genomes. Within virions, only the (–) strands of the genomes (3.2 kb) are complete, whereas the (+) strands are incomplete. The genomes replicate via the reverse transcription of genomic RNA intermediates. These pregenomes are packaged into nucleocapsids and degraded during the synthesis of the DNA (–) strand *(5)*. Upon completion of (–) strand DNA synthesis, the capsids mature into the enveloped virions (Dane particles), which are found in the sera of infected individuals *(6)*. Subgenomic viral transcript RNAs do exist but are not packaged into nucleocapsids *(5)*. Based on these observations, there should be no replication-related release of HBV–RNA from hepatocytes into the blood. However, damage to liver cells may discharge viral RNA contained in nucleocapsids or as free forms.

Köck et al. *(7)* were the first to detect serum HBV–RNA considered to be associated with a virus particle in sera used for in vitro infection of leukocytes from uninfected individuals. The recent identification of serum HBV–RNA molecules not capable of entering replicative processes indicated the existence of circulating viral RNA, which is free of cells and particles. Here, methods are described to extract and characterize HBV–RNA from serum and plasma. They make it possible to monitor HBV expression profiles and to describe the transition from replicative to nonreplicative infection stages known to occur late during chronic infection. To perform the individual assays described below, a laboratory setup for work in molecular biology is required.

2. Materials

1. High Pure Viral Nucleic Acid Kit (Roche, cat. no. 1858874).
2. Ribosomal RNA (Roche, cat. no. 206938).

From: *Methods in Molecular Medicine, vol. 95: Hepatitis B and D Protocols, volume 1*
Edited by: R. K. Hamatake and J. Y. N. Lau © Humana Press Inc., Totowa, NJ

3. Amplification grade DNase I (Invitrogen, cat. no. 18068-015).
4. T4 polynucleotide kinase (New England Biolabs, cat. no. M0201S).
5. Hybond-N+ (Amersham, cat. no. RPN 303B)
6. Hybridization buffer: 5X standard sodium citrate (SSC), 0.5 *M* sodium phosphate pH 6.8, 1X Denhardt's, 1% sodium dodecylic sulfate (SDS), and 0.1 mg/mL tRNA.
7. Washing buffer: 2X SSC, 0.1% SDS.
8. Digoxigenin-11-2'-deoxy-uridine-5'- triphosphate (Roche, cat. no. 1093088).
9. DIG Nucleic Acid Detection Kit (Roche, cat. no. 1175041).
10. Taq DNA polymerase (Invitrogen, cat. no. 18038-018).
11. Titan One Tube RT/PCR System (Roche, cat. no. 1855476).
12. Plasmid pCRII-TOPO (Invitrogen, cat. no. K4550-01).
13. For the analysis of discernible 3' end regions of viral RNA ***(8, 9)***, anchored oligo(dT) antisense primers are used in conjunction with the same upstream sense primer to differentiate between full-length (f) and truncated (tr) RNA. Other primer pairs are used to recognize corresponding regions on DNA. **Table 1** shows a list of suitable primers for PCR and RT–PCR and primers for establishing probes, together with a scheme showing their relative position on viral RNA. *Xho*I coordinates ***(10)*** are used for the designation of primers and to indicate their respective 5' ends.

3. Methods

3.1. Sample and Reagent Preparations

3.1.1. Collection of Serum Samples

1. Up to 5 mL of blood are taken intravenously and transferred into DNase- and RNase-free tubes.
2. Tubes are centrifuged at low speed (2000*g*) at 4°C to separate serum from other blood components.
3. The supernatant is transferred to a new tube and recentrifuged under the same conditions (*see* **Note 1**). Average yield is 2–3 mL of serum.
4. Purified serum is immediately portioned into aliquots of 200 μL and stored in a deep freeze at –80°C. It is also possible to process serum samples prefrozen at –20°C, thawed once, and refrozen at –70°C. Repeated thawing and freezing should be avoided, however, because they lead to a gradual loss of RNA. For information on sending samples to other laboratories (*see* **Note 2**).

3.1.2. Extraction of DNA/RNA

1. Immediately after the samples are defrosted, serum nucleic acids are extracted using the High Pure Viral Nucleic Acid Kit (*see* **Note 3**). As a modification, poly(A) RNA as a carrier is replaced by ribosomal RNA, which is added at half the amount of poly(A) RNA (*see* **Note 4**). After binding to a glass fiber fleece, nucleic acids are eluted in a 50-μL volume and are either processed or stored at –70°C for later analysis.
2. In case PCR and RT–PCR yield identical amplification products from DNA and RNA (*see* **Subheadings 3.2.1.** and **3.2.2.**), nucleic acids are subjected to (DNase) I treatment. Digestion is carried out using amplification grade DNase I.

3.1.3. Hybridization Probes

Two types of probes are used for verification of amplification products obtained in PCR and RT–PCR assays described below; one that recognizes sequences common to

Table 1
Oligonucleotides Primers and Probes[a]

No.	Designation[b]	Sequence
1.	1434 +	TCTCATCTGCCGGACCGTGT
2.	1445 +	GGACCGTGTGCACTTCGCTT
3.	1454 +	GCACTTCGCTTCACCTCTGC
4.	1464 +	TCACCTCTGCACGTCGCATG
5.	1485 –	TCCATGCGACGTGCAGAGGTGAAGC
6.	1561 +	GACCGACCTTGAGGCATACTTCAAAGACTG
7.	1574 –	CCTCAAGGTCGGTCGTTGAC
8.	1590 –	CAGTCTTTGAAGTATGCCTCAAGGTCGGTC
9.	1668 –	AATTTATGCCTACAGCCTCC
10.	1678 +	ACCAGCACCATGCAACTTTT
11.	1683 **a**	$(T)_{15}$ GCTGG
12.	1752 +	GTGCCTTGGGTGGCTTTAGGGCATGGACAT
13.	1806 **a**	$(T)_{15}$ AGCTC
14.	1808 **a**	$(T)_{15}$ GAAGC
15.	1824 –	AGAGAGTAACTCCACAGAAG

[a] Oligonucleotides in relation to f and tr RNA

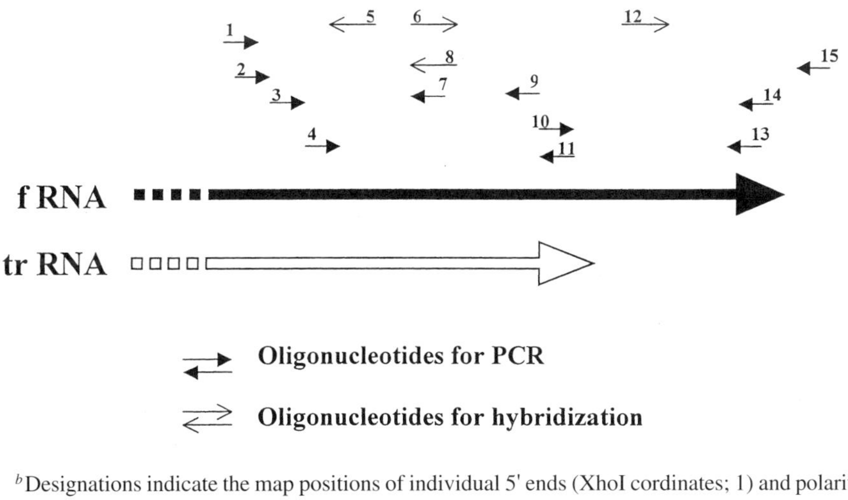

[b] Designations indicate the map positions of individual 5' ends (XhoI cordinates; 1) and polarities. **a** denotes the anchor of oligo(dT) primers.

both full-length and truncated RNA and another that recognizes sequences represented only on full-length RNA (**Fig. 2A**).

3.1.3.1. Preparation of Radiolabeled Primer Probes and Hybridization

1. For establishing ^{32}P primer probes (1561+, 1752+, 1485–, 1590–), primers are subjected to the T4 kinase reaction. This enzyme transfers the phosphate from the γ position of ATP to the 5' OH terminus of the primer, resulting in ^{32}P end labeling. The reaction is performed in

a T4 polynucleotide kinase buffer [70 m*M* Tris-HCl, 10 m*M* $MgCl_2$, 5 m*M* dithiothreitol (DTT), pH 7.6] at 37°C in a final volume of 20 µL following the manufacturer's instructions. As radiolabeled, 1.85 MBq γ ^{32}P ATP is added at a specific activity of 185 TBq/mmol.

2. For hybridization, amplification products are transferred onto a nylon membrane via the capillary method ***(11)*** and cross-linked by ultraviolet (UV) light according to the supplier's instructions. Hybridization conditions are essentially as described ***(11)***, with the following details regarding time and temperature.
3. Prehybridization for 2–4 h at 68°C.
4. Hybridization for 16 h at 68°C.
5. Washing is performed two to four times for 20 min at 68°C.

3.1.3.2. Preparatin of Digoxigenin-Labeled Probes and Hybridization

1. As an alternative to radiolabeled probes, digoxygenin (DIG) probes are produced via PCR. The following primer pairs are used: 1454+/1668– recognizing a sequence segment represented on tr and f HBV-RNA; and 1678+/1824– recognizing a sequence segment represented only on f HBV–RNA.
2. In these PCR reactions, DIG-11-dUTP partially replaces dTTP as a substrate for *Taq* polymerase. As standard, the following nucleotide concentrations are used: 200 µ*M* dATP, dGTP, dCTP; 180 µ*M* dTTP; and 20 µ*M* DIG-11-dUTP. A DIG-11-dU/dT ratio of 1:10 in the probes is favorable for the analysis of the amplification products of serum RNA via PCR. Synthesis of DIG probes is performed according to the manufacturer's instructions.
3. Hybridization and visualization are performed according to instructions of the "The Dig Application Manual for Filter Hybridization" (Roche Diagnostics).
4. To visualize bound DIG-labeled probes, an anti-DIG antibody conjugated to alkaline phosphatase is used. During the enzymatic cleavage of the substrate BCIP, the product reacts with NBT resulting in an insoluble purple-brown precipitate directly on the membrane.

3.2. Serum HBV–DNA and RNA Assays

The analysis of HBV nucleic acids focuses on the X gene 3' region as a region common to all HBV transcripts. PCR and RT–PCR are performed using both conventional primer pairs and primer pairs that are targeted to the transition site of transcript sequences into the poly (A) tails by inclusion of an anchored oligo (dT) primer.

3.2.1. PCR Assay with Conventional Primer Pairs

HBV DNA of the X gene region spanning the positions 1445+ and 1574– is amplified via PCR using the respective primers (**Table 1**).

1. For each reaction, add the following components to a PCR tube:
   34.75 µL H_2O (distilled, autoclaved), 2.0 µL nucleic acid extract, 0.75 µL primer 1455+ (100 ng/µL), 0.75 µL primer 1574– (100 ng/µL), 5.0 µL dNTP mixture (10 m*M*), 1.5 µL $MgCl_2$ (50 m*M*), 5.0 µL PCR buffer (200 m*M* Tris-HCl [pH 8.4], 500 m*M* KCl), 0.25 µL *Taq* DNA polymerase.
2. Tubes are incubated in a thermal cycler at 93°C for 1 min 40 s.
3. A table of 35 amplification cycles are run: 90°C 40 s, 58°C 50 s (annealing), 70°C 40 s (DNA amplification).
4. Cycling is followed by incubation at 70°C for 15 min and cooling down to 4°C.
5. Amplification products are separated by electrophoresis on a 3% agarose gel.

3.2.2. RT–PCR Assay with Conventional Primer Pairs

HBV RNA of the X gene region spanning the positions 1445+ and 1574– is amplified using the Titan One Tube RT–PCR System. This system uses AMV RT combined with an Expand High Fidelity Enzyme Mix consisting of *Taq* DNA polymerase and a proofreading polymerase. Both DNA and RNA sequences are amplified. Instructions of the manufacturer are followed strictly.

1. If it is desired to amplify RNA exclusively, the samples are subjected to DNase I digestion prior to PCR. DNase I digestion protocol:
   a. 16.0 μL serum nucleic acids.
   b. 2.0 μL DNase I buffer (200 m*M* Tris-HCl [pH 8.4], 20 m*M* $MgCl_2$).
   c. 2.0 μL DNase I (1 U/μL).
   d. Incubate at 25°C for 15 min.
   e. Stop reaction by adding 2 μL ethylenediaminetetraacetic acid (EDTA) (25 m*M*).
   f. Inactivate enzyme at 65°C for 10 min.
2. In the one step RT–PCR, reverse transcription as well as PCR are performed without changing reagents between cDNA synthesis and amplification. To the reaction mixture, 1.5 μL (100 ng/μL) each of the primers 1445+ and 1574– is added, with a final volume of 50 μL.
3. Incubate tubes in a thermocycler at 50°C for 20 min (reverse transcription).
4. Subsequent steps in the cycler correspond to the PCR protocol as described above.
5. PCR and RT–PCR can also be carried out using the primer pair 1434+ and 1668–, resulting in the amplification of a larger segment shared by both f and tr transcripts. Here, the annealing temperature is 56°C.

3.2.3. f RNA Assay

RT–PCR involving anchored oligo (dT) primers recognizing full-length transcripts terminating at the polyadenylation signal downstream of the X reading frame is carried out in two rounds. In the first round, the primer 1434+ is combined with two anchored oligo (dT) primers, representing poly(A) addition sites at positions 1806 and 1808 (**Table 1**), respectively. In the second round (seminested PCR), the same anchored oligo(dT) primers are combined with the primer 1454+ (*see* **Note 5**).

1. The first round is performed using the Titan One Tube RT–PCR System. The manufacturer's instructions are strictly followed. The following amounts of primers are added to the reaction mixture: 1.5 μL 1434+ (100 ng/μL) and 3 μL each of the anchored primers 1806a and 1808a (100 ng/μL), with a final volume of 50 μL.
2. Incubate tubes as described above at 50°C for 20 min (reverse transcription).
3. Incubate tubes at 93°C for 1 min 40 s.
4. A total of 35 amplification cycles are run: 90°C 40 s, 53°C 50 s (annealing), 70°C 40 s (DNA amplification).
5. Cycling is followed by incubation at 70°C for 15 min.
6. Finally, store tubes at 4°C.
7. Amplification products are separated by electrophoresis on a 3% agarose gel.
8. Second-round PCR parameters are identical to ones used in the first round. To the reaction mixture are added 5 μL first-round products, 0.75 μL (100 ng/μL) of primer 1454+ and 0.75 μL each of the anchored oligo (dT) primers 1806a and 1808a (100 ng/μL), with a final volume of 50 μL.

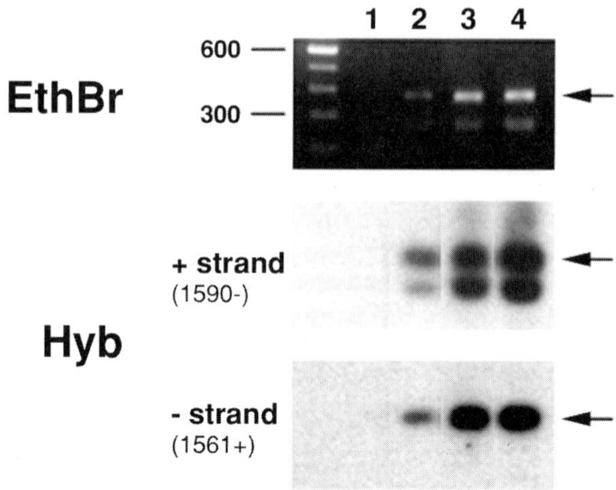

Fig. 1 f RNA assay. (**Top Panel**) Second-round amplification products separated on a 3% agarose gel and stained with ethidium bromide (EthBr, rearranged lanes of the same gel). Visible marker bands (left outer lane) belong to a 100-bp ladder and range from 300 to 600 bp. RNA from sera of chronically HBV-infected patients (1, 2, 3, 4) was analyzed. Arrow points to the predicted amplification product (370 bp). (**Middle panel**) Blotted amplification products hybridized to ^{32}P-labeled primer 1590– Arrow points to the 370 bp signal. (**Bottom Panel**) Hybridization to primer 1561+.

Typical results obtained in the f RNA assay are shown in **Fig. 1**. Agarose gel electrophoresis displays the expected signals for amplification products of 370 bp in size (priming by 1808a is more frequent than priming by 1806a). A second signal is observed for amplification products of a higher mobility. Hybridization with strand-specific primer probes (1561+ for –strand, 1590– for +strand) reveals positive strand specificity of the faster migrating DNA product due to asymmetric amplification **(Fig. 2A,** positive strand hybridization panel). A similar asymmetry of amplification applies for the tr RNA assay.

Fig. 2. Comparison of f RNA and tr RNA assay. (**A**) Central Panel: Agarose gel documenting second-round product profiles obtained in the f and tr RNA assays (f, tr) from serum RNA of an HBV carrier. Filled triangle points to 370 bp f-product. Open triangle points to the 235 bp tr-product. Left and Right Panels: Hybridization of the blotted products to the primer-probes 1561+ and 1752+, respectively. (**B**) Transitions into the poly(A) tail (A_n) of f RNA amplification products obtained by anchored primers 1806a, 1808a, and 1683a. The pentanucleotide sequences of these primers are highlighted by gray shadings, light gray for 1806a and 1880a used as primer for the f RNA assay and dark gray for 1683a used as primer for the tr RNA assay. Use of 1683a causes an artificial 3' addition of its five anchor bases and a variation in product length. The 3' end regions of amplified cDNA are shown in relation to the relevant segment of the HBV genome (Top). (**C**) Scheme depicting primers in relation to f and tr RNA and primer probes to differentiate between tr (1561+) and f (1752+) amplification products.

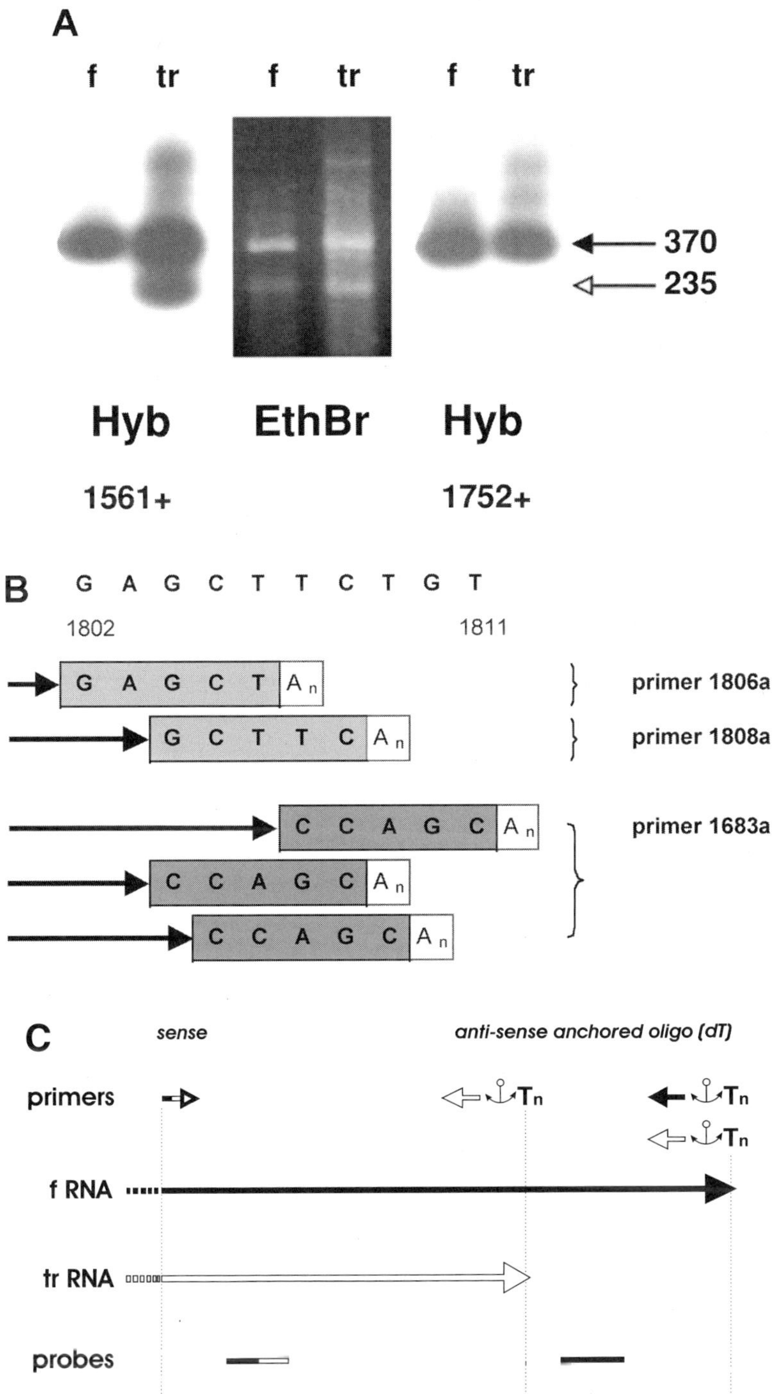
A
f tr f tr f tr
370
235
Hyb EthBr Hyb
1561+ 1752+
B
G A G C T T C T G T
1802 1811
G A G C T A n
G C T T C A n
C C A G C A n
C C A G C A n
C C A G C A n
primer 1806a
primer 1808a
primer 1683a
C
sense
anti-sense anchored oligo (dT)
primers
Tn
Tn
Tn
f RNA
tr RNA
probes

3.2.4. tr RNA Assay

RT–PCR for truncated transcripts involves an anchored oligo (dT) primer (1683a, **Table 1**), recognizing polyadenylation at the signal within the X reading frame. It is also carried out in two rounds using the conditions in **Subheading 3.2.3.** In the first round, the oligo (dT) primer is combined with primer 1445+, in the second round, it is combined with primer 1464+.

Figure 2A documents a representative result obtained with the tr RNA assay. The signal indicative of tr RNA corresponds to the expected 235-bp product (tr lanes in left and central panels). A second signal corresponding to 370 bp is observed when samples also contain f RNA, as is the case for the example shown (f lanes in all panels). Cloning into plasmid pCRII-TOPO and sequencing reveal that the anchored primer 1683a recognizes 3' termini one to three bases distant from the position 1806 or two to five bases distant from position 1808 (**Fig. 2B**)

3.2.5. tr RNA Assay for Both f and tr RNA (f/tr RNA Assay)

The results gained by the tr RNA assay suggest that it is possible to detect both RNA species in one assay (f/tr RNA assay) in terms of molecular weight. To further discriminate f and tr RNA in terms of sequence content, a primer probe specific for sequences present only on f RNA is used (**Fig. 1A**, compare left and right panels). The scheme in **Fig. 2C** demonstrates the principle of differential identification. **Figure 3** documents representative results obtained with the f/tr RNA assay for a series of chronically HBV-infected hepatitis B surface antigen (HBsAg) seropositive patients differing in hepatits B e antigen (HBeAg) expression (*see* **Notes 6** and **7**).

3.3. Quantitation of HBV Serum RNA Molecules

The number of HBV serum RNA molecules of a given type is quantified by adding various amounts of competitor cDNA (plasmids carrying inserts of the respective cDNA). The competitor spans the region targeted by the individual PCR assay and contains either an insertion or a deletion, leading to amplification products with a migration behavior different from that of the unaltered target sequence. Assuming the same amplification efficiency of target sequence and competitor, comparison of signal intensities allows one to quantify the target sequence (competitive PCR). At a 1:1 ratio of signal intensities of competitor and target sequence the known number of competitor molecules equals that of the target sequence. **Table 2** shows a list of control and competitor cDNA plasmids and their allocation to individual assays.

1. The protocols for competitive PCR and RT–PCR simply require the addition of the competitor to the assay mixture. As an example for quantification of tr RNA (two amplification cycles, *see* **Subheading 3.2.4.**), three tubes containing a constant amount of tr target sequence receive 1 μL 100 fg/μL, 1 μL 10 fg/μL, and 1μL 1fg/μL of competitor plasmid J166 ***(16)*** (*see* **Table 2**). The amounts of competitor chosen are calculated to correspond to 2×10^6 to 2×10^4 tr RNA molecules per mL blood, respectively (*see* **Note 8**).
2. Amplification products are then separated by electrophoresis on a 3% agarose gel and detected both by ethidium bromide staining and hybridization (**Fig. 4**).

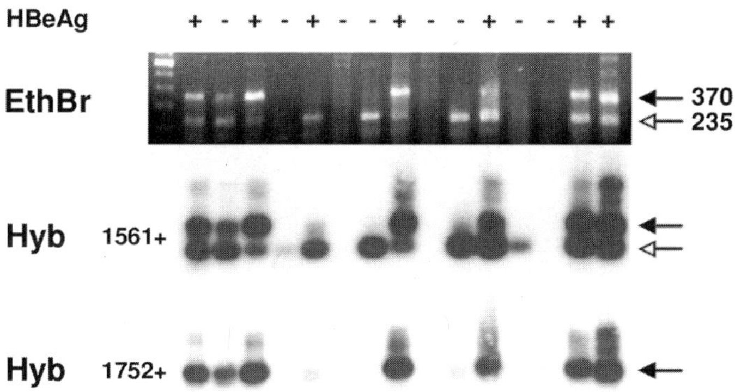

Fig. 3. Application of f/tr RNA assay to a series of serum samples. (**Top Panel**) Serum RNA second-round PCR products obtained in the f/tr RNA assay separated on a 3% agarose gel. The HBe serostatus of the chronically infected patients (all HBs seropositive) is indicated. Outermost left lane 100 bp ladder, the 600 bp signal being the brightest. Filled and open triangles point to the 370 and 235 bp amplification products. (**Middle and Bottom Panels**) Hybridization to the primer probes 1561+ and 1752+.

Table 2
cDNA Plasmids Used as Competitors and as Control Targets in PCR Assays

Designation [a]	Map position of cloned HBV cDNA	Assay
J166 (50) [b]	1445–1808+ $(T)_{15}$ [c]	x DNA and xRNA
J166 (16)	1445–1656+ 71bp [d]	tr RNA
19L27	1434–1808+ $(T)_{15}$ [e]	f RNA
9T40A [f]	1434–1808+ $(T)_{15}$	f RNA (control target)
9T41A [f]	1445–1683+ $(T)_{15}$	tr RNA (control target)

[a] cDNA amplification products are cloned into pCRIITOPO, length 3950 bp (Invitrogen, cat. no. K4550-01).
[b] Before addition to PCR assay, the plasmids are cut by *Eco*RI.
[c] 31-bp tandem repeat of the sequence 1487 to 1517; deleted from 1626–1644 and 1682–1696.
[d] 51 cellular bases joined to 1683 a.
[e] Deleted from 1689 to 1746.
[f] Derived from HBx expression vectors pMT9T40A and pMT9T41A *(12)*.

Ethidium bromide visualizes the decrease of the competitor and the corresponding increase of the target sequence (left panels, first three lanes). Hybridization, in addition, verifies the sequence identity of competitor and target sequences (right panels). In line with the fact that the tr RNA assay also detects f RNA, f RNA also participates in competition. **Figure 4** shows three examples: one without f RNA, one with comparatively low levels of f RNA, and one with high levels of f RNA. Therefore, it is possible to estimate the f RNA copy number. However, an exact quantification of f RNA requires an especially adjusted competitive f RNA RT–PCR using plasmid 19L27 as a competitor (**Table 2**).

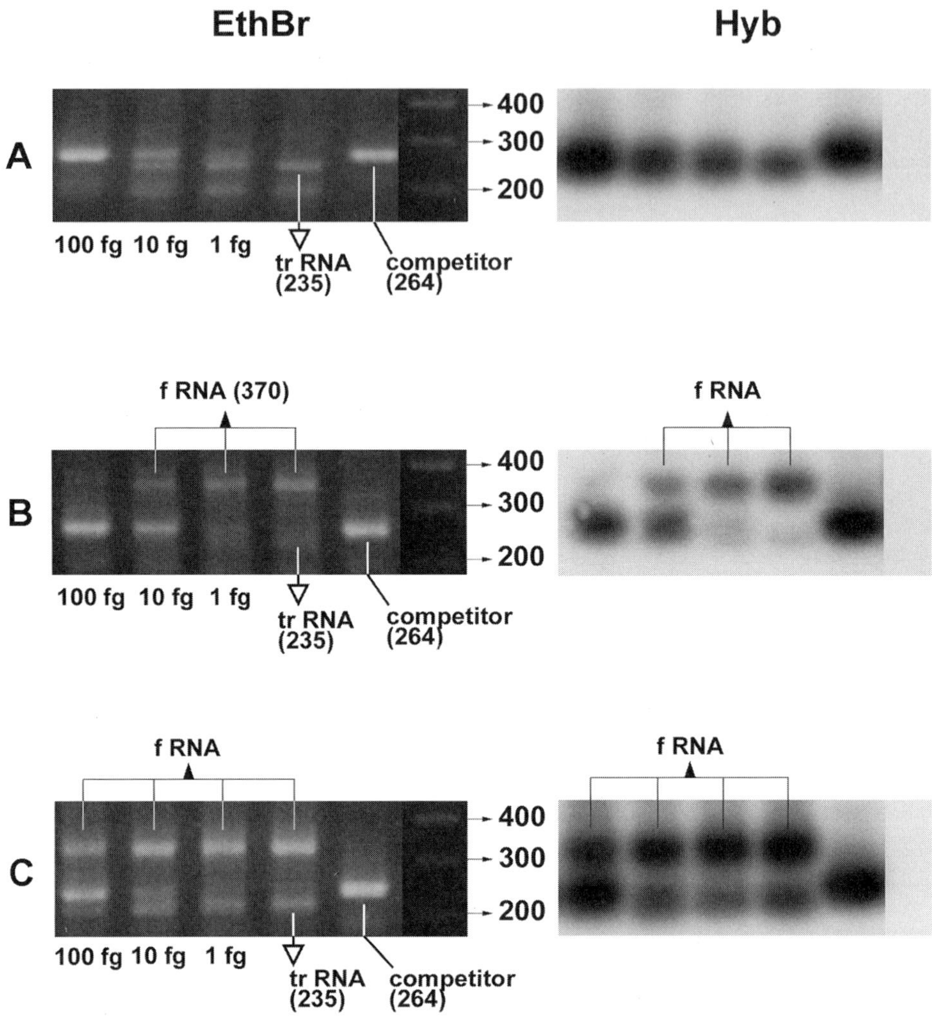

Fig. 4. Quantitation of tr RNA. Serum RNA from patients with only tr RNA (**A**), with tr RNA plus low (**B**) and high levels (**C**) of f RNA subjected to competitive tr RNA RT–PCR. Panels to the left (ethidium bromide patterns, marker lanes of the same gel rearranged): First three lanes, addition of competitor J166(16) at indicated amounts. Following lanes, no competitor, competitor alone, and marker. In **A**, the positions of the wild-type tr (235 bp) and the competitor (264 bp) amplification products are indicated. In **B** and **C**, the position of the wild-type f amplification product (370 bp) is shown in addition. Panels to the right: Hybridization patterns obtained with the primer probe 1561+ detecting both tr and f amplification products. Based on the EthBr patterns, tr RNA copy numbers per mL of blood are about 1×10^5 (**A**), 2×10^4 (**B**) and 4×10^5 (**C**).

4. Notes

1. It is likely that circulating cell free nucleic acids (particularly cell- and virus particle-free [nonencapsidated] viral RNA molecules) are protected by complex formation with lipoprotein, the true nature of which has yet to be elucidated. Therefore, any manipulation of serum such as filtering or high-speed centrifugation may remove significant amounts of target material.
2. Samples can be delivered conveniently by mail to cooperating laboratories following the addition of guanidinium buffer, for example, after addition of the lysis buffer from the High Pure Viral Nucleic Acid Kit.
3. If a supplier introduces a new version of its kit, its efficiency should be tested before extractions are performed on a larger scale; addition of a carrier is unnecessary in our hands based on comparative quantitation with and without a carrier. When a carrier is used, about 50% is recovered in the final nucleic acid preparation.
4. The analysis of 3' end regions by anchored oligo(dT) primers may be influenced by the high background of competing poly(A) plus RNA.
5. The primer 1454+ functions well despite the facts that its 3' part corresponds to the 11 bp direct repeat of HBV DNA and that both copies of the repeat DR I (position 1697) and DR II (position 1463) are located on the target sequence.
6. The principle of verification of PCR products by probes recognizing sequences common to different amplification products and sequences present only on one product can be applied for tailoring probes used in corresponding f/tr RNA real-time PCR protocols.
7. In laboratories not equipped with radioactive isotopes, radiolabeled probes can be replaced by the DIG probes described here, according to our own experience. A conclusive interpretation of the amplification patterns is possible, although it is complicated to a certain degree by signals due to asymmetric amplification. If it is desired to work with DIG probes exclusively, strand-specific probes should be developed.
8. Calculation of RNA copy numbers assumes a one-to-one conversion of RNA into DNA and should be performed with some caution. Dilution intervals of the competitor by a factor of 10 (e.g., 100 fg, 10 fg, 1 fg) are sufficient for many questions. However, if one is interested in the exact amount of the target, dilution series with narrower intervals are recommended.

5 References

1. Kamm, R. C., and Smith, A. G. (1972) Nucleic acid concentrations in normal human plasma. *Clin. Chem.* ***18***, 519–522.
2. Kopreski, M. S., Benko, F. A., Kwak, L.W., and Gocke, C.D. (1999) Detection of tumor messenger mRNA in the serum patients with malignant melanoma. *Clin. Cancer Res.* ***5***, 1961–1965.
3. Chen, X. Q., Bonnefoi, H., Pelte, M. F., et al. (2000) RNA telomerase as a detection marker in the serum of breast cancer patients. *Clin Cancer Res.* ***6***, 3823–3826.
4. Su, Q., Wang, S.-F., Chang, T.-E., et al. (2001) Circulating hepatitis B virus nucleic acids in chronic infection: representation of differently polyadenylated viral transcripts during progression to nonreplicative stages. *Clin. Cancer Res.*, 7, 2005–2015.
5. Nassal, M., and Schaller, H. (1996) Hepatitis B replication—an update. *J. Viral Hepat.* ***3***, 217–226.
6. Gerelsaikhan, T., Tavis, J. E., and Bruss, V. (1996) Hepatitis B virus nucleocapsid development does not occur without genomic DNA synthesis. *J. Virol.* ***70***, 4269–4274.

7. Köck, J., Theilmann, L., Galle, P., and Schlicht, H.-J. (1996) Hepatitis B virus nucleic acids associated with human peripheral blood mononuclear cells do not originate from replicating virus. *Hepatology* ***23***, 405–413.
8. Kairat, A., Beerheide, W., Zhou, G., Tang, Z.-Y., Edler, L., and Schröder, C. H. (1999) Truncated hepatitis B virus RNA in human hepatocellular carcinoma: its representation in patients with advancing age. *Intervirology* ***42***, 228–237.
9. Schutz, T., Kairat, A., and Schröder, C. H. (2000) Anchored oligo(dT) primed RT/PCR: identification and quantification of related transcripts with distinct 3'-ends. *J. Virol. Methods* ***86***, 167–171.
10. Loncarevic, I. F., Zentgraf, H., and Schröder, C. H. (1990) Sequence of a replication competent hepatitis B virus genome with a preX open reading frame. *Nucl. Acids Res.* ***18***, 4940.
11. Sambrook, J., Fritsch, E.F., and Maniatis, T. (eds.) (1990) *Molecular Cloning*, Cold Spring Harbor Laboratory Press, NY, 9.31–9.62.
12. Hilger, C., Velhagen, I., Zentgraf, H., and Schröder, C. H. (1991) Diversity of hepatitis B virus X gene-related transcripts in hepatocellular carcinoma: a novel polyadenylation site on viral DNA. *J. Virol.* **65**, 4284–4291.

5

Quantification of HBV Covalently Closed Circular DNA from Liver Tissue by Real-Time PCR

Scott Bowden, Kathy Jackson, Margaret Littlejohn, and Stephen Locarnini

1. Introduction

Hepadnaviruses utilize an unusual replication strategy. On infection, the partially double-stranded open circular genomic DNA is transported to the hepatocyte nucleus, where host-cell enzymes convert it to a relaxed circular fully double-stranded molecule. From this replicative form is generated a covalently closed circular (ccc) DNA, which associates with cellular histones to form a viral minichromosome *(1,2)*. The HBV (hepatitis B virus) ccc DNA remains in the cell nucleus and serves as the transcriptional template for HBV–RNA production.

Viral replication proceeds by the production of multiple copies of a terminally redundant replicative RNA, known as the pregenome. Viral mRNAs, including those that code for the multifunctional polymerase protein, core protein, and envelope proteins, are transported to the cytoplasm for translation. The pregenomic RNA is encapsidated in precursors of the virion core particle and are reverse transcribed by the viral polymerase to form a minus-sense single-strand DNA *(3)*. Subsequently, the pregenome is degraded, and the minus-strand DNA acts as a template for synthesis of a plus-strand DNA of variable length.

At this stage, the assembled nucleocapsids can follow either of two pathways. They can associate with the envelope proteins to produce virions and be secreted from the cell or they can be recycled back to the nucleus as part of a regulatory pathway to maintain a pool of ccc DNA molecules *(4)*. These two pathways result in the formation of a steady-state population of 5–50 ccc DNA molecules per infected hepatocyte *(5)*.

This reservoir of HBV ccc DNA in the nucleus poses a difficult hurdle for antiviral therapy to overcome. As HBV replication does not employ a semiconservative mechanism, any nucleotide analog-based therapy would not be expected to affect directly the preexisting ccc DNA template. This expectation has been borne out by clinical experience. A major reason for the relapse seen after completion of antiviral therapy for hepatitis B infection

From: *Methods in Molecular Medicine, vol. 95: Hepatitis B and D Protocols, volume 1*
Edited by: R. K. Hamatake and J. Y. N. Lau © Humana Press Inc., Totowa, NJ

was recognized more than 18 yr ago by Omata and colleagues ***(6)***, who demonstrated that this ccc DNA form was not eliminated by treatment with interferon alpha.

Similarly, in animal models of HBV infection, hepadnaviral ccc DNA appears to be relatively unaffected by nucleoside analog therapy ***(7,8)***, despite the reduction of all other viral DNA forms in the liver. A contributing reason for this failure could be a long intrahepatic half-life of viral ccc DNA, which under normal circumstances may be as stable as host-cell DNA. A relatively short half-life of 3–5 d for duck HBV ccc DNA has been reported ***(9)***; however, this study was in vitro, and the half-life in vivo remains undetermined. Furthermore, Newbold and colleagues ***(2)*** have demonstrated that duck HBV ccc DNA exists as different topoisomers *in situ*, which may have functional and structural implications.

Overall, current evidence suggests that the eradication of chronic HBV infection probably requires the elimination of the viral ccc DNA species ***(10)***. This result can occur by cytokine-mediated clearance of intracellular virus or by T-cell–mediated destruction of infected cells ***(11,12)***. The role of antiviral chemotherapy with nucleoside analogs may therefore lie in reducing the viral load sufficiently to let the host immune mechanisms eradicate the remaining infection.

In patients receiving long-term nucleoside analog therapy for chronic HBV infection, monitoring for the presence and level of intrahepatic ccc DNA may provide a useful guide to the efficacy of treatment and the likelihood of long-term response, and may aid in the decision of when to cease therapy. Quantification of HBV ccc DNA by conventional techniques such as Southern hybridization is difficult because of the limited amount of clinical material available and the low copy number of ccc DNA molecules that may be in the cell.

To overcome these difficulties, assays employing selective HBV ccc DNA polymerase chain reaction (PCR) have now been described ***(13,14)***. The strategy of the selective PCR to differentiate intracellular HBV ccc DNA from virion open circular DNA and other HBV replicative intermediates was originally devised by Kock et al. ***(13)*** (**Fig. 1**). The strategy exploits the unusual feature of the HBV genome in that it is not fully double-stranded. The genomic DNA has a gap in the minus-strand and an incomplete plus-strand of variable length. In the intrahepatic HBV ccc DNA molecule, these regions are continuous and complete. Thus, selective ccc DNA primers can be designed to amplify the region that corresponds to the gap and incomplete region in the partially double-stranded virion DNA. For the HBV ccc DNA, amplification proceeds unhindered; however, for the other HBV–DNA forms that lack continuity in this region, amplification will be inefficient.

The selectivity of the HBV ccc DNA primers is not absolute. Partial elongation products can be generated from the PCR of non-ccc forms of HBV–DNA, which can provide a template for further amplification. The specificity of the selective ccc DNA PCR can be further enhanced by the addition of Plasmid-Safe adenosine triphosphate (ATP)-dependent deoxyribonuclease DNase (Epicentre Technologies), which hydrolyzes linear double-stranded DNA as well as linear and closed circular single-stranded DNA. Addition of DNase after extraction generally produces another log reduction in the background amplification. Under these conditions, a thousandfold excess of non-ccc

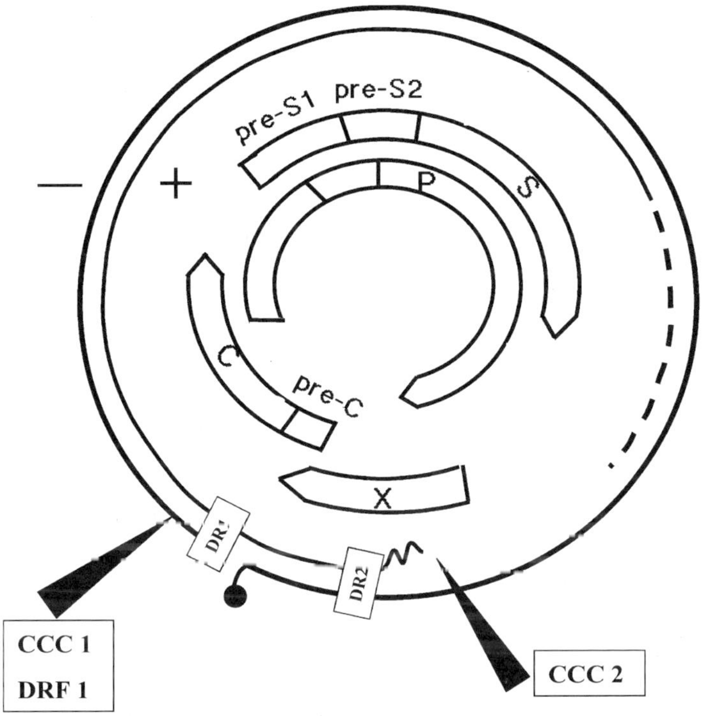

Fig. 1. The structural and genetic organization of the genome of HBV. The outer bold circles represent the DNA genome as present in the virion. The plus (+) and minus (–) strands are shown with the capped oligoribonucleotide (√) and terminal protein (•) attached to the 5' end of the receptive DNA strands; the four major open reading frames (precore/core, pre-S1/pre-S2/S, P, and X) as shown in the center. The cohesive overlap region lies between the direct repeat (DR) DR1 and DR2. The primers for selective amplification of ccc DNA are indicated on either side of DR1 and DR2.

HBV–DNA would be needed before there could be any significant contribution to the quantitative HBV ccc DNA assay *(15)*.

Most of the PCR assays described for measuring levels of HBV ccc DNA have relied on end-point measurement, which has been the standard method of quantifying low levels of DNA. However, such procedures usually rely on coamplification of an internal standard of known copy number and require post-PCR manipulation, which increases the risk of contamination. A recent innovation in the quantification of DNA has been the development of real-time PCR, in which PCR product is detected as it accumulates. In this case, quantification is based on the reaction kinetics of PCR, where there is an inverse logarithmic relationship between the cycle of PCR in which the product is first detected and the initial level of target DNA.

A prerequisite for real time PCR is a detection chemistry that will generate a signal in proportion to the amount of PCR product accumulated and an instrument capable of detecting the signal throughout the thermal cycling process. These items have been provided by the development of suitable fluorescent chemistry and instruments capable of monitoring fluorescence, such as the Roche LightCycler™ (see Roche LightCycler™ website).

The LightCycler™ is a microvolume fluorimeter combining high-speed thermal cycling with real-time on-line fluorescent measurement. The fluorescent chemistry is provided by SYBR Green 1 dye, which binds preferentially to double-stranded DNA. Upon excitation, the dye gives a fluorescent signal proportional to the amount of newly synthesized DNA. When SYBR Green 1 dye is used, specificity of the PCR product needs to be verified by melting-curve analysis after the amplification. Specific product is detected by a characteristic melting at the appropriate T_m, whereas artifacts melt at lower temperatures. Alternatively, for more specific detection, juxtaposed hybridization probes, which are internal to the amplification primers, can be used to monitor the accumulation of PCR product.

The LightCycler™ system has been designed to monitor fluorescence resonance energy transfer (FRET), where the 3' end of one probe is labeled with a donor fluorophore and the 5' end of the other probe has an acceptor fluorophore. Upon excitation from an external source, the donor fluorophore transfers energy to the acceptor fluorophore which in turn emits a signal of a specified wavelength for detection. FRET will only occur if the two probes hybridize successfully, thus achieving the desired specificity.

2. Materials

2.1. Solutions and Kits

1. Nuclease-free water. Store at –20°C (Promega Corporation, Sydney, Australia, cat. no. P1193).
2. QIAamp DNA mini kit [QIAGEN, Melbourne, Australia, cat. no. 51306 (250X)].
3. Plasmid-Safe ATP-dependent DNase (10 U/μL). Store at –20°C (Epicentre Technologies, cat. no. E3105K).
4. LightCycler™-FastStart DNA master SYBR Green 1. Store at –20°C [Roche Molecular Biochemicals, cat. no. 3003 230 (96X)].
5. LightCycler™-FastStart DNA master hybridization probes. Store at –20°C, [Roche, cat. no. 3 003 248 (96X)].
6. LightCycler™-control kit DNA. Store at –20°C [Roche, cat. no. 2 158 833 (50X)].
7. HBV ccc DNA hybridization probes. Store at –20°C and avoid exposure to light (TIB MOLBIOL, Berlin, Germany).
8. Primers (Geneworks, Adelaide, Australia).

2.2. Primers

The selective HBV ccc DNA primers designed by Kock et al. ***(13)*** proved to be unsuitable for use in the LightCycler™ because the rapid cycling kinetics do not allow the generation of such a large PCR product. In their place, we modified the primers DRF1 and DRR3 deduced by Mason et al. ***(14)*** to overcome HBV genotype and strain differences. Optimal sensitivity was obtained by combining two upstream primers (safety primers), CCC1 and DRF1, with a new antisense primer, CCC2.

CCC1 5' GCG GWC TCC CCG TCT GTG CC 3'
DRF1 5' GTC TGT GCC TTC TCA TCT GC 3'
CCC2 5' GTC CAT GCC CCA AAG CCA CC 3'

1. Make 100 μ*M* stock solution with nuclease-free water and store at –20°C.
2. For working stock, dilute 2 μL each of upstream primers CCC1 and DRF1 and 4 μL of downstream primer CCC2 with 32 μL of nuclease-free water and store at –20°C.

2.3. Equipment

1. Filtered pipet tips (10F μL, 20 μL, 200 μL βT aerosol barrier tips, Continental Lab Products, distributed through Integrated Sciences, cat. nos. βT10Fμl, βT20μl, βT200μl).
2. Unskirted Sarstedt microtubes, 1.5 mL with cap [Biocorp cat. no. EV-7161 (500 X)].
3. LightCycler™ capillaries (Roche, cat. no. 1 909 339 [8 × 96]).
4. LightCycler™ centrifuge adapters [Roche, cat. no. 1 909 312 (32)].
5. LightCycler™ sample carousel (Roche, cat. no. 1 909 282).
6. LightCycler™ carousel centrifuge (Roche).
7. LightCycler™ (Roche).
8. Microcentrifuge.
9. Water bath/heat block.

2.4. Tissue Samples

Only a section of the liver biopsy is required, but samples should preferably be around 5–10 mg. Sections should be placed in Sarstedt tubes and stored at –70°C as soon as possible before the next step of DNA extraction.

3. Methods (*see* Note 1)

3.1. Controls for Assay

1. Reagent control. This control contains all the PCR mastermix reagents with nuclease-free water in place of any extracted DNA.
2. Two negative controls. If available, one negative control should comprise liver tissue from a patient known to be HBV-negative that has undergone the same extraction procedure as the samples to be assayed. A second negative control, which acts as a specificity control, can comprise genomic HBV–DNA extracted from a suitable serum sample.
3. A positive control. One positive control should comprise liver tissue from a patient known to be HBV-positive, which gives a detectable signal in the HBV ccc DNA assay. From a single extraction, small aliquots of eluted DNA should be stored at –70°C and subsequently thawed and added for each PCR assay. With this procedure, reproducibility of the assay can be determined.

3.2. HBV Standards

The quantification of the HBV ccc DNA relies on the direct comparison to external standards that have been amplified in parallel reactions. However, the choice of an appropriate HBV external standard is problematic because there is no widely available HBV ccc DNA reference reagent. A suitable alternative is to use a plasmid containing a fully double-stranded copy of the HBV genome and titrate it against a standard of known titer in a commercial assay. As several HBV clones have been constructed with greater than genome length, it is important to ascertain whether the plasmid has a monomeric form of HBV or not, because this may influence the final calculation of sample copy number. We use a series of four dilutions of a single copy HBV genome containing plasmid to achieve final concentrations of around 10^2–10^5 copies/μL.

3.3. Sample Preparation

All steps are to be performed in the extraction area. The procedure followed is essentially as described in the tissue protocol of the QIAGEN QIAamp DNA mini kit.

1. Place 5–10 mg of tissue into a Sarstedt tube and add 180 μL buffer ATL. For pieces of tissue larger than 10 mg, cut into smaller pieces using a sterile scalpel.
2. Add 20 μL of 20 mg/mL proteinase K (or appropriate volume to achieve equivalent concentration).
3. Mix by vortexing and incubate overnight at 56°C to achieve complete lysis. Vortex occasionally during incubation to enhance the lysis process.
4. Continue with the protocol outlined in the QIAGEN notes with the following modifications; the RNase step is not necessary, and in the final step, elute with only 50 μL of the supplied elution buffer.
5. For each sample, prepare reaction mix: 2 μL 10X Plasmid-Safe reaction buffer, 0.8 μL 25 m*M* adenosine triphosphate (ATP), 1 μL Plasmid-safe ATP-dependent DNase (10 U/μL) (*see* **Note 2**), 11.2 μL nuclease-free water
6. Add 5 μL extracted liver sample. Mix and spin briefly.
7. Incubate at 37°C for 30 min.
8. Inactivate enzyme by incubating at 70°C for 30 min.

If samples are not to be used immediately, they should be stored at –20°C.

3.4. SYBR Green 1 Procedure

3.4.1. Preparation of Master Mixture (*see* **Note 3**)

1. Thaw reagents and spin tubes at 16,000*g* for 10–15 s. Protect LightCycler™ reaction mix from light.
2. Add contents of vial 1b (colorless cap) to vial 1a (green cap). Mix by tapping tube, then briefly centrifuge and keep in dark. This combined reaction mix may be stored at 4°C in the dark for several weeks.
3. Prepare the master mixture in a Sarstedt tube. For each reaction: 11.8 μL nuclease-free water, 3.2 μL $MgCl_2$ (5 m*M*), 1 μL primers (10 μ*M* each), 2. μL SYBR Green 1 reaction mix. For large numbers of samples, prepare an additional reaction volume to allow for losses during aliquotting. The $MgCl_2$ concentration may need to be varied (see LightCycler™-FastStart DNA master SYBR Green 1 instructions).
4. Mix tube by tapping, and then spin briefly.

3.4.2. Template Addition (*see* **Note 4**)

1. Place the required number of capillaries in numerical order in precooled centrifuge adaptors. Avoid touching the bottom of the capillaries.
2. Aliquot 18 μL of master mix into each capillary.
3. Add 2 μL of reagent control, negative controls, samples, standards, and positive control into appropriate capillaries in that order.
4. Put caps on capillaries, and then transfer them to clean rack for transportation to the amplification area.

3.4.3. LightCycler™ Amplification and Quantification (see **Note 5**)

1. Load capillaries into the LightCycler™ carousel in numerical order. It is recommended that goggles be worn because of possible capillary breakage.
2. Spin the carousel in the special centrifuge until it reaches 735*g* and transfer to the LightCycler™.
3. Program the LightCycler™ as follows:

		Temperature Transition	Acquisition Mode
Denature –95°C for 10 min (1 cycle) (Analysis mode–none)		20°C/s	None
Cycling	–95°C for 15 s (45 cycles) (Analysis mode–quantification)	20°C/s	None
	–63°C for 10 s	20°C/s	None
	–72°C for 25 s	10°C/s	None
	–82°C for 2 s	20°C/s	Single
Melt	–95°C for 10 s	20°C/s	None
	–65°C for 15 s	20°C/s	None
	–95°C for 10 s	0.1°C/s	Continuous
Cool –40°C for 30 s			
Mode F1/1			
Fluorimeter gains 5, 15, 30			

4. Run assay and analyze results as per manufacturer's instructions.

3.5. Master Hybridization Probes Procedure

3.5.1. Preparation of Master Mixture (see **Note 3**)

1. Thaw reagents and spin tubes at 16,000*g* for 10–15 s (protect hybridization probes from light).
2. Add contents of vial 1b (colorless cap) to vial 1a (red cap). Mix by tapping tube, and then briefly centrifuge and keep in dark. This combined reaction mix may be stored at 4°C for several weeks.
3. Prepare the master mixture in a Sarstedt tube. For each reaction: 11.4 μL nuclease-free water, 3.2 μL Mg Cl_2 (5 m*M*), 1 μL primers (10 μ*M*), 0.4 μL hybridization probes (10 μ*M*), 2 μL hybridization probe mix. For large numbers of samples prepare an additional reaction volume. The $MgCl_2$ concentration may need to be varied. (See LightCycler™-FastStart DNA master hybridization probes instructions.)
4. Mix by tapping, and then spin briefly.
5. Proceed with aliquotting and sample addition in amplification area as per SYBR Green 1 procedure.

3.5.2. LightCycler™ Amplification and Quantification (see **Note 5**)

1. Load capillaries into LightCycler™ carousel in numerical order.
2. Spin the carousel in the special centrifuge until it reaches 735*g* and transfer to the LightCycler™.

3. Program the LightCycler™ as follows:

		Temperature Transition	Acquisition Mode
Denature (1 cycle) (Analysis mode–none)	–95°C for 10 min	20°C/s	None
Cycling (45 cycles) (Analysis mode–quantification)	–95°C for 10 s	20°C/s	None
	–63°C for 10 s	20°C/s	Single
	–72°C for 20 s	20°C/s	None
Cool	–40°C for 30 s	20°C/s	None
Mode F2/F1			
Fluorimeter gains 1, 15, 30			

4. Run assay and analyze the results as per manufacturer's instructions.

3.6. β-Globin Amplification and Quantification

As there is variation in the amount of liver tissue among samples, quantifying the amount of the housekeeping gene, β-globin, allowed for the standardization of the extracted DNA and expression of HBV ccc DNA as copies per genome equivalent. A commercial kit, specifically designed to amplify a 110-kb fragment of the human β-globin gene, is available from Roche for use in the LightCycler™ (DNA control kit). The kit includes human genomic DNA of known concentration, which allows construction of a standard curve for comparison of the unknown liver samples. Specific hybridization probes for β-globin are also included in the kit.

The control kit DNA contains a stock of 15 ng/μL human genomic DNA. An aliquot of 2 μL contains approximately 10^4 genome equivalents. Serial 1:10 dilutions of the stock solution are made to achieve the following final concentrations:

1.5 ng/μL = 10^3 genome equivalents/2 μL;
150 pg/μL= 10^2 genome equivalents/2 μL;
15 pg/μL = 10^1 genome equivalents/2 μL;
1.5 pg/μL = 10^0 genome equivalents/μL.

These concentrations are then used as standards and tested with the liver samples either by the SYBR Green 1 method or with the master hybridization probes. In our experience, the extracted liver samples need to be diluted 1:10 prior to testing with the β-globin primers.

3.7. Quantification of HBV ccc DNA

The HBV ccc DNA copy number for the extracted liver samples is calculated by dividing the copies/μL determined in **Subheadings 3.4.** or **3.5.** by the genome equivalents/μL (**Subheading 3.6.**) and the result expressed as HBV ccc DNA copies/genome equivalent.

Presently, the significance of a particular level of ccc DNA in relationship to the natural history of the disease is unknown. To derive meaning, the end of treatment level would need to be compared with the pretreatment load. It is envisaged that the undetectable end of treatment ccc DNA by PCR would be a significant step toward the successful control of HBV infection by antiviral therapy.

4. Notes

1. As the technique involves a nucleic acid amplification technology, it is important that three physically separate areas be used to reduce the risk of contamination: a dedicated clean area for the preparation of PCR mastermix and other reagents, an area for the extraction of DNA from samples, and a contained area for the amplification and concomitant detection. In addition, the work flow should be designed to reduce the possible risk of contamination.
2. Extracted liver samples should be digested with Plasmid-Safe ATP-dependent DNase to reduce the amount of non-ccc forms of HBV–DNA.
3. These steps should be performed in the clean area.
4. These steps should be performed in the extraction area.
5. These steps should be performed in the amplification area.

Acknowledgments

The method described here evolved from informal discussions with several interested parties. Carolyn Luscombe and Madhu Singh from VIRIDAE (Vancouver, Canada) made important contributions in the early phase of development. Craig Gibbs from Gilead Sciences (Foster City, CA) provided substantial funding, which allowed the assays to progress from a research test to a research tool, and encouraged participation and contributions of other scientists. Of these, special thanks must go to Bettina Werle and Fabien Zoulim from INSERM (Lyon, France), who had great input into modifyng the assay to a real-time format.

References

1. Bock, C.T., Schranz, P., Schroder, C. H., and Zentgraf, H. (1994) Hepatitis B virus genome is organized into nucleosomes in the nucleus of the infected cell. *Virus Genes* **8**, 215–229.
2. Newbold, J. E., Xin, H., Tencza, M., et al. (1995) The covalently closed duplex form of the hepadnavirus genome exists in situ as a heterogeneous population of viral minichromosomes. *J. Virol.* **69**, 3350–3357.
3. Summers, J., and Mason, W. S. (1982) Replication of the genome of a hepatitis B-like virus by reverse transcription of an RNA intermediate. *Cell* **29**, 403–415.
4. Tuttleman, J. S., Pourcel, C., and Summers, J. (1986) Formation of the pool of covalently closed circular viral DNA in hepadnavirus-infected cells. *Cell* **47**, 451–460.
5. Jilbert, A. R., Wu, T. T., England, J. M., et al. (1992) Rapid resolution of duck hepatitis B virus infections occurs after massive hepatocellular involvement. *J. Virol.* **66**, 1377–1388.
6. Yokosuka, O., Omata, M., Imazeki, F., Okuda, K., and Summers, J. (1985) Changes of hepatitis B virus DNA in liver and serum caused by recombinant leukocyte interferon treatment: analysis of intrahepatic replicative hepatitis B virus DNA. *Hepatology* **5**, 728–734.
7. Dean, J., Bowden, S., and Locarnini, S. (1995) Reversion of duck hepatitis B virus DNA replication in vivo following cessation of treatment with the nucleoside analogue ganciclovir. *Antiviral Res,* **27**, 171–178.
8. Moraleda, G., Saputelli, J., Aldrich, C. E., Averett, D., Condreay, L., and Mason, W. S. (1997) Lack of effect of antiviral therapy in nondividing hepatocyte cultures on the closed circular DNA of woodchuck hepatitis virus. *J. Virol.* **71**, 9392–9399.

9. Civitico, G. M., and Locarnini, S.A. (1994) The half-life of duck hepatitis B virus supercoiled DNA in congenitally infected primary duck hepatocyte cultures. *Virology* **203**, 81–89.
10. Locarnini, S. A., Civitico, G. M., and Newbold, J. E. (1996) Hepatitis B: new approaches for antiviral chemotherapy. *Antiviral Chemistry Chemotherapy* **7**, 1–12.
11. Guidotti, L. G., Rochford, R., Chung, J., Shapiro, M., Purcell, R., and Chisari, F. V. (1999) Viral clearance without destruction of infected cells during acute HBV infection. *Science* **284**, 825–829.
12. Guo, J., Zhou, H., Liu, C., et al. (2000) Apoptosis and regeneration of hepatocytes during recovery from transient hepadnavirus infections. *J. Virol.* **74**, 1495–1505.
13. Kock, J., Theilmann, L., Galle, P., and Schlicht, H. J. (1996) Hepatitis B virus nucleic acids associated with human peripheral blood mononuclear cells do not originate from replicating virus. *Hepatology* **23**, 405–413.
14. Mason, A. L., Xu, L., Guo, L., Kuhns, M., and Perrillo, R. (1998) Molecular basis for persistent hepatitis B virus infection in the liver after clearance of serum hepatitis B surface antigen. *Hepatology* **27**, 1736–1742.
15. Littlejohn, M., Bowden, S., Jackson, K., Angus, P., and Locarnini, S. (2001) Selective PCR for hepatitis B virus ccc DNA: validation of real-time assays. *Hepatology* **34**, 311A.

6

In Situ Hybridization for the Detection and Localization of HBV DNA in Liver Sections

Vicky C. H. Lai and Johnson Y. N. Lau

1. Introduction

The technique of *in situ* hybridization was first developed to localize specific DNA sequences on chromosomes *(1)*. This technique has subsequently been modified to detect viral nuclear acids in tissue sections. Information gathered from this type of study can help us to identify the site of viral replication at the subcellular level and to understand the relationship between viral expression and disease activity.

In this chapter, a nonradioisotopic *in situ* hybridization procedure, optimized to detect hepatitis B virus HBV DNA in formalin-fixed, paraffin-embedded liver tissues, is described *(2)*. Briefly, the traditional radioactive-labeled HBV DNA probe is replaced by the nonradioactive digoxigenin (DIG)–labeled DNA probes. The DNA probe labeled by DIG has been shown to have the same sensitivity as a ^{32}P-labeled DNA probe and is able to detect HBV DNA between 1 and 3 ng in a spot hybridization *(3)*. The viral DNA probe hybrids are then traced by anti-DIG antibody conjugated with alkaline phosphatase and visualized by alkaline phosphatase–based enzymatic reaction. This procedure was initially developed by Drs. Naoumov and Lau and was subsequently modified and extensively used in the laboratory of Professor Wu and Dr. Lai. By using this procedure, we have shown that positive HBV DNA staining is mainly confined in the cytoplasm and the nucleus of infected hepatocytes **(Fig. 1)**.

2. Materials

1. Plasmid pHBV130.4 containing the full-length HBV DNA (kindly provided by Professor Murray). Any HBV DNA probe is useful for the experiments described here.
2. DIG-High Prime kit (Roche Molecular Biochemicals, Indianapolis, IN).
3. DIG Quantification Teststrips and DIG Control Teststrips (Roche Molecular Biochemicals).
4. Poly-L-lysine-coated microscope slides: Poly-L-lysine with concentration of 0.1% (Sigma Chemicals Co., St. Louis, MO) is layered onto glass microscope slides and allowed to dry.

From: *Methods in Molecular Medicine, vol. 95: Hepatitis B and D Protocols, volume 1*
Edited by: R. K. Hamatake and J. Y. N. Lau © Humana Press Inc., Totowa, NJ

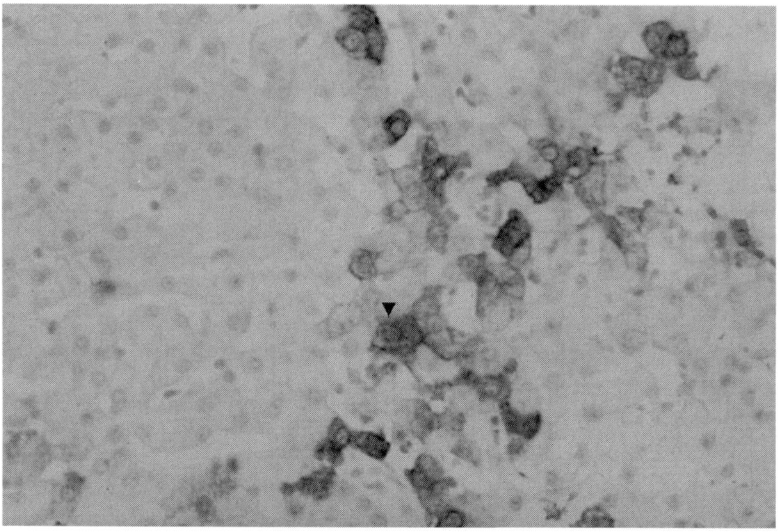

Fig. 1. HBV DNA was detected in the cytoplasm (mainly) and nucleus of infected hepatocytes by using nonradioisotopic *in situ* hybridization. Some infected hepatocytes showed the presence of HBV DNA in both the cytoplasm and nucleus (arrowhead).

5. Analytical-grade xylene and absolute ethanol (Fisher Scientific, Pittsburgh, PA).
6. Phosphate-buffered saline (PBS): a 10X PBS stock is 1.37 *M* NaCl, 27 m*M* KCl, 43 m*M* Na_2HPO_4, 14 m*M* KH_2PO_4 (pH 7.3).
7. Protease (Type XXXIV, Sigma).
8. 50 m*M* Tris-HCl, pH 7.4 (Fisher Scientific).
9. PBS with 26 m*M* glycine (Sigma).
10. 4% paraformaldehyde in PBS: Dissolve 8 g of paraformaldehyde (Sigma) in 100 mL deionized water and heat up to 50°C; add 10 *N* NaOH until the white powder dissolves, mix with 100 mL of 2X PBS, adjust the pH to 7.4 with concentrated HCl, and store at 4°C.
11. Deionized formamide: Mix 500 mL of formamide (Sigma) with 50 g of resin (AG 501-X8, 20–50 mesh, Bio-Rad, Glattsbrugg, Switzerland); stir for 30 min at room temperature; filter through Whatman 2, and store in 5-mL aliquots at –20°C, protected from light.
12. 50% Dextran sulfate: Dissolve dextran sulfate (Sigma) in deionized water and store in aliquots at –20°C.
13. 10 mg/mL herring sperm DNA (Type XIV, Sigma).
14. 50X Denhardt's solution: Dissolve 50 mg Ficoll 400, 50 mg polyvinylpyrrolidone, and 50 mg bovine serum albumin (Sigma) in 5 mL of deionized water, and store in aliquots at –20°C.
15. Standard saline citrate (SSC): 20X stock is 3 *M* NaCl, 0.3 *M* Na_3 citrate, pH 7.0.
16. Tris-buffered saline (TBS): 10X stock is 1 *M* Tris-HCl, pH 7.5, 1.5 *M* NaCl.
17. Tween-20 (Sigma).
18. Normal sheep serum (Dako, Carpinteria, CA).
19. Bovine serum albumin (Sigma).

20. Sheep polyclonal anti-DIG antibody conjugated with alkaline phosphatase (Roche Molecular Biochemicals).
21. TNM buffer: 100 m*M* Tris-HCl, pH 9.5, 100 m*M* NaCl, 50 m*M* $MgCl_2$.
22. Substrate solution: Add 45 µL of nitroblue tetrazolium (100 mg/mL in dimethylformamide, Roche Molecular Biochemicals), 35 µL of 5-bromo-4-chloro-3-indoyl-phosphate (50 mg/mL in dimethylformamide, Roche Molecular Biochemicals), and 0.024% levamisole (Sigma) in 10 mL of TNM buffer. Prepare immediately before use.
23. 0.1% nuclear fast red solution: Dissolve 0.1 g of nuclear fast red (Sigma) in 100 mL deionized water.
24. Mounting medium: Permount (Fisher Scientific).
25. Coplin jars and humidified slide chambers.

3. Methods

3.1. Preparation of DIG-Labeled HBV DNA Probes

1. Transfer 300 ng of the plasmid pHBV130.4 containing full-length HBV DNA to a 1.5-mL microcentrifuge tube; add deionized water to a final volume of 16 µL.
2. Denature the DNA at 95°C for 10 min and quickly chill the sample on ice.
3. Add 4 µL of DIG-high prime reaction mixture to the tube (*see* **Note 1**).
4. Incubate at 37°C for 16 h.
5. Heat the tube at 65°C for 10 min to stop the reaction.
6. Quantitate the amount of DIG-labeled DNA probe by using the DIG quantification teststrips.
7. Aliquot the labeled probe and store at –20°C.

3.2. In situ *Hybridization and Detection of HBV DNA on Paraffin Sections*

1. Place 5-µm thick paraffin sections on poly-L-lysine–coated glass slides, air-dry, and store at room temperature.
2. Deparaffinize tissue sections in xylene twice for 10 min.
3. Rehydrate to PBS through a standard ethanol series (absolute ethanol, twice for 5 min, then 95% ethanol for 5 min and 70% ethanol for 5 min).
4. Protease digestion: Treat each section with 100–200 µL of protease (0.5 mg/mL in 50 m*M* Tris-HCl, pH 7.4) and place them in a humidified slide chamber. Incubate the sections for 10 min at 37°C (*see* **Note 2**).
5. Stop the protease activity by transferring the slides to a Coplin jar containing freshly prepared PBS with 26 m*M* glycine and wash twice for 5 min.
6. Rinse the tissue sections in PBS twice for 2 min.
7. Gently fix the sections by 4% paraformaldehyde in PBS for 5 min at room temperature.
8. Block the fixation in freshly prepared PBS with 26 m*M* glycine twice for 5 min.
9. Rinse the tissue sections in PBS twice for 2 min.
10. Dehydrate the sections through a standard ethanol series (70% ethanol for 5 min, 95% ethanol for 5 min, and then absolute ethanol, twice for 5 min) and air-dry for 1.5 h.
11. Add 10 µL of hybridization mixture to each section: 50% deionized formamide, 10% (w/v) dextran sulfate, 0.4 mg/mL herring sperm DNA, 5X Denhardt's solution, 2X SSC, and 0.4 µg/mL DIG-labeled probe.
12. Cover the sections with plastic cover slip, remove gas bubbles, and seal with nail polish.
13. Denature the DNA on the sections by placing the slides in an oven at 95°C for 10 min.
14. Cool the slides for 5 min on a wet paper towel.

15. Place the slides in a humidified slide chamber and incubate in an oven overnight at 37°C.
16. Remove the cover slips and wash the sections two times for 5 min at room temperature in 2X SSC, two times for 3 min at 62°C in 2X SSC, 3 min at 62°C in 0.1X SSC, and 5 min at room temperature in 2X SSC.
17. Rinse the sections in TBS with 0.1% Tween-20, three times for 5 min at room temperature, followed by two 5-min washes in TBS.
18. Overlay the sections with 100–200 μL of TBS containing 10% normal sheep serum and 3% bovine serum albumin. Incubate for 15 min at room temperature.
19. Remove excess buffer and overlay the sections with 200 μL of TBS containing 0.2% sheep anti-DIG antibody and 1% bovine serum albumin. Incubate for 2 h at 37°C (*see* **Note 3**).
20. Wash the sections in TBS with 0.1% Tween-20 five times for 3 min.
21. Rinse the sections twice in TBS.
22. Place the slides in TNM buffer for 5 min.
23. Apply the substrate solution and leave in the dark for 1 h (*see* **Note 4**).
24. Check the intensity of positive staining under an inverted microscope. Do not allow the sections to dry (*see* **Note 5**).
25. Rinse the sections with tap water.
26. Counterstain with 0.1% nuclear fast red solution for 5 min.
27. Briefly rinse the sections with tap water to remove excess nuclear fast red solution.
28. Dehydrate the sections through a standard ethanol series, clear through xylene and mount the slides (*see* **Note 6**).
29. Remember that controls are critical for this experiment (*see* **Note 7**).
30. Results from one of the experiments are illustrated in **Fig 1.**

4. Notes

1. The DIG-labeled DNA probe described in this protocol is synthesized by a random primed labeling method in the presence of DIG-11-dUTP. This labeling method produces a heterogeneous population of probe strands, ranging from 200 to 1000 basepairs. Many of these probe strands have overlapping complementary regions, which may lead to signal amplification in *in situ* hybridization.
2. Protease treatment on the tissue sections is to digest the surrounding proteins of the target to expose the viral DNA for binding to the labeled DNA probe. The concentration of protease used should be optimized to prevent overdigestion of the tissue sections. Optimization parameters for this treatment include the concentration of protease, incubation temperature, and incubation time. Excessive digestion of the tissue sections may result in loss of cellular organization of the tissue and also cellular morphology.
3. It is important to avoid drying of the solution on the sections during immunochemical detection, which may significantly increase the background staining. A wet paper towel is placed in the slide chamber during incubation with antibody.
4. Levamisole is added to the substrate solution to block the endogenous alkaline phosphatase in liver.
5. Development of a color signal should be carefully monitored to avoid understaining or overstaining on the sections. We usually monitor the color signal every 15 min under an inverted microscope.
6. After the sections are counter stained, the dehydration steps through a standard ethanol series should be performed quickly to avoid loss of the positive staining.

7. Positive and negative controls should be included in all experiments to monitor the assay performance. Negative controls can be performed by removing the HBV DNA probe in the hybridization mixture and testing on liver sections from patients with non-HBV disease.

References

1. Gall, J. G., and Pardue, M. L. (1971) Nucleic acid hybridization in cytological preparations. *Meth. Enzymol.* **38** 470–480.
2. Wu, P. C., Fang, W. S., Lai C. L., et al. (1996) Hepatic expression of hepatitis B virus genome in chronic hepatitis B virus infection. *Am. J. Clin. Pathol.* **105** 87–95.
3. Naoumov, N. V., Lau, J. Y., Daniels, H. M., Alexander, G. J., and Williams, R. (1991) Detection of HBV-DNA using a digoxigenin-labelled probe: a rapid technique without loss of sensitivity. *J. Hepatol.* **12** 382–385.

7

Quantitative Assay of Hepatitis B Surface Antigen in Serum or Plasma Using Laurell Electrophoresis

Wolfram H. Gerlich, Ulrike Wend, and Dieter Glebe

1. Introduction

1.1. Clinical Significance

Hepatitis B virus (HBV) leads to an overexpression of its surface antigen (HBsAg) in the infected hepatocytes. HBsAg is constitutively secreted as pleomorphic particles, predominantly spherical and partly filamentous. Their diameter appears in negatively stained electron micrographs as approx 20 nm. HBsAg typically reaches serum concentrations between 30 and 100 µg/mL during the incubation phase before acute hepatitis B; in immunotolerant hepatitis B e antigen (HBeAg)-positive HBV carriers and immunosuppressed carriers, HBsAg reaches serum concentrations up to 1000 µg/mL, corresponding to 2×10^{13} or 2×10^{14} particles/mL, respectively ***(1)***. A high HBsAg concentration reflects both a large number of HBsAg-expressing cells and a low elimination rate of HBsAg.

With the onset of the immune defense, the HBsAg concentration starts to decrease, albeit slowly, because of its long half-life and the low levels of antibody against HBsAg (anti-HBs). Resolving acute hepatitis is characterized by a decrease of more than 50% in the HBsAg concentration within 4 wk after its onset, whereas chronic HBV infection is characterized by a lesser decrease or even an increase ***(2–4)***.

In patients with HBeAg-positive chronic hepatitis B, the level of HBsAg is inversely correlated with the response to interferon. Most patients with HBsAg levels <30 µg/mL respond, whereas patients with higher HBsAg levels do not ***(5,6)***. Anti-HBe positive patients with persistent HBV infection generally have lower HBsAg levels <30 µg/mL, irrespective of disease activity or viremia. Nevertheless, a relatively high HBsAg concentration (>1 µg/mL) would reflect a relatively large number of HBsAg-expressing and -secreting hepatocytes. Whether this finding has any impact on the long-term prognosis of chronic HBV carriers is not known.

From: *Methods in Molecular Medicine, vol. 95: Hepatitis B and D Protocols, volume 1*
Edited by: R. K. Hamatake and J. Y. N. Lau © Humana Press Inc., Totowa, NJ

1.2. Heterogeneity of HBsAg

Use of the term HBsAg is not clearly defined. Originally, HBsAg was considered to be the surface antigen of HBV. Later, it was determined that HBsAg existed in various subtypes with the exclusive determinants d or y, w or r, and w1–w4. Furthermore, HBV genotypes A through H have been identified. Besides the genetic heterogeneity, HBsAg contains three distinct co-carboxyterminal polypeptides within one particle. The large HBsAg protein (LHBs) contains the three domains preS1, preS2, and S; the middle HBs protein (MHBs) contains preS2 and S; and the small HBs protein (SHBs) contains only the S domain *(1)*.

SHBs was the first identified HBsAg protein in the early 1970s, whereas MHBs and LHBs, including the preS domains, were unknown until 1983. Most workers still consider only SHBs as HBsAg, and indeed SHBs may form secreted HBsAg particles in the absence of MHBs or LHBs. SHBs particles are the only component of the commonly used hepatitis B vaccines, and natural HBsAg particles contain SHBs as the major antigenic component *(7)*.

Nevertheless, it should be kept in mind that natural HBsAg from patients with or carriers of HBV contains preS1 and preS2, and antisera against natural HBsAg particles will contain anti-preS1 and anti-preS2 in addition to anti-SHBs, which is usually considered to be identical with anti-HBs. Anti-preS antibodies usually detect denaturation-resistant sequential epitopes, whereas anti-HBs epitopes are predominantly conformational *(1,7,8)*.

In this chapter we describe a technique for quantitation of natural HBsAg particles in serum or plasma, which may also be used for purified or "recombinant" HBsAg particles. However, the quantitative calibration is only valid for similar types of HBsAg particles.

1.3. Principle of the Technique

The technique invented by C. B. Laurell is a combination of electrophoresis and immune precipitation in agarose gels. Immune precipitation lines are generated in zones where antigen and antibody meet at equivalent stoichiometric amounts. The antibody is mixed with liquid agarose solution and then spread out on a slide. The antigen is placed in small wells in the antibody/agarose layer and thereafter transported by electrical forces through the agarose. At the edges of the migrating antigen spot, the immune precipitate forms until the antigen is used up, resulting in a precipitation "arch" or "rocket" (*see* **Fig. 3**). The length or the area of the arches is proportional to the amount of antigen applied in the well. The technique described below is a modification of a previously described method *(9)*.

The antiserum we used was generated in a way to provide optimal crossreactivity with all HBV genotypes available to us (A, C, and D). For this purpose, a sheep was immunized first with 100 μg highly purified natural HBsAg from HBeAg-positive carriers of genotype A, thereafter with D, and thereafter with C, and finally with a mix of all three antigens. Any high titered antiserum against SHBs or HBsAg may be used (*see* below), but approx 40% of the antibodies raised with only one HBsAg subtype are subtype-specific.

Alternative methods are enzyme-linked immunosorbent assays (ELISAs). Today's commercially available ELISAs for HBsAg are very sensitive, with a detection limit of down to 0.1 ng/mL. Signal strength of these ELISAs reaches saturation at concentrations around 5–100 ng/mL. However, the typical range of HBsAg concentration is between 1000 and 100,000 ng/mL. Thus, reliable quantitation by ELISA requires dilution series. Furthermore, ELISAs are usually not calibrated in quantitative units.

1.4. Definition of HBsAg Units

There is much confusion about units of HBsAg reactivity. Many workers avoid quantitation completely or provide sample to cutoff ratio (S/CO) units. Occasionally, these units are converted to ng HBsAg, but most communicated ng/mL values are too high, because the HBsAg used for calibration had partially lost reactivity.

We recommend the use of the original Paul Ehrlich unit (PEU), which is equivalent to 1 ng of native HBsAg protein of either genotype A or D ***(9)***. Reference samples are available from the authors. The PEU has been correlated to the IU of anti-HBs ***(10)***. A total of 1 IU anti-HBs can remove 900 PEU or 0.9 ng HBsAg from a strongly HBsAg-positive serum; this amount was measured by the technique described below.

1.5. Other Hepadnaviruses

The technique has also been successfully applied to the surface-antigen particles of woodchuck hepatitis viruses ***(11)*** and duck hepatitis B virus (W. H. Gerlich, unpublished).

2. Materials

2.1. Reagents

1. A polyvalent high-titer antiserum with $>10^5$ IU/L anti-HBs, preferably with 10^6 IU/L. The antiserum must be rich in group-specific antibodies against determinant a (and possibly conserved preS epitope). It may be achieved by immunizing animals, preferably sheep, with 100–1000 μg purified HBsAg particles from a virus carrier with an HBV genotype (A or D) and boosted with 100 μg HBsAg from a carrier with a different HBV genotype (D or A or another type). The HBV carrier should preferably have a high titer and test positive for preS-Ag and HBeAg. The antiserum should be adsorbed with glutaraldehyde-crosslinked gel of human plasma particles to remove antibodies against human serum proteins.
2. A reference serum (or plasma) with 50 μg HBsAg/mL. This serum is available from the Institute of Medical Virology (IMV) at 100 μg/mL.
3. Standard low mr agarose (e.g., Biorad cat. no. 162-0100) 1.2 g per 100 mL.
4. 2X buffer: 17.7 g Tris-HCl; 0.15 g $CaCl_2$, adjust with HCl to about pH 9.4; 9.0 g 5,5-diethylbarbital acid; double-distilled H_2O to 1000 mL; pH adjustment to 8.6. **Caution!** Barbital may not be freely available because it is a narcotic substance.
5. Serum or plasma samples containing HBsAg, 10 μL per run.
6. For dilutions: negative human or fetal calf serum or plasma. Do not mix serum with plasma.

2.2. Equipment and Disposables

1. Glass slides 2 × 3 in. (5.0 × 7.5 cm) with smooth edges to avoid cuts. Glass slides should be fat free. If insufficient adherence of the agarose to the glass is a problem, the slides should be precoated by dipping them into 0.1% hot agarose solution in hot water.

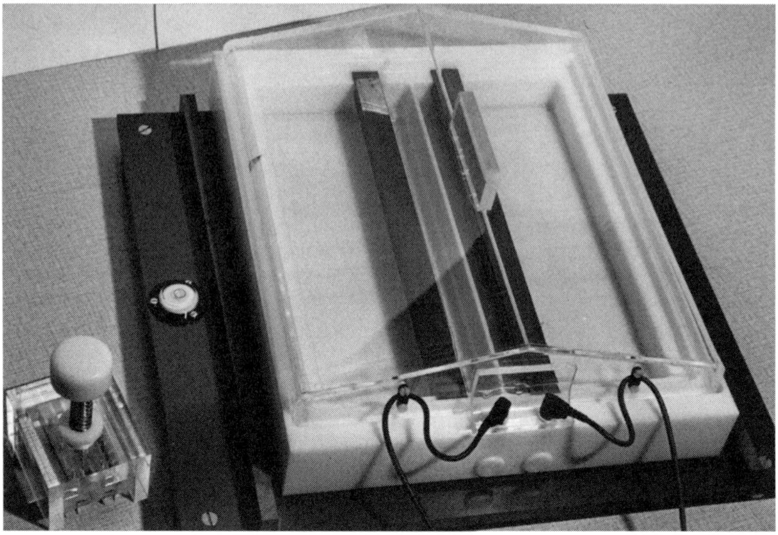

Fig. 1. The electrophoresis chamber and the gel punch built at the workshop of the Institute of Medical Virology.

2. Thick filter paper pieces (e.g., Schleicher and Schuell cat. no. 2668/8). Cut them to 7.5 × 10.0 cm.
3. An electrophoresis chamber for three or four slides with large buffer tanks of 450 mL each and a semipermeable chamber for the platinum electrodes (*see* **Fig. 1**).
4. A punching/cutting device for the agarose gels (**Fig. 2**).
5. A power supply delivering constant current at 4.5 mA per slide.
6. A leveling table for pouring the agarose gel onto the slides.
7. Water bath at 56°C ± 1°C.
8. Accurate Eppendorf pipet for applying 10 μL.
9. Dark-field illumination of immune precipitates with white (cold) light from below above a dark background and a measuring device with a scale (producer in Germany: Eschenbach).

3. Methods

Read the entire procedure completely before starting. Staff must be anti-HBs-positive!

1. Select and arrange samples, write a pipetting plan (**step 14**), and calibrate the technique first (*see* **Note 1**).
2. Melt 1.2 g agarose in 100-mL double-distilled H_2O by heating and mixing in a microwave oven or in a boiling water bath to a clear solution; mix well. Cool down this solution in the 56°C water bath for 5–10 min.
3. Put 4.5 mL of 2X buffer in a 10-mL glass tube and transfer into the 56°C water bath for at least 10 min.
4. Put the required number of slides (three or four) on the leveling table.

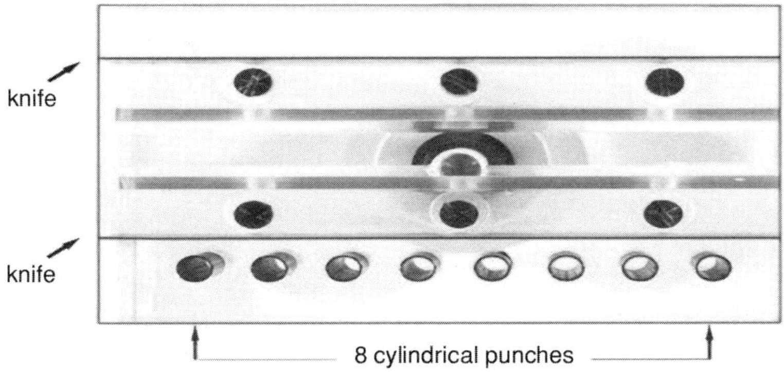

Fig. 2. Punching/cutting pattern for agarose slides.

5. Transfer 4.5-mL agarose solution to the prewarmed 2X buffer and mix by pipetting up and down.
6. Take 6 mL out of the mix and put into a prewarmed 10-mL glass pipet; distribute it swiftly and evenly onto one glass slide. Repeat this step without break for the other slides, and let the slides rest for 10 min to solidify.
7. Apply the punching/cutting device to the gel slides to generate the pattern shown in **Fig. 3**.
8. Aspirate the gel cylinders from the hole with a narrow-bore pipet tip and mild vacuum. Edges of the hole must not be damaged. (*see* **Note 2**).
9. Remove the center layer of the agarose gel from the slide by pushing it to the side with a spatula.
10. Add a suitable amount of anti-HBs antiserum (e.g., 25 μL of sheep antiserum as described in **Subheading 2.1.1.**, with 1 IU/μL anti-HBs) into the 3 mL of 0.6% agarose solution in 56°C warm 1X buffer left from step 6; swirl and pour this mix rapidly and evenly onto the free center area of the slide.
11. Let the slides rest for 10 min. Avoid drying them out. If the slides cannot be used immediately, put them into a moist chamber, but do not store them longer than a few hours.
12. Fill 450 mL 1X buffer into both chambers of the electrophoresis tank.
13. Place the slides on the supports in the chamber, the eight holes being at the cathode (minus pole). Place the filter paper, prewetted with 1X buffer at the edges of the slides with an overlap of 4 mm on the gel on both sides. The filter must not touch the hole. The filters should hang into the buffer chambers and be separated from the electrode compartments.
14. Slowly fill 10 μL of each sample into a hole according to the pipetting plan. The samples should be arranged in a rack according to the pipetting plan, with the eight samples in one row. Each slide must include one positive control with a defined amount of HBsAg/mL, e.g., 30 μ/mL preferably in the center holes nos. 4 or 5. Before this method is used routinely, a calibration line must be established (*see* **Note 1**).
15. Close the electrophoresis chamber by the cover and start electrophoresis at a constant current of 4.5 mA per slide and the holes at the minus pole. Use a timer that shuts off power after 15 h. Do not extend the electrophoresis time! (*See* **Note 3**.)
16. Take out the slides with gloves (the samples, slides, filters, and electrophoresis buffer may be potentially infectious). Wipe the bottom of the slides with paper towels.

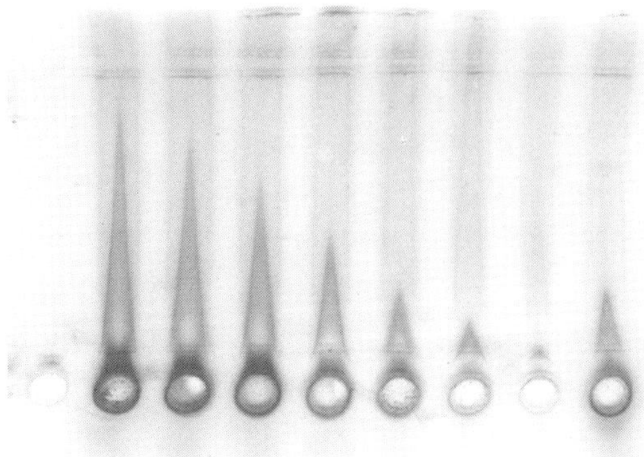

Fig. 3. Pattern resulting from the punching/cutting device and precipitation arches generated by decreasing amounts of HBsAg added to the holes.

17. Put the slide into the measuring device with dark-field illumination and measure the distance between the tip of the precipitation arch and the edge next to the holes of the antibody-containing agarose layer (*see* **Fig. 1**).
18. Once the calibration curve is established, the lengths of the arches produced by each sample are measured and then multiplied with the correction factor (c. f.) for each slide. (c. f. = actual length of the reference/length of reference in the calibration function. c. f. should be between 0.8 and 1.2, preferably 1.0. Samples with small precipitation arches below the antibody agar are estimated to have 0.2 μg/mL if weak and 0.5 μg/mL if somewhat stronger. Samples with open precipitation figures or length above 110% of the 30 μg/mL reference sample should be repeated in suitable dilution to produce a result in the range of 10–35 μg/mL.

4. Notes

1. For calibration, run a dilution series in duplicate or triplicate in the eight holes of the reference plasma with 0.5; 1; 2; 5; 10; 20; 30; 40; 50 μg HBsAg/mL diluted in negative plasma. Determine the length of the precipitation arch for each sample and establish the regression line or function using the mean values from two or three runs. Variation coefficients should not exceed 10% for samples containing ≥ 10 μg/mL; the length should be 15–24 mm for 30 μg/mL. If the length is too short, use less antiserum; if it is too long or the arches are open at the top, use more antiserum.
2. Uneven or disrupted holes should not be used.
3. The slides may rest after electrophoresis in the closed chamber for 2 d.

References

1. Kann, M., and Gerlich, W. H. (1998). Hepatitis B. In: *Topley & Wilson's Microbiology and Microbial Infections,* 9th ed. Arnold, London, vol. 1, 745–773.
2. Gerlich, W. H., Stamm, B., and Thomssen, R. (1977) Prognostische Bedeutung des quantitativen HBsAg-Nachweises bei der akuten Hepatitis B. *Verh. Dtsch. Ges. Inn. Med.* **83**, 554–557.
3. Frösner, G. G., Schomerus, H., Wildmann, K. H., et al. (1982) Diagnostic significance of quantitative determination of hepatitis B surface antigen in acute and chronic hepatitis B infection. *Eur. J. Clin. Microbiol.* 1, 52–58.

4. Chulanov, V. P., Shipulin, G. A., Schaefer, S., and Gerlich, W. H. (2003) Kinetics of HBV DNA and HBsAg in acute hepatitis B patients with and without coinfection by other hepatitis viruses. *J. Med. Virol,* **69**, 313–323.
5. Burczynska B., Madalinski K., Pawlowska J., et al., (1994) The value of quantitative measurement of HBeAg and HBsAg before interferon-α treatment of chronic hepatitis B in children. *J. Hepatol.* **21**, 1097–1102.
6. Erhardt, A., Reineke, U., Blondin, D., et al. (2000) Mutations of the core promoter and response to interferon treatment in chronic replicative hepatitis B. *Hepatology* **31**, 716–725.
7. Heermann K. H., Kruse F., Seifer M., and Gerlich W. H. (1987) Immunogenicity of gene S and pre-S domains in hepatitis virions and HBsAg filaments. *Intervirology* **28**, 14–25.
8. Deepen R., Heermann K.-H., Uy A., Thomssen R., and Gerlich W. H. (1990) Viral preS1 hepatocyte receptor and its antibody in hepatitis B virus infected persons and in recipients of hepatitis B vaccines. *Med. Microbiol. Immunol.* **179**, 49–60.
9. Gerlich W. H., and Thomssen R. (1975) Standardized detection of hepatitis B surface antigen: determination of its serum concentration in weight units per volume. *Dev. Biol. Stand.* **30**, 78–87.
10. Stamm, B., Gerlich W., and Thomssen R. (1980) Quantitative determination of antibody against hepatitis B surface antigen: measurement of its binding capacity. *J. Biol. Stand.* **8**, 59–68.
11. Lu, M., Klaes, R., Menne, S., et al. (2003) Induction of antibodies to the PreS region of surface antigens of woodchuck hepatitis virus (WHV) in chronic carrier woodchuck by immunizations with WHV surface antigens. *J. Hepatol.* **39**, 405–413.

8

In Situ Detection of Hepatitis B Viral Antigens

An Immunohistochemical Approach

Jane W. S. Fang and Johnson Y. N. Lau

1. Introduction

Hepatitis B virus (HBV) infection is the most common type of viral hepatitis, affecting more than 350 million people worldwide. To understand in detail the pathogenetic mechanisms involved and assess the value of antiviral therapy, the detection of HBV antigens and genome in the target organ, the liver, is essential.

One of the approaches to study HBV viral antigen expression in the liver is by *in situ* immunohistochemical detection in cryostat or formalin-fixed liver biopsy sections. This simple and time-honored method has greatly enhanced our knowledge of the pathogenesis of HBV. The localization of HBV viral antigen expression in liver in relation to the natural history of chronic HBV infection has helped to define the evolution of the viral infection in liver at different stages of the disease process ***(1)***. Moreover, colocalization of HBV antigens and human leukocyte antigens and cytokines has also helped to identify host immune-mediated response as a key factor in the pathogenesis of liver diseases ***(2–4)***. Immunohistochemical detection has been used to characterize a unique disease process in HBV infection—fibrosing cholestatic hepatitis ***(5)***.

In this chapter, the authors outline the materials and methods of performing immunohistochemical detection for hepatitis B surface antigens (pre-S1, pre-S2, HBsAg), hepatitis B core antigen (HBcAg), and hepatitis B e antigen (HBeAg). Notes in **Subheading 4** highlight common pitfalls and provide suggestions on techniques for better results ***(3–5)***.

2. Materials

2.1. Solutions and Reagents

1. Deparaffinization and rehydration series: 100% xylene (Fisher Scientific), 80% xylene/20% alcohol (95%, Fisher Scientific), 50% xylene/50% alcohol, 20% xylene/80% alcohol, 95% alcohol.
2. Methanol (≥99.9%, Fisher Scientific).

From: *Methods in Molecular Medicine, vol. 95: Hepatitis B and D Protocols, volume 1*
Edited by: R. K. Hamatake and J. Y. N. Lau © Humana Press Inc., Totowa, NJ

3. Hydrogen peroxide (30%, Fisher Scientific).
4. Isopentane (≥99.5%, Sigma, St. Louis, MO).
5. Chloroform (≥99.5%, Fisher Scientific).
6. Acetone (≥99.5%, Fisher Scientific).
7. Tissue-freezing medium (Fisher Scientific).
8. Poly-L-lysine (Sigma).
9. Tris-buffered saline (TBS), pH 7.4–7.6 (Sigma).
10. Bovine serum albumin (BSA; ≥98% pure, Sigma).
11. Rabbit or swine serum consistent with the secondary antibody type (Sigma; Dako; Boeringer Manheim).
12. Diaminobenzidine (DAB, Sigma).
13. Fast red TR salt (Sigma).
14. Naphthol AS-MX phosphate (Sigma).
15. Levamisole (Sigma).
16. 0.1 M Tris-HCl, pH 8.2 (Sigma).
17. Counterstain: hematoxylin stain (Fisher Scientific).
18. Glycerol (≥99.5%, Fisher Scientific).
19. Clear nail polish.
20. Primary antibodies (*see* **Notes 1** and **2**).
    a. HBsAg: mouse monoclonal antibody D2H5 (this source is from Drs. Tedder and Ferns, London, UK), working dilution 1:100 to 1:200.
    b. HBeAg: mouse monoclonal antibody E2E6 (from Drs. Tedder and Ferns, London, UK), working dilution 1:5.
    c. preS1: monoclonal mouse antibody MA18/7 (provided by Prof. W. H. Gerlich and Dr. K. H. Heermann, Gottingen, Germany), working dilution 1:100.
    d. preS2: mouse monoclonal antibody 5535 (provided by Prof. A. Alberti, Padova, Italy), working dilution 1:50.
    e. HBcAg: rabbit polyclonal antibody (Dako), working dilution 1:200.

    Dilutions are made with 1% animal serum (same as secondary antibody) in 1% BSA/TBS.
21. Secondary antibodies conjugated to either peroxidase or alkaline phosphatase (*see* **Notes 3** and **4**).
    a. HBsAg/HBeAg/preS1/preS2: rabbit antimouse antibody (Sigma).
    b. HBcAg: swine antirabbit antibody (Dako).

    Dilute 1:30 in 1% BSA/TBS.

2.2. Equipment/Tools

1. Slide-staining dishes: vertical and horizontal (Fisher Scientific).
2. Slide racks and trays (Fisher Scientific).
3. Positively charged slides (Fisher Scientific).
4. PAP pen (Dako).
5. Permount (Fisher Scientific) or any mounting agent.
6. Glass cover slip (Fisher Scientific).
7. Light microscope.

2.3. Tissues for Study

2.3.1. Preparation of Cryostat Liver Sections

The specimens obtained by percutaneous liver biopsy will be divided into two parts: one part is fixed in 10% formaldehyde saline and processed for routine histological studies, and the other part is embedded in tissue-freezing medium on a cardboard mount and snap-frozen in liquid nitrogen–cooled isopentane. Cryostat liver tissue sections are cut at 5 μm thickness using a cryotome and placed on slides previously coated with 0.01% poly-L-lysine to enhance attachment (*see* **Note 5**). The sections are dried at room temperature, wrapped individually with aluminum foil, and stored at –20°C. Immediately before sections are stained, they should be thawed at room temperature. After thawing, the sections should be fixed in chloroform-acetone (1:1 vol/vol) for 5 min and extensively washed with TBS, pH 7.6 (*see* **Note 6**).

2.3.2. Preparation of Formalin-Fixed, Paraffin-Embedded Liver Sections

Formalin-fixed, paraffin-embedded liver biopsy sections are cut at 5 μm thickness using a standard microtome. In a warm water bath about 55°C, floating paraffin liver sections are gently adhered to positively charged slides or slides that have been previously coated with 0.01% poly-L-lysine to enhance attachment (*see* **Note 5**).

3. Methods

1. *Paraffin sections*. Deparaffinize and rehydrate liver biopsy section slides by going through the xylene/alcohol series. Allow slides to soak at each station for about 2 min. *Cryostat sections*. Proceed to Step 2.
2. If peroxidase is being used as the tracer, soak the sections in 10% hydrogen peroxide/methanol for 15 min for quenching the endogenous peroxidase activity. If peroxidase is not used, this step can be omitted.
3. Rinse slides in TBS.
4. Lay slides across horizontal slide trays for drying.
5. Circle the tissue with a PAP pen (*see* **Note 7**).
6. Apply premixed 10% animal serum (as used for secondary antibody) in 3% BSA/TBS to cover the tissue section, about 250 μL per slide (*see* **Note 8**). Soak for 15 min at room temperature (*see* **Note 9**).
7. Flick off BSA/TBS.
8. Apply primary antibody to cover the tissue section, at least 100 μL per slide, for 30 min at room temperature.
9. Rinse slide in TBS three times.
10. Apply secondary antibody to cover the tissue section, at least 100 μL per slide, for 30 min at room temperature.
11. Rinse slide in TBS three times.
12. Staining for peroxidase system. Add DAB solution (either freshly made by mixing 6 mg DAB in 10 mL TBS pH 7.6 and 3 μL of 30% hydrogen peroxide or by using DAB tablets available through Sigma) to cover the tissue for 5–10 min at room temperature (*see* **Note 10**).

    Staining for alkaline phosphatase system. Premix 9 mL naphthol solution (4 mg in 18 mL 0.1 *M* Tris-HCl pH 8.2) and 10 mg fast red TR salt and 1 mL levamisole (24 mg in 10 mL 0.1 *M* Tris-HCl pH 8.2) to block endogenous alkaline phosphatase activity. Filter and apply to cover tissue for 10–20 min at room temperature (*see* **Note 11**).
13. Rinse slide in TBS three times.
14. Counterstain with hematoxylin for about 5–10 min at room temperature.
15. Rinse with water.
16. Flick off excess fluid on tissue.

17. Mounting cryostat sections/alkaline phosphatase. Apply a drop of glycerol/TBS (1:1) to cover tissue. Float glass cover slip on top and remove all bubbles under the slip. Apply nail polish around edges of cover slip.

    Mounting formalin sections (stained with peroxidase). Dehydrate tissue by going through graded alcohol series (50%→80%→95%); soak for about 2 min per station. Apply a drop of Permount to cover tissue. Float glass cover slip on top and remove all bubbles under the slip.
18. View under microscope when slides are dry.
19. The expression of HBV viral antigen is scored independently by two observers. We propose a 0 to 4+ scale corresponding to positivity in 0%, 1–5%, 5–30%, 30–60%, and >60% of hepatocytes examined (*see* **Note 12**).

4. Notes

1. Most primary antibodies against HBV viral antigens are now commercially available. It is recommended that manufacturer's instructions be followed for dilutions and selection of secondary antibodies. Primary monoclonal antibodies against different epitopes of the same viral antigens may be combined to optimize the readout.
2. Specificity controls, e.g., mouse monoclonal anti-rubella antibody (from Drs. R. Tedder and B. Ferns, London, UK) or any commercially available antibody that is known not to crossreact with tissue protein, could be used instead of the HBV-specific antibody.
3. To enhance signals, additional layers of antibodies conjugated with a suitable enzyme system may be used. For example, if a primary mouse monoclonal antibody and a secondary rabbit anti-mouse antibody conjugated with peroxidase or alkaline phosphatase are used, a third layer of mouse monoclonal antibody conjugated to peroxidase or alkaline phosphatase may be added for amplification of the signal.
4. For colocalization, precautions need to be taken to use two different enzyme systems for the differential readout, e.g., peroxidase–DAB and alkaline phosphatase–fast red TR salt can be used concurrently. In addition, the two secondary antibodies should be from different animals and have no cross-activity against each other or the other primary antibody. Finally, to ensure that the detection of the antigens was maximal, single staining for HBsAg and HBcAg should be performed out for all patients; in each case, detection of the HBV antigens should be optimized to maximal.
5. Adhesives may not be necessary for routine immunohistochemical staining. However, they are recommended for procedures that involve more vigorous washing, e.g., in multiple antigen staining and combined immunohistochemistry and *in situ* hybridization. We chose to use 0.01% poly-L-lysine as an adhesive based on the positive charge of this compound. Alternative adhesives have also been used by others.
6. Fixing solutions involving other combinations of organic solvents, e.g., acetone, chloroform, methanol, and ethanol, have all been used. We found that a combination of chloroform and acetone in 1:1 ratio was the best in our hands.
7. The wax circle introduced by the PAP pen will reduce the dispersion of the antibody solutions.
8. The mixture of animal serum and BSA in TBS provides a blocking solution to reduce the background signal. Proportions may vary for the best result. It is important to select the appropriate animal serum, which should be consistent with the animal source for the secondary antibody.
9. Liver contains a significant amount of biotin. If an avidin–biotin system is used, adequate blocking using extra avidin is needed. In our experience, ready-to-use kits with premixed

secondary antibodies and staining reagents often produce much false-positive signal with cryostat liver sections, probably because it is difficult to quench all the endogenous biotin.

10. Optimal signal detection should be monitored closely at the staining step by viewing the signal under a microscope. In our experience, DAB staining for HBsAg and HBcAg usually takes 1–2 min, whereas staining for HBeAg takes 8–10 min. Staining beyond this duration leads to high background and inaccurate grading of positively stained cells.
11. Other enzyme substrates, e.g., BCIP/NBT liquid substrate system (Sigma; follow manufacturer's instructions), may be used for an alkaline phosphatase system. The selection of appropriate substrates may be important in colocalization experiments to differentiate signals for different viral antigens. Other popular alternatives for tracers are fluorescent labels (with the aid of fluorescent microscopy). We have used FITC and Evans blue as counterstain, with good results.
12. The liver section should contain at least five intact hepatic lobules to be applicable for this grading purpose.

References

1. Lau, J. Y. N. and Wright, T. L. (1993) Molecular virology and pathogenesis of hepatitis B. *Lancet* **342**, 1335–1340.
2. Lau, J. Y. N., Bird, G. L., Naoumov, N. V., and Williams, R. (1993) Hepatic HLA antigen display in chronic hepatitis B virus infection: relation to hepatic expression of HBV genome/gene products and liver histology. *Dig. Dis. Sci.* **38**, 888–895.
3. Fang, J. W. S., Wu, P. C., Lai, C. L., Lo, C. K., Meager, A, and Lau, J. Y. L. (1994) Hepatic expression of interferon-α in chronic hepatitis B virus infection. *Dig. Dis. Sci.* **39**, 2014–2021.
4. Fang, J. W. S., Shen, W. W., Meager, A., and Lau, J. Y. N. (1996) Activation of the tumor necrosis factor-a system in the liver in chronic hepatitis B virus infection. *Am. J. Gastroenterol.* **91**, 748–753.
5. Lau, J. Y. N., Davies, S. E., Bain V. G., et al. (1992) High level expression of hepatitis B viral antigens in fibrosing cholestatic hepatitis. *Gastroenterology* **102**, 956–962.

9

Detection of Hepatitis B Virus X Antigen by Immunohistochemistry and Western Blotting

Jie Liu and Mark A. Feitelson

1. Introduction

The genome of hepatitis B virus (HBV) is a partially double-stranded DNA molecule within virus particles that is approx 3.2 kbp long *(1,2)*. It has four open reading frames, all on one strand, that encode the surface antigen or envelope polypeptides, core or nucleocapsid polypeptide, the viral polymerase, and the so-called "X" protein *(1,2)*.

The hepatitis B surface antigen (HBsAg) consists of a family of integral membrane proteins within the envelope of virus and subviral particles that are found in the blood of infected patients *(3,4)*. Within the envelope of the virus particles is the nucleocapsid of HBV, which is an icosahedron made up of the hepatitis B core antigen (HBcAg) polypeptide *(5,6)*. A proteolytic fragment of the core polypeptide, known as e antigen or HBeAg, is secreted into the blood of patients and is a surrogate marker of infectivity and viral replication *(7,8)*.

The viral polymerase, encoded by the largest open reading frame, has DNA-dependent DNA polymerase activity, RNA-dependent DNA polymerase (reverse transcriptase), and RNase H activity *(9–11)*, reflecting the fact that HBV is a DNA virus that replicates by the reverse transcription of a pregenomic RNA replication intermediate *(12)*. The amino-terminal portion of the polymerase also serves as a primer for viral replication *(13)*. Together, these proteins are required for virus replication and assembly of mature viral particles.

The fourth open reading frame, located at the extreme 3' end of the HBV genome, encodes a small polypeptide of about 17 kDa known as the hepatitis B x antigen (HBxAg) *(1)*. HBxAg has been shown to be a promiscuous *trans*-activating protein that may alter the expression of both viral and cellular genes *(14)*. Further work has shown that HBxAg stimulates HBV gene expression and replication *(15,16)*, which is important to help maintain the chronic carrier state *(17,18)*. In addition, it has been proposed

From: *Methods in Molecular Medicine, vol. 95: Hepatitis B and D Protocols, volume 1*
Edited by: R. K. Hamatake and J. Y. N. Lau © Humana Press Inc., Totowa, NJ

that HBxAg alterations in the patterns of cellular gene expression play important roles in the pathogenesis of hepatocellular carcinoma (HCC) ***(19,20)***, which is a late sequela of chronic HBV infection.

Interestingly, the carrier state, which is characterized by the persistence of viral particles and/or subviral HBsAg particles in blood for years or decades, is an important risk factor for the development of HCC ***(21,22)***. The development and progression of chronic liver disease (CLD) are important risk factors for the development of HCC ***(21,22)***. If HBxAg contributes centrally to both of these risk factors, which increasingly seems to be the case, then it may help to explain the very high risk of carriers with liver disease developing HCC ***(21,22)***. The facts that there are an estimated 350 million HBV carriers worldwide who are at risk for the development of CLD and HCC ***(23)***, that up to 1 million new cases of HCC appear each year, that HCC is rapidly fatal (<3% survival over 5 yr), and that there are very few treatment options ***(24,25)*** suggest that the detection and characterization of HBxAg are important for elucidating some of the mechanisms whereby chronic HBV infection gives rise to HCC.

1.1. Detection of HBxAg

Based upon the HBV genome, the X gene would be expected to encode a polypeptide of approx 17 kDa, so it was surprising that the first observations on HBxAg from infected tissue yielded a polypeptide of 28 kDa and a polypeptide of about 24 kDa from infected cells ***(26)***. Based on a computer analysis, HBxAg contains several potential protein kinase C or casein kinase II sites, and there is some evidence that HBxAg becomes phosphorylated in HepG2 cells ***(27)***, although phosphorylation does not seem to account for the appearance of a 24- or 28-kDa polypeptide. On the other hand, HBxAg phosphorylation has not been observed in human embryonic 293 cells ***(28)***. HBxAg also has several potential myristylation sites, although there is no evidence thus far that HBxAg is myristylated. In addition, since HBxAg was initially identified as a *trans*-activating protein, it was expected that HBxAg expression levels in the liver would be low, and initial observations seemed to confirm this ***(29)***.

Based upon these initial observations, a number of population-based cross-sectional studies were designed to detect anti-HBx in the hope that the antibody marker would provide indirect evidence that HBxAg was actually made during infection. Accordingly, anti-HBx was detected in the sera of patients with fulminant and acute hepatitis ***(30)*** and more frequently in patients with chronic hepatitis ***(30,31)***, cirrhosis ***(30,32)***, and HCC ***(26,30,32)***. Anti-HBx was also found in patients with high ***(30,33,34)*** or low levels ***(26)*** of viral replication.

When longitudinal studies were performed in carriers, anti-HBx developed in HBeAg-positive sera several weeks or months prior to the clearance of virus and often persisted until the development of anti-HBe, suggesting that anti-HBx may be an early marker of viral clearance ***(35)***. This finding was followed closely by reports that HBxAg was present in the serum of carriers as a 17-kDa polypeptide and sometimes as an additional 13-kDa polypeptide in the sera of patients with other markers of viral replication ***(36,37)***. Independent work showed that HBxAg staining in the liver biopsies from carriers costained with hepatitis B core antigen (HBcAg) ***(38,39)***.

Since intrahepatic HBcAg staining, especially in the cytoplasm of infected hepatocytes, correlates strongly with viral replication, the coexpression of HBxAg further supports a role for HBxAg in supporting viral replication. In addition, the finding of HBxAg staining in 12 of 36 patients with chronic hepatitis (33%), in nontumor liver from 23 of 29 patients with HCC (79%), and in the tumor cells from 36 of the same patients (78%) ***(40)*** suggested that HBxAg was a common marker in the livers of carriers. Similar observations were made elsewhere ***(39)***.

The findings that the X gene integrates frequently into host-cell DNA during hepatocellular regeneration that accompanies bouts of chronic liver disease ***(41)***, that the X-region transcripts are frequently overexpressed from these integrated templates ***(42–44)***, and that the distribution and intensity of staining increase with the extent and severity of lesions in chronically infected livers ***(45–47)*** suggest that HBxAg is made from integrated HBV-DNA templates independent of viral replication. These observations also provide an explanation for the direct relationship between HBxAg expression and chronic liver disease.

Even after all this work, there was considerable variability in the presence, frequency, and distribution of HBxAg among different studies. This variability was highlighted in a comparative study, where 11 different antibodies from 5 different laboratories produced somewhat different results ***(48)***. Although not all the variables were explored, the nature of the antibody (monoclonal or polyclonal), the antigen to which each antibody was raised (synthetic peptides or full-length HBxAg), the stage of disease in which liver tissue was procured, the different tissue fixation methods, and various staining methods (immunohistochemistry or immunofluorescence) probably underscore some of the differences seen in the literature. In addition, it has recently been reported that HBxAg may be mutated in HCC ***(43)***, which may also result in variability of detection.

A major challenge in understanding the contribution of HBxAg to viral replication and/or to the development of HCC has been the difficulty in detecting HBxAg in cells transfected with recombinant plasmids and in some strains of X transgenic mice. When cells are transfected with an expression plasmid containing a strong promoter, and the cells are then selected for drug resistance over a few weeks, the resulting cultures produce little or no detectable HBxAg. This finding may reflect the fact that HBxAg is proapoptotic ***(49,50)*** and that selection of HBxAg-positive cells under conditions dependent upon cell growth results in cultures that have the least amount of HBxAg. Low levels of HBxAg may also result from the short half-life of the protein, the majority (70%) of which has a $t_{1/2}$ of 15 min ***(27)***.

Furthermore, the ability to detect HBxAg may depend on the type of cell line used for expression. For example, HBxAg was detected by Western blotting in transfected NIH3T3 cells ***(51)***, but these cells are mostly transformed, and the apoptotic pathways usually triggered by HBxAg may be inoperative in the parental cell line. HBxAg expression has been documented by immunofluorescence or Western blotting among cells in which the protein was introduced by scrape loading ***(52)*** or transient transfection ***(53–55)*** where drug resistance was not used for the selection of HBxAg-positive cells. Similarly, when HBx was placed under control of the inducible tetracycline promoter and stably transfected into HepG2 cells, easily detectable levels of HBxAg were observed by Western blotting following induction, although expression was then lost as these cells underwent apoptosis ***(49)***.

HBxAg-triggered apoptosis was also observed in HepG2 cells stably transfected with a recombinant plasmid in which X-gene expression was produced by the Cre/*lox*P recombination system ***(56)***. More recently, HBxAg has been stably expressed in a mouse hepatoma cell line (Hepa 1-6) transfected with a recombinant retroviral plasmid encoding the X gene, in part as a result of the failure of HBxAg to trigger apoptosis in these cells ***(57)***. Interestingly, when recombinant retroviruses encoding HBx were used to infect HepG2 cells, and the cultures were then briefly selected in neomycin to kill uninfected cells, sustained high levels of HBxAg were observed ***(58)***. In contrast, some of the studies with stably transfected cell lines required ^{35}S-methionine radiolabeling to detect HBxAg ***(59)***. Other studies aimed at functionally characterizing HBxAg have not demonstrated HBxAg expression in the systems under study ***(60–63)***. Interestingly, many of these studies use cell lines stably transfected with HBx- or HBV-expression plasmids, which after selection may only express low levels of HBxAg.

HBxAg expression is also quite variable in transgenic mice, with some animals showing high levels of protein expression ***(64,65)***, and other strains of mice showing little ***(66)*** or no ***(67,68)*** expression of HBxAg. The variability in these results may involve the use of different X-expression plasmids, as well as the facts that they integrate at different host sites and that differences include the strains of mice used, and the antibodies available for detection. Hence, the detection of HBxAg is really dependent on the type of system created to study the structure and biological function of this protein. With this in mind, the following protocols are presented to provide an outline for the detection of HBxAg in tissue and tissue culture cells.

2. Materials

2.1. Solutions

1. 1 *M* Tris-HCl: Dissolve 121.14 g of Tris base (cat. no. Bp152-5, Fisher Scientific) in 800 mL of Milli-Q water. Adjust the pH to 7.6, 6.8, or 8.8 by adding concentrated HCl (cat. no. A144-212, Fisher Scientific) and then adjust the volume to 1 L with Milli-Q water.
2. 0.05 *M* Tris-HCl, 0.15 *M* NaCl, pH 7.6: Mix 50 mL of 1 *M* Tris-HCl stock solution (pH 7.6) and 150 mL of 1 *M* NaCl (cat. no. S640-3, Fisher Scientific) stock solution together. Adjust the final volume to 1 L with Milli-Q water.
3. Tissue lysis buffer: 50 m*M* Tris-HCl, pH 8.0, 150 m*M* NaCl, 0.1% sodium dodecyl sulfate (SDS), 1% NP-40, 0.1 mM phenylmethanesulfonyl fluoride PMSF, 0.2 m*M* ethylenediaminetetraacetic acid (EDTA), and 1 mg/mL aprotinin.
4. 0.1% Trypsin: Dissolve 0.1 g of $CaCl_2$ (cat. no. C-3306, Sigma) in 90 mL of Milli-Q water; adjust the pH to 7.8 by adding diluted NaOH (cat. no. S320-500, Fisher Scientific). Add 100 mg of trypsin (cat. no. T8003, Sigma). Adjust the volume to 100 mL with water.
5. 4% paraformaldehyde (PFA), pH 7.0: Dissolve 40 g of PFA (cat. no. O4042-500, Fisher Scientific) in 800 mL of 0.01 *M* phosphate-buffered saline (PBS) by heating to 60°C and by adjusting the pH to 7.0 with 1 *N* NaOH (cat. no. S320-500, Fisher Scientific). Adjust the volume to 1 L with 0.01 *M* PBS.
6. 0.2% Triton X-100: Preheat Triton X-100 (cat. no. T9284, Sigma) in a 37°C water bath. Add 0.2 mL of preheated Triton X-100 to 99.8 mL of 0.01 *M* PBS.

7. 0.2 *M* NaH_2PO_4: Dissolve 27.6 g of $Na.H_2PO_4{\cdot}H_2O$ (cat. no. S369-1, Fisher Scientific) in 1 L of water.
8. 0.2 *M* Na_2HPO_4: Dissolve 28.4 g of Na_2HPO_4 (cat. no. S374-1, Fisher Scientific) in 1 L of water.
9. 0.2 *M* phosphate buffer, pH 7.4 (100 mL): Mix 19 mL of 0.2 *M* NaH_2PO_4 and 81 mL of 0.2 *M* Na_2HPO_4.
10. 0.01 *M* PBS (1X PBS) (1 L): Dissolve 8.7 g of NaCl (cat. no. S640-3, Fisher Scientific) in 500 mL Milli-Q water. Add 50 mL of 0.2 *M* phosphate buffer. Adjust the volume to 1 L with Milli-Q water.
11. 10% sodium dodecyl sulfate (SDS): Dissolve 100 g of SDS (cat. no. L6026, Sigma) in 900 mL of Milli-Q water. Warm to 67°C. Adjust to pH 7.2 by adding concentrated HCl. Adjust volume to 1 L with water.
12. 1 *M* dithiothreitol (DTT): Dissolve 1.54 g of DTT (cat. no. 15046-0, Sigma) in 10 mL of 0.01 *M* sodium acetate (cat. no. 71179, Sigma), pH 5.2. Aliquot and store at –20°C after filtration.
13. 200 m*M* PMSF: Dissolve PMSF (cat. no. P7626, Sigma) in 2-propanol (cat. no. 442369, Sigma) at a concentration of 34.8 mg/mL (200 m*M*). Aliquot this solution and store at –20°C.
14. 0.5 *M* EDTA: Dissolve 186.1 g of EDTA (cat. no. E5134, Sigma) in Milli-Q water preheated to 60°C. Add 1 *N* NaOH to pH 8.0. Adjust volume to 1 L with water. Aliquot and autoclave.
15. 10% ammonium persulfate (freshly prepared): Dissolve 0.1 g of ammonium persulfate (cat. no. A1433, Sigma) in 1 mL of Milli-Q water.
16. Xylene: cat. no. 011831-36, Fisher Scientific.
17. Ethanol: dehydrated 200 (Pharmco).
18. Paraffin: Tissue prep paraffin, melting point 56–57°C, cat. no. T565 (Fisher Scientific).
19. NP-40: cat. no. P128324 (Fisher Scientific).
20. Aprotinin: cat. no. A3886 (Sigma).
21. Bromophenol blue: cat. no. B0126 (Sigma).
22. Glycerol: cat. no. G5516 (Sigma).
23. Acrylamide/Bis (40% stock, 37.5:1): cat. no. 161-0148, Bio-Rad.
24. TEMED: cat. no. 161-0800, Bio-Rad.
25. Glycine: cat. no. Bp381-1, Fisher Scientific.
26. Methanol: cat. no. 022917-36, Fisher Scientific.
27. Tween-20: cat. no. Bp337-50, Fisher Scientific.
28. Bovine serum albumin (BSA): cat. no. A-2153, Sigma.
29. 30% Hydrogen peroxide: cat. no. H325-500, Fisher Scientific.
30. Peroxidase-labeled polymer: cat. no. K4010, DAKO Envision+.
31. Diaminobenzidine (DAB) chromogen solution: cat. no. K3467, DAKO.
32. Hematoxylin solution: cat. no. GHS-2-16, Sigma.
33. Mounting medium: 8310-4, Stephens Scientific.
34. OCT compound: Tissue freezing medium, (Tissue-Tek, OCT compound 4538).
35. HRP-labeled anti-rabbit antibody: cat. no. PI-1000, Vector.

2.2. Equipment

1. Cryostat: Reichert HistoStat Cryostat Microtome, Model 976C.
2. Microtome: Leits, Model 1512.
3. Disposable pellet pestle: cat. no. K749520-0590, Fisher Scientific.
4. Cordless motor: cat no. K749540-0000, Fisher Scientific.

5. Electrophoresis: Mini-protein 2 electrophoresis and blotting apparatus, cat. no. 165-4130 (Bio-Rad).
6. Microscope slides: Charged and precleaned, cat. no. 15-188-52 (Fisher Scientific).
7. Microscope: Olympus, BH-2.
8. Cytospin: cytospin3, Shardon.
9. Heating block: Lab-line slide warmer, Model No.26005 (Lab-line Instruments).
10. Microscope cover glass: cat. no. 12-545E, Fisher Scientific.
11. Immobilon-P transfer membrane: cat. no. IPVH00010, Millipore.

3. Methods

3.1. Detection of HBxAg in Formalin-Fixed, Paraffin-Embedded Tissues (Fig. 1A, B)

3.1.1. Embedding

Each tissue sample is placed inside a labeled cassette. The lid is snapped into place and then processed as follows: 50% ethanol for 30 min; 80% ethanol (twice) for 30 min each (*see* **Note 1**); 90% ethanol (twice) for 30 min each (*see* **Note 1**); 100% ethanol (twice) for 30 min each (*see* **Note 1**); 100% ethanol/xylene (1:1 v/v) for 30 min.; xylene (twice) for 30 min each (*see* **Note 1**); paraffin (twice) for 30 min each (*see* **Notes 1** and **2**).

3.1.2. Slide Preparation

1. Tissue samples (5 μm thick) were cut on a microtome.
2. Two consecutive tissue sections were placed upon each slide, and the slides were then put on a heating block at 37°C overnight.

3.1.3. Immunostaining Protocol for Tissue

1. Each of the slides was then rehydrated as follows: Xylene (twice) for 10 min each; 100% ethanol (twice) for 5 min each; 95% ethanol for 5 min; 85% ethanol for 5 min; running water for 5 min.
2. Slides are then incubated with 0.1% trypsin in 0.1% $CaCl_2$ (pH 7.8) (preheated to 37°C) at room temperature for 10 min.
3. Rinse gently with distilled water or buffer solution (0.05 *M* Tris-HCl, 0.15 *M* NaCl, pH 7.6).
4. Block the endogenous peroxidase in the tissue by adding 1% H_2O_2 (from 30% H_2O_2 stock [Fisher Scientific cat. no. 001823]) to each tissue slide at room temperature for 15 min.
5. Rinse gently with running water.
6. Gently blow-dry slides.
7. Add 1% BSA in buffer (0.05 *M* Tris-HCl, 0.15 *M* NaCl, pH 7.6) to the tissue samples for 20 min at room temperature.
8. Add primary antibody (anti-X99) or negative control (preimmune serum) (dilution for each is 1:4000). Tap off excess buffer and wipe the slides (but do not dry). Incubate slides with primary antibody overnight at 4°C in a humidified chamber.
9. Rinse each slide gently with washing buffer (0.05 *M* Tris-HCl, 0.15 *M* NaCl, pH 7.6) twice for 5 min each.
10. Incubate each sample in peroxidase-labeled polymer (Dako Envision+, cat. no. K4010) for 30 min at room temperature.
11. Add the substrate by washing slides as in **step 9**. Add prepared liquid DAB-chromogen solution (DAKO) to cover specimens. Incubate for 2–10 min.

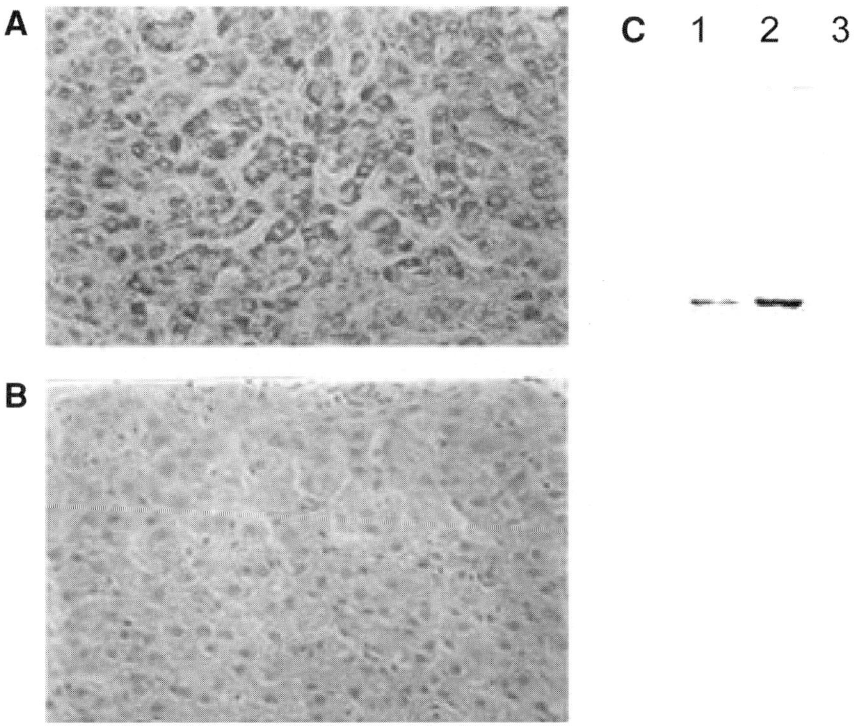

Fig. 1. Immunohistochemical detection of HBxAg in the liver of a patient chronically infected with HBV **(A)** or in the liver of an uninfected patient **(B)**. A dark cytoplasmic staining is the HBxAg signal (×200). In **C**, homogenates from two different HBV-infected livers (lanes 1 and 2) and an uninfected liver (lane 3) are analyzed on sodium dodecyl sulfate gels, and the Western blot is performed with anti-HBx. A single band at 17 kDa was observed only in homogenates from infected liver.

12. To counterstain, immerse slides in a bath of hematoxylin (Sigma) 15 times (dip in and out). Rinse gently with running tap water for 5 min. Decolorize by putting slides in 70% ethanol containing 1% HCl for a 1 s and then quickly transferring slides to running tap water for 10 min.
13. The samples are then dehydrated through alcohol to xylene as follows: 85% ethanol for 5 min; 95% ethanol for 5 min; 100% ethanol for 5 min; 100% ethanol for 5 min; xylene (twice) for 5 min each.
14. For mounting, specimens were covered by microscope cover glass (Fisher Scientific) with mounting medium (Stephens Scientific).
15. Slides were then viewed under the microscope.

3.2. Staining of HBx–Transfected Cells (Fig. 2)

1. Collect the cells following standard trypsinization by centrifugation and resuspend them (at 1×10^7 cells/mL) in a serum-free medium. Perform a cytospin (1000*g* 3 min) to collect cells on slides (Fisher Scientific).

A

B

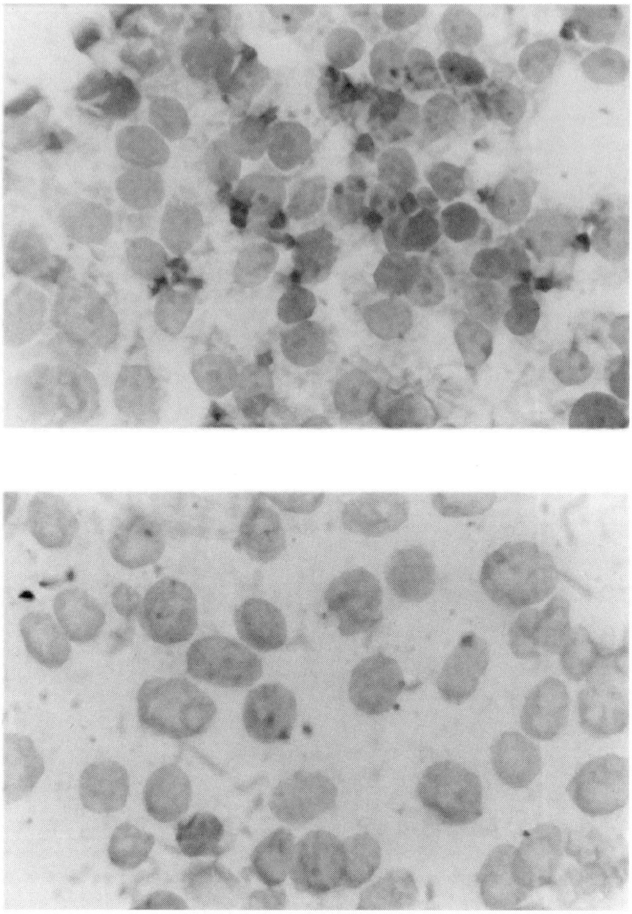

Fig. 2. Staining for HepG2 cells stably transfected with the HBV X gene and probed with the anti-HBx **(A)** or preimmune serum **(B)**. The cytoplasmic staining is HBxAg in the transfected cell line.

2. Air-dry slides for 30 min.
3. Put slides in 4% PFA, pH 7, for 20 min. Alternatively, cells can be grown directly on slides and fixed with 4% PFA for 20 min followed by PBS washing.
4. Wash the slides (with cells) in 3X PBS for 2 min.
5. Wash the slides in 1X PBS twice, 2 min each.
6. Incubate cells in 0.2% Triton X-100 in PBS for 30 min at 37°C.
7. Rinse gently with washing buffer (0.05 *M* Tris-HCl, 0.15 *M* NaCl, pH 7.6).
8. Block the endogenous peroxidase for 5 min in 1% H_2O_2 (in H_2O).
9. Follow the subsequent steps listed for the processing of paraffin slides (*see* **Subheading 3.1.3., step 5**).

3.3. Staining HBxAg on Frozen Sections

All the tissue specimens must be stored in either liquid nitrogen or at –70°C.

1. The samples are sectioned by cryostat at 5–10 μm thickness. Before cutting the tissue specimens, place them in a cryostat chamber and mount on cutting chucks with a thin layer of an OCT compound.
2. Cut sections slowly (2–3 s to traverse the cut face).
3. Collect sections by gently touching each one to a warm slide (Fisher Scientific).
4. Blow-dry slides.
5. Fix slides in 4% PFA for 20 min.
6. Rinse slides with 3X PBS using a squirt bottle, and incubate for 5 min.
7. Repeat **step 6** twice with 1X PBS.
8. Alternatively, the slides can be treated with 40%, 75%, 95%, and 100% ethanol and stored at –70°C in an airtight box for later use.
9. Block endogenous peroxidase for 10 min with 1% H_2O_2 in H_2O.
10. Follow the remaining steps outlined for the processing of paraffin sections (*see* **Subheading 3.1.3., step 5**).

3.4. Western Blotting to Detect HBx Protein (Fig. 1C)

3.4.1. Monolayer Cultures

1. Remove medium and wash cells thoroughly with PBS.
2. Put 1 mL of ice-cold cell lysis buffer into a 100-mm dish. (Cell lysis buffer: 50 m*M* Tris-HCl, pH 8.0, 150 m*M* NaCl, 1% NP-40, 0.1 m*M* PMSF, and 0.2 m*M* EDTA.)
3. Scrape plate with a rubber policeman. Pass the lysate through a 21-gauge needle to shear the DNA.
4. Microcentrifuge cell lysate at 3550*g* for 10 min at 4°C. Keep all lysates on ice for immediate use or store at –20°C.

3.4.2. Suspension Cultures

1. Collect 10^6–10^8 cells by centrifugation at 3,000*g* for 5 min.
2. Remove medium and wash the pellet with ice-cold PBS thoroughly.
3. Add 1 mL of ice-cold cell lysis buffer (as in protocol for preparation of monolayer cultures). Mix gently with a pipet and incubate on ice for 30 min.
4. Collect the cell lysate as described in the protocol for monolayer cultures.

3.4.3. Tissue Samples

1. Cut fresh tissue into small pieces in a plate on ice. Tissue can be frozen and thawed in lysis buffer. Use ice-cold tissue lysis buffer at 1:6 (w/v tissue:buffer ratio) to lyse tissue.
2. Homogenize tissue with a Dounce homogenizer on ice.
3. Transfer the homogenate to microcentrifuge tubes. Centrifuge at 3550*g* for 20 min at 4°C.
4. Perform protein quantitation in the supernatant. At this point, the lysate can be processed or stored at –20°C.

3.4.4. Electrophoresis

1. Mix 40–60 μg of whole-cell lysate with an equal volume of 2X SDS gel-loading buffer. Loading buffer: 100 m*M* Tris-HCl (pH 6.8), 200 m*M* DTT, 4% SDS, 0.2% bromophenol blue, 20% glycerol.

2. Place the sample in a boiling water bath for 5 min.
3. Load samples onto a 12% SDS-polyacrylamide gel (*see* **Note 3**).
4. Run the gel using constant voltage (100 V) for 1.5–2.0 h, or until the bromophenol blue reaches the bottom of the resolving gel.
5. Transfer proteins from the gel to nitrocellulose by constant current 100 mA (20–30 V) in transfer buffer for 1–2 h using an electroblotting apparatus (Bio-Rad). Transfer buffer: 40 m*M* glycine, 50 m*M* Tris-HCI base, 0.04% SDS, 20% methanol, pH 8.3.

3.4.5. Immunoblotting

1. Block nonspecific binding by incubating membrane in 5% nonfat dry milk for 1 h at room temperature.
2. Incubate anti-HBx antibody X-99 (1:500) in buffer (0.05 *M* Tris-HCl, 0.15 *M* NaCl, 5% nonfat dry milk, pH 7.6) at 4°C overnight.
3. Rinse and wash the membrane in fresh changes of wash buffer: quick rinses: once for 15 min, twice for 5 min each. Washing buffer: 0.05 *M* Tris-HCl, 0.15 *M* NaCl, 0.1% Tween-20, pH 7.6.
4. Incubate membrane in HRP-labeled second antibody diluted 1:1600 (HRP-labeled antirabbit Ig) in buffer (0.05 *M* Tris-HCl, 0.15 *M* NaCl, pH 7.6) for 1 h at room temperature.
5. Repeat washing as in **step 3**.
6. Incubate membrane in an equal volume of detection reagent 1 and detection reagent 2 provided by the manufacturer (Amersham/Pharmcia Biotech; ECL Western blotting detection regents). Drain off detection reagent and wrap blots in plastic wrap. Expose and develop with X-ray film (1 s to 3 min) to see 17-kDa band (HBxAg).

4. Notes

1. Each incubation is in a fresh batch of reagent.
2. Tissue prep paraffin, melting point 56–57°C (Fisher).
3. The separating gel (10 mL of a 12% gel) is made by adding the following agents in sequential order: distilled water (3.15 mL), 1 *M* Tris-HCl (pH 8.8) (3.75 mL), acrylamide/bis (40% stock, 37.5:1) (3 mL), and 10% ammonium persulfate (freshly prepared for each gel) (50 µL). Mix gently but thoroughly, degas under vacuum, and then add 10% SDS (w/v) and TEMED (7 µL). Mix gently and pour within gel mold to desired height. Gently overlay with distilled water and allow to polymerize (15–20 min). Before the stacking gel is poured (*see* below), remove the water from the top of the running gel.

   The stacking gel (10 mL of a 4% gel) is made by adding the following agents in sequential order: (7.675 mL) distilled water, (1.25 mL) 1 *M* Tris-HCl (pH 6.8), 100 µL 10% SDS (w/v), (0.975 mL) acrylamide/bis (40% stock, 37.5:1), and (50 µL) ammonium persulfate (freshly prepared for each gel). Mix gently but thoroughly, degas under vacuum, and then add 100 µL of 10% SDS (w/v) and then 10 µL TEMED. Mix and pour on top of separating gel until the level reaches the top of the teeth in the comb. Allow to polymerize (should be 15–20 min). Remove the comb, rinse the wells with running buffer (25 m*M* Tris-HCl base, 200 m*M* glycine, 0.1% SDS), fill the top-half and bottom-half cells with running buffer, and then underlay the samples in each well below the running buffer. *Note:* Make sure that no air bubbles lodge between the gel and the running buffer.

References

1. Galibert, F., Mandart, E., Fitoussi, F., Tiollais, P., and Charnay, P. (1979) Nucleotide sequence of the hepatitis B virus genome (subtype *ayw*) cloned in *E. coli. Nature* **281**, 646–650.

2. Valenzuela, P., Quiroga, M., Zaldivar, J., Gray, P., and Rutter, W. J. (1980) The nucleotide sequence of the hepatitis B viral genome and the identification of the major viral genes. In: Fields, B. N., Jaenisch, R., and Fox, C. F. (eds.), *Animal Virus Genetics*, Academic Press, New York, 57–70.
3. Bayer, M. E., Blumberg, B. S., and Werner, B. (1968) Particles associated with Australia antigen in sera of patients with leukemia, Down's syndrome and hepatitis. *Nature* **218**, 1057–1059.
4. Dane, D. S., Cameron, C. H., and Briggs, M. (1970) Virus-like particles in serum of patients with Australia antigen-associated hepatitis. *Lancet* **2**, 695–698.
5. Almeida, J. D., Rubenstein, D., and Stott, E. J. (1971) New antigen-antibody system in Australia antigen-positive hepatitis. *Lancet* **2**, 1225–1227.
6. Budkowska, A. (1977) Immunochemical and morphological studies of hepatitis B core antigen isolated from the nuclei of hepatocytes. *J. Infect. Dis.* **135**, 463–467.
7. Maynard, J. E., Barret, D. H., Murphy, B. L., Bradley, D. W., Berquist, K. R., and Bender T. R. (1976) Relation of e antigen to hepatitis B virus infection in an area of hyperendemicity. *J. Infect. Dis.* **133**, 339–342.
8. Okado, K., Kamiyama, I., Inomata, M., Imai, M., Miyakawa, Y., and Mayumi, M. (1976) e Antigen and anti-e in the serum of asymptomatic carrier mothers as indicators of positive and negative transmission of hepatitis B virus to their infants. *N. Engl. J. Med.* **294**, 746 749
9. Bavand, M., Feitelson, M., and Laub, O. (1989) The hepatitis B virus-associated reverse transcriptase is encoded by the viral *pol* gene. *J. Virol.* **63**, 1019–1021.
10. Oberhaus, S. M., and Newbold, J. E. (1993) Detection of DNA polymerase activities associated with purified duck hepatitis B virus core particles by using an activity gel assay. *J. Virol.* **67**, 6558–6566.
11. Radziwill, G., Tucker, W., and Schaller, H. (1990) Mutational analysis of the hepatitis B virus P gene product: domain structure and RNase H activity. *J. Virol.* **64**, 613–620.
12. Summers, J., and Mason, W. (1982) Replication of the genome of a hepatitis B-like virus by reverse transcription of an RNA intermediate. *Cell* **29**, 403–415.
13. Bartenschlager, R., and Schaller, H. (1988) The amino-terminal domain of the hepadnavirus P-gene encodes the terminal protein (genome-linked protein) believed to prime reverse transcription. *EMBO J.* **7**, 4185–4192.
14. Rossner, M. T. (1992) Hepatitis B virus X-gene product: a promiscuous transcriptional activator. *J. Med. Virol.* **36**, 101–117.
15. Nakatake, H., Chisaka, O., Yamamoto, S., Matsubara, K., and Koshy, R. (1993) Effect of X protein on transactivation of HBV promoters and on viral replication. *Virology* **195**, 305–314.
16. Colgrove, R., Simon, G., and Ganem, D. (1989) Transcriptional activation of homologous and heterologous genes by the hepatitis B virus X gene product in cells permissive for viral replication. *J. Virol.* **63**, 4019–4026.
17. Chen, H. S., Kaneko, S., Girones, R., et al. (1993) The WHV X gene is important for establishment of virus infection in woodchucks. *J. Virol.* **67**, 1218–1226.
18. Zoulim, F., Saputelli, J., and Seeger, C. (1994) Woodchuck hepatitis virus X protein is required for viral infection *in vivo*. *J. Virol.* **68**, 2026–2030.
19. Henkler, F., and Koshy, R. (1996) Hepatitis B virus transcriptional activators: mechanisms and possible role in oncogenesis. *J. Viral Hepat.* **3**, 109–121.
20. Arbuthnot, P., Capovilla, A., and Kew, M. (2000) Putative role of hepatitis B virus X protein in hepatocarcinogenesis: effects on apoptosis, DNA repair, mitogen-activated protein kinase and JAK/STAT pathways. *J. Gastroenterol. Hepatol.* **15**, 357–368.

21. Beasley, R. P., Hwang, L. Y., Lin, C. C., and Chien, C. S. (1981) Hepatocellular carcinoma and hepatitis B virus: a prospective study of 22,707 men in Taiwan. *Lancet* **2**, 1129–1133.
22. Beasley, R. P., and Hwang, L. Y. (1994) Epidemiology of hepatocellular carcinoma. In: Vyas, G. N., Dienstag, J. L., and Hoofnagle, J. H. (eds.), *Viral Hepatitis and Liver Disease*, Grune and Stratton, New York, 209–224.
23. Maddrey, W. C. (2001) Hepatitis B—an important public health issue. *Clinica y Laboratorio* **47**, 51–55.
24. Lok, A. S., Heathcote, E. J., and Hoofnagle, J. H. (2001) Management of hepatitis B: 2000—summary of a workshop. *Gastroenterology* **120**, 1828–1853.
25. Hilleman, M. R. (2001) Overview of the pathogenesis, prophylaxis and therapeutics of viral hepatitis B, with focus on reduction to practical applications. *Vaccine* **19**, 1837–1848.
26. Moriarty, A. M., Alexander, H., and Lerner, R. A. (1985) Antibodies to peptides detect new hepatitis B antigen: serological correlation with hepatocellular carcinoma. *Science* **227**, 429–433.
27. Schek, N., Bartenschlager, R., Kuhn, C., and Schaller, H. (1991) Phosphorylation and rapid turnover of hepatitis B virus X protein expressed in HepG2 cells from a recombinant vaccinia virus. *Oncogene* **6**, 1735–1744.
28. Levrero, M., Jean-Jean, O., Balsano, C., Will, H., and Perricaudet, M. (1990) Hepatitis B virus (HBV) X gene expression in human cells and anti-HBx antibodies detection in chronic HBV infection. *Virology* **174**, 299–304.
29. Ke-qin, H., Jian-jie, H., and Will, H. (1988) A preliminary study on localization of HBxAg in liver tissue of patients with chronic liver disease and its significance. *Chinese Med. J.* **101**, 671–674.
30. Vitvitski-Trepo, L., Kay, A., Pichoud, C., et al. (1990) Early and frequent detection of HBxAg and/or anti-HBx in hepatitis B virus infection. *Hepatology* **12**, 1278–1283.
31. Levrero, M., Jean-Jean, O., Balsano, C., Will, H., and Perricaudet, M. (1987) Hepatitis B virus (HBV) X gene expression in human cells and anti-x antibodies detection in chronic HBV infection. In: Robinson, W. S., Koike, K., and Will, H. (eds.), *Hepadna Viruses*, Alan R. Liss, New York, 237–252.
32. Pfaff, E., Salfeld, J., Gmelin, K., Schaller, H., and Theilmann, L. (1987) Synthesis of the X-protein of hepatitis B virus *in vitro* and detection of anti-X antibodies in human sera. *Virology* **158**, 456–460.
33. Haruna, Y., Hayashi, N., Katayama, K., et al. (1991) Expression of X protein and hepatitis B virus replication in chronic hepatitis. *Hepatology* **13**, 417–421.
34. Suzuki, K., Uchida, T., Shikata, T., et al. (1990) Expression of pre-S1, pre-S2, S and X peptides in relation to viral replication in livers with chronic hepatitis B. *Liver* **10**, 355–364.
35. Feitelson, M. A., and Clayton, M. M. (1990) The X antigen/antibody markers in hepadnavirus infections. II. Antibodies to the X gene product(s). *Gastroenterology* **99**, 500–507.
36. Feitelson, M. A., and Clayton, M. M. (1990) X antigen polypeptides in the sera of hepatitis B virus infected patients. *Virology* **177**, 367–371.
37. Feitelson, M. A., Clayton, M. M., and Blumberg, B. S. (1990) The X antigen/antibody markers in hepadnavirus infections. I. Presence and significance of the hepadnavirus X gene product(s) in serum. *Gastroenterology* **98**, 1071–1078.
38. Vitvitski, L., Meyers, M. L., Sninsky, J. J., et al. (1988) Expression of the X gene product of hepatitis B virus and WHV in infected livers and transfected 3T3 cells: evidence for cross-reactivity and correlation with core/e gene expression. In: Zuckerman, A. J. (ed.), *Viral Hepatitis and Liver Disease*, Alan R. Liss, New York, 341–344.

39. Katayama, K., Hayashi, N., Sasaki, Y., et al. (1989) Detection of hepatitis B virus X gene protein and antibody in type B chronic liver disease. *Gastroenterology* **97**, 990–998.
40. Zentgraf, H., Herrmann, G., Klein, R., et al. (1990) Mouse monoclonal antibody directed against hepatitis B virus X protein synthesized in *Escherichia coli*: detection of reactive antigen in liver cell carcinoma and chronic hepatitis. *Oncology* **47**, 143–148.
41. Takeuchi, M., Fujimoto, J., Niwamoto, H., Yamamoto, Y., and Okamoto, E. (1997) Frequent detection of hepatitis B virus X-gene DNA in hepatocellular carcinoma and adjacent liver tissue in hepatitis B surface antigen-negative patients. *Dig. Dis. Sci.* **42**, 2264–2269.
42. Diamantis, I. D., McGandy, C. E., Chen, T. J., Liaw, Y. F., Gudat, F., and Bianchi, L. (1992) Hepatitis B X-gene expression in hepatocellular carcinoma. *J. Hepatol.* **15**, 400–403.
43. Poussin, K., Dienes, H., Sirma, H., et al. (1999) Expression of mutated hepatitis B virus X genes in human hepatocellular carcinoma. *Int. J. Cancer* **80**, 497–505.
44. Schluter, V., Meyer, M., Hofschneider, P. H., Koshy, R., and Caselmann, W. H. (1994) Integrated hepatitis B virus X and 3' truncated preS/S sequences derived from human hepatomas encode functionally active transactivators. *Oncogene* **9**, 3335–3344.
45. Wang, W., London, W. T., Lega, L., and Feitelson, M. A. (1991) Hepatitis B x antigen in liver from carrier patients with chronic hepatitis and cirrhosis. *Hepatology* **14**, 29–37.
46. Wang, W., London, W. T., and Feitelson, M. A. (1991) Hepatitis B x antigen in hepatitis B virus carrier patients with liver cancer. *Cancer Res.* **51**, 4971–4977.
47. Feitelson, M. A., Lega, L., Duan, L.-X., and Clayton, M. (1993) Characteristics of woodchuck hepatitis X antigen in the livers and sera from chronically infected animals. *J. Hepatol.* **17**, S24–S34.
48. Su, Q., Schroder, C. H., Hofmann, W. J., Otto, G., Pichlmayr, R., and Bannasch, P. (1998) Expression of hepatitis B virus X protein in HBV-infected human livers and hepatocellular carcinomas. *Hepatology* **27**, 1109–1120.
49. Kim, H., Lee, H., and Yun, Y. (1998) X-gene product of hepatitis B virus induces apoptosis in liver cells. *J. Biol. Chem.* **273**, 381–385.
50. Pollicino, T., Terradillos, O., Lecoeur, H., Gougeon, M. L., and Buendia, M. A. (1998) Pro-apoptotic effect of the hepatitis B virus X gene. *Biomed. Pharmacother.* **52**, 363–368.
51. Shirakata, Y., Kawada, M., Fujiki, Y., et al. (1989) The X gene of hepatitis B virus induced growth stimulation and tumorigenic transformation of mouse NIH3T3 cells. *Jpn. J. Cancer Res.* **80**, 617–621.
52. Jameel, S., Siddiqui, A., Maguire, H. F., and Rao, K. V. S. (1990) Hepatitis B virus protein produced in *Escherichia coli* is biologically functional. *J. Virol.* **64**, 3963–3966.
53. Takada, S., Kaneniwa, N., Tsuchida, N., and Koike, K. (1997) Cytoplasmic retention of the p53 tumor suppressor gene product is observed in the hepatitis B virus X gene transfected cells. *Oncogene* **15**, 1895–1901.
54. Kuzhandaivelu, N., Cong, Y. S., Inouye, C., Yang, W. M., and Seto E. (1996) XAP2, a novel hepatitis B virus X-associated protein that inhibits X transactivation. *Nucleic Acids Res.* **24**, 4741–4750.
55. Becker, S. A., Lee, T. H., Butel, J. S., and Slagle, B. L. (1998) Hepatitis B virus protein interferes with cellular DNA repair. *J. Virol.* **72**, 266–272.
56. Shintani, Y., Yotsuyanagi, H., Moriya, K., et al. (1999) Induction of apoptosis after switch-on of the hepatitis B virus X gene mediated by the Cre/*lox*P recombination system. *J. Gen. Virol.* **80**, 3257–3265.
57. Lee, Y. H., and Yun, Y. (1998) HBx protein of hepatitis B virus activates Jak1-STAT signaling. *J. Biol. Chem.* **273**, 25,510–25,515.

58. Lian, Z., Pan, J., Liu, J., et al. (1999) The translation initiation factor, SUI1, may be a target of hepatitis B x antigen in hepatocarcinogenesis. *Oncogene* **18**, 1677–1687.
59. Su, F., and Schneider, R. J. (1997) Hepatitis B virus HBx protein sensitizes cells to apoptotic killing by tumor necrosis factor α. *Proc. Natl. Acad. Sci. USA* **94**, 8744–8749.
60. Blum, H. E., Zhang, Z. S., Galun, E., et al. (1992) Hepatitis B virus X protein is not central to the viral life cycle *in vitro*. *J. Virol.* **66**, 1223–1227.
61. Shin, E. C., Shin, J. S., Park, J. H., Kim, H., and Kim, S. J. (1999) Expression of Fas ligand in human hepatoma cell lines: role of hepatitis B virus X (HBx) in induction of Fas ligand. *Int. J. Cancer* **82**, 587–591.
62. Lara-Pezzi, E., Majano, P. L., Gomez-Gonzalo, M., et al. (1998) The hepatitis B virus X protein up-regulates tumor necrosis factor a gene expression in hepatocytes. *Hepatology* **28**, 1013–1028.
63. Doong, S. L., Lin, M. H., Tsai, M. M., Li, T. R., Chuang, S. E., and Cheng, A. L. (1998) Transactivation of the human MDR1 gene by hepatitis B virus X gene product. *J. Hepatol.* **29**, 872–878.
64. Ueda, H., Ullrich, S. J., Ngo, L., et al. (1995) Functional inactivation but not structural mutation of p53 causes liver cancer. *Nat. Genet.* **9**, 41–47.
65. Koike, K., Moriya, K., Iino, S., et al. (1994) High-level expression of hepatitis B virus HBx gene and hepatocarcinogenesis in transgenic mice. *Hepatology* **19**, 810–819.
66. Schmitteckert, E. M., and Schlicht, H. J. (1999) Detection of the human hepatitis B virus X-protein in transgenic mice after radioactive labeling at a newly introduced phosphorylation site. *J. Gen. Virol.* **80**, 2501–2509.
67. Slagle, B. L., Lee, T. H., Medina, D., Finegold, M. J., and Butel, J. S. (1996) Increased sensitivity to the hepatocarcinogen diethylnitrosamine in transgenic mice carrying the hepatitis B virus X gene. *Mol. Carcinog.* **15**, 261–269.
68. Lee, T. H., Finegold, M. J., Shen, R. F., DeMayo, J. L., Woo, S. L., and Butel, J. S. (1990) Hepatitis B virus transactivator X protein is not tumorigenic in transgenic mice. *J. Virol.* **64**, 5939–5947.

10

Detection of Serum HDV RNA by RT-PCR

Antonina Smedile, Maria Grazia Niro, and Mario Rizzetto

1. Introduction

The cloning and sequencing of the hepatitis D virus (HDV) genome in 1986 established the peculiar features that make HDV the only genus of the Deltaviridae family *(1)*. HDV is a defective negative-strand RNA virus that requires concurrent infection with the hepatitis B virus (HBV) to complete its replicative cycle. The 36-nm virion consists of the delta antigen (HDV Ag) and the RNA genome of 1.6 kb within an envelop of surface antigen (HBsAg), provided by the HBV infecting the host (*2*, **Fig. 1**). The structure and biological properties and replication mechanism of HDV are similar to those of plant RNA viruses such as the viroids and satellite RNAs *(3)*.

HDV contains one open reading frame encoding a single protein (HDV-Ag) that is translated from a 0.8-kb mRNA transcribed from the genomic RNA *(4)*. There are two isoforms of HDVAg: the small HDV-Ag (p24) and the large HDV-Ag (p27); the latter is generated by post-transcriptional RNA editing *(5)*. This process involves a nucleotide change at position 1012, referred to as the amber/W site, and requires a highly conserved base-paired structure within the unbranched rod structure of HDV RNA. HDV-Ag p24 promotes HDV replication, whereas HDV-Ag p27 inhibits HDV replication and is essential for virion assembly *(6)*.

The cloning of HDV RNA has provided genetic probes for the measurement of HDV RNA in serum and liver by nucleic acid hybridization methods *(7)*. A cDNA fragment containing a short nucleotide segment (153 bp) provided in the mid-1980s the first prototype for DNA hybridization assays that was used in early studies to measure HDV RNA in sera of chimpanzees and chronically infected patients *(8)*. The sensitivity of HDV RNA detection has further improved in the 1990s with the development of different cDNA and RNA probes of various genome lengths (**Fig. 2**). Sensitivity improved first when using a full-length cDNA probe, with detection ranging from 0.1 to 10 pg/mL *(8)*, and has further increased 100- to 1000-fold with the subsequent introduction of RNA–RNA hybridization (RNA probe) *(9)*.

From: *Methods in Molecular Medicine, vol. 95: Hepatitis B and D Protocols, volume 1*
Edited by: R. K. Hamatake and J. Y. N. Lau © Humana Press Inc., Totowa, NJ

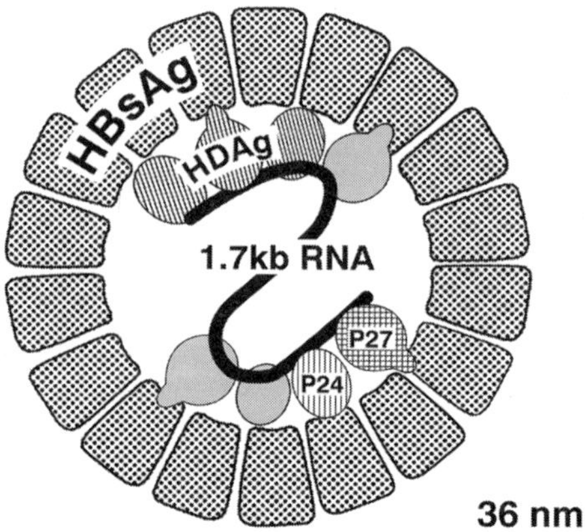

Fig. 1. Schematic virion of HDV.

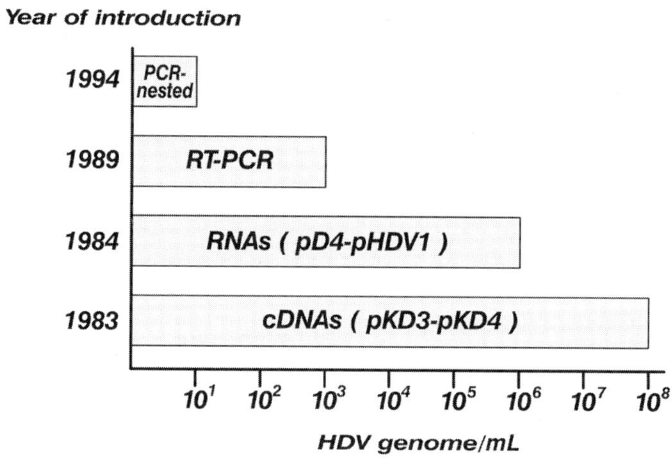

Fig. 2. Increased sensitivity of HDV RNA assay by using cDNA, RNA hybridization assay, and PCR (I and nested).

In the 1990s, the introduction of reverse transcriptase–polymerase chain reaction (RT–PCR) ***(10)*** techniques has led to the detection of as few as 1000 genomes (10^3)/μL in serum for single PCR and fewer than 10 HDV genomes/μL for nested PCR; both assays allow a semiquantitative analysis of the viral load ***(11)***.

Three genotypes of HDV were identified in sera from patients with HDV infection ***(12)***. A 357-nt semiconserved region, with a high degree of sequence conservation (containing functional domains), has been used for genetic analysis. Isolates were studied worldwide ***(13, 14)***. Genotype I, found in Europe, North America, North Africa, the Middle East, and East Asia, is predominant. Genotype II is present only in East Asia (Taiwan

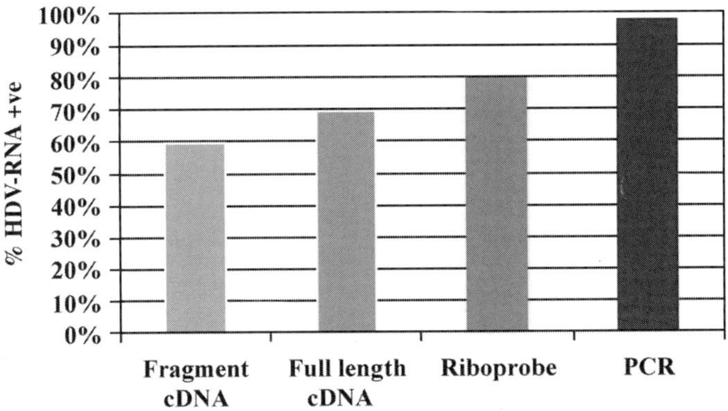

Fig. 3. Rate of HDV RNA positivity in chronic hepatitis D with different assays.

and Japan). Genotype III is exclusively associated with HDV infection in northern South America *(15)*.

HDV RNA in serum is the earliest diagnostic marker of acute HDV infection and the indicator of viral replication in chronic liver disease *(16)*. Testing for HDV RNA is particularly helpful in immunosuppressed individuals and in monitoring treated patients with very low initial or residual viral titers, respectively, before and at the end of therapy *(11–17)*. The percentages of HDV RNA-positive patients, achieved with a blot-hybridization assay and the more sensitive PCR methods, are reported in **Fig. 3**.

Because of the high sensitivity of the assay, the determination of HDV RNA by PCR presently represents the best analytical tool in the clinical setting. There is a high potential infectivity of HDV sera in HBV-positive subjects, so caution is required in all steps during the procedure; HBsAg-positive laboratory personnel who are at high risk of HDV superinfection should not work with HDV-infected sera. Separate laboratory working stations are recommended to avoid PCR contamination as well as interspaced negative controls between testing samples *(13)*. The use of sterile material and aliquots of reagents for PCR testing is generally advised.

We report here an RT-PCR assay for the detection of HDV RNA standardized for clinical use in the sera of patients with HDV disease. The pairs of HDV primers used for PCR I and nested PCR were recommended as the most efficient and reliable *(13,18,19)*; they amplify a semiconserved region of the HDV (**Table 1**), including the C-terminal portion of the HDV-Ag gene, the RNA editing site, and the polyadenylation signal (**Fig. 4**).

2. Materials

2.1. Extraction Reagents

1. 2X lysis buffer: Prepare a 500-mL stock solution using the following reagents: 100 mL 0.5 *M* ethylenediaminetetraacetic acid (EDTA), 50 mL 1 *M* HEPES, pH 7.2, 50 mL 4 *M* NaCl; 200 mL 10% sodium dodecyl sulfate (SDS). The solution can be stored at 37°C.

Table 1
HDV Primer Sequences

Primer	Sequence	Location
5413	5'sI–GCC CAG GTG GGA CCG CGA GGA GGT – 3'sI	858–881 nt
8276	5'sI–ACA AGG AGA GGC AGG ATC ACC GAC – 3'sI	1312–1289 nt
5414	5'sI–GAG ATG CCA TGC CGA CCC GAA GAG – 3'sI	883–906 nt
5415	5'sI–GAA GGA AGG CCC TCG AGA ACA AGA – 3'sI	1288–1265 nt

The final solution used for master mix shall contain 0.1 *M* EDTA, 0.1 *M* HEPES, pH 7.2, 0.4 *M* NaCl, 4.0% SDS (*see* **Note 1**).

2. Proteinase K (Invitrogen, Carlsbad, CA, USA): Dissolve 20 mg in 100 mL of distilled water. Aliquot and store at –20°C.
3. tRNA yeast 10 mg/mL (Invitrogen): Dissolve 25 mg in 2.5 mL of distilled water and store at –20°C (*see* **Note 1**).
4. 0.5 *M* EDTA: Dissolve 93.6 g of EDTA (MW 372.24) in 400 mL of distilled water. Adjust to pH 8 with NAOH. Add distilled water to a final 500-mL volume.
5. Buffered saturated phenol, pH 4.5 (Invitrogen): Store at 4°C. Handle with care. Be aware that phenol can cause severe chemical burns on skin and will damage clothing. This reagent should be used under a chemical cabinet while wearing safety glasses.
6. Aliquot 15 mL of phenol/chloroform (50/50%, v/v) in Falcon tubes to be used once. Store at 4°C.
7. 3 *M* sodium acetate, pH 5.2: Dissolve 24.61 g of sodium acetate anhydrous (MW 82.035) in 80 mL of distilled water. Adjust pH to 5.2 with glacial acetic acid. Add distilled water to a final 100-mL volume. Sterilize by autoclaving in aliquots. Store at room temperature.
8. 70% Ethanol: Add 30 mL distilled water to 70 mL absolute ethanol. Aliquot and store at –20°C.
9. Isopropanol: Aliquot and store at –20 C.

2.2. PCR Reagents

1. M-MLV RT (Invitrogen): 40,000 U, 200 U/μL. PCR reaction buffer 5X with 15 m*M* $MgCl_2$ and 0.1 *M* dithiothreitol (DTT). Store at –20°C.
2. 100 m*M* dNTP set (Finnzymes, Expoo, Finland): Each nucleotide is supplied as 100-m*M* solution in water, pH 7.5. Mix each 1:10 and pool. Aliquot in tubes of 200 μL amounts. Store at –20°C.
3. Hexanucleotide mix 10X conc (Boehringer-Roche); 50 U. Dilute in 1.25-mL distilled water. Store at –20°C.
4. RNAsin RNAse Inhibitor (Promega); 10,000 U, 40 U/μL. Store –20°C.
5. Hot StarTaq (Taq DNA-polymerase 250 U [QIAGEN]): Supplied PCR reaction buffer 10X (with 15 m*M* $MgCl_2$).
6. Q-Solution 5X: 25 m*M* $MgCl_2$. Store –20°C.
7. PCR primers are listed in **Table 1**.

2.3. Other Reagents

1. 50X TAE buffer, stock solution for agarose gel electrophoresis: Combine 193.6 g Tris-HCl base, 108.9 g sodium acetate·$3H_2O$, 15.2 g Na_2 EDTA·2 H_2O, and 700 mL water. Dissolve

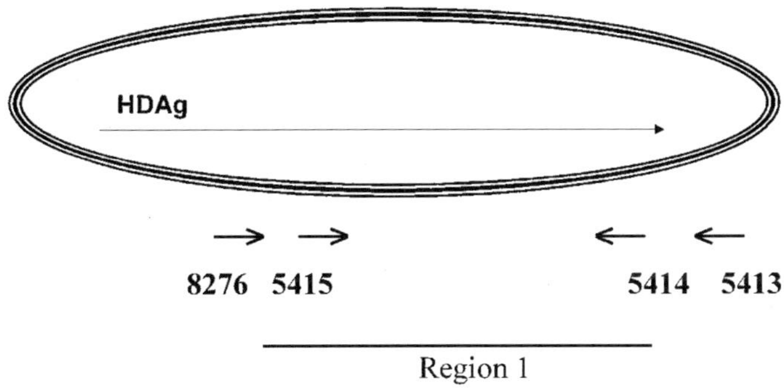

Fig. 4. Primer locations in HDV–RNA rod structure.

and adjust pH to 7.2 with acetic acid. Add water to a final volume of 1 L and autoclave. Store at room temperature.

2. 20X TBE buffer: Combine 121 g Tris base, 61.7 g boric acid, 7.44 g Na_2 EDTA·2 H_2O, and water to a final volume of 1 L (*see* **Note 2**).
3. Ethidium bromide (10 mg/mL): Add 0.2 g ethidium bromide to 19.8 mL water to dissolve. Store solution at room temperature in a foil-wrapped bottle to prevent exposure to light. Handle with care, ethidium bromide is a mutagen. (This solution can be purchased from GIBCO BRL, Rockville, MD.)
4. Gel-loading buffer, DNA (glycerol) 5X: Combine 5 mL glycerol, 1 mL 10X TBE, 1 mL 10% bromophenol blue, 1 mL 10% xylene cyanol, 2 mL water. Mix and store at –20°C. Aliquot in Eppendorf tubes.
5. 100-bp DNA ladder marker, 50 μL (Invitrogen): Dilute adding 100 μL blue dye 6X and 850 μL TAE 1X. Use 10 μL of this solution.

3. Methods

3.1. Isolation of Nucleic Acids from Serum (see **Note 3**)

We suggest the use of a separate room for nucleic acid extraction and thereafter two separate working stations: one for dispensing reagents for RT-PCR and first-step PCR and the other for nested PCR. Caution is recommended during the extraction procedure to avoid sample contamination. Powder-free gloves should be changed between sample handling. It is suggested to test only a few samples on each occasion (no more than 12, including negative controls). Disposable cotton-plugged pipet tips and autoclaved microtubes should be used.

1. Prepare a master mix containing the following reagents for each sample: 220 μL 2X H-lysis buffer, 22 μL proteinase K (20 mg/mL), 5.5 μL tRNA (10 mg/mL), 152.5 μL water for total volume of 400 μL. To each sample tube, add 350 μL of the master mix. A repeating pipettor may be convenient for dispensing the master mix.
2. Add 50 μL of serum for each sample. Gloves should be changed between handling of each sample.

3. Incubate at 37°C for at least 2 h, preferably overnight.
4. Add 400 µL of phenol; vortex and spin in a microfuge at 4000*g* for 10 min at room temperature.
5. Prepare 400 µL of phenol/chloroform and 40 µL of 3 *M* sodium acetate (pH 5.2) in a fresh tube.
6. After microfuging the samples, transfer the aqueous (upper) phase to the tube from **step 5**. Vortex and spin at 4000*g* in a microfuge for 10 min at room temperature.
7. Prepare 400 µL of cold isopropanol in fresh tubes.
8. After microfuging the samples, transfer the aqueous (upper) phase to the tube from **step 7**.
9. Incubate at 80°C for at least 1 h.
10. Pellet RNA in a microfuge at 8000*g* for 30 min at 4°C. Carefully remove the supernatant and recover the pellet.
11. Wash the pellet by adding 250 µL of 70% ethanol, spinning for 15 min at 8000*g* at 4°C in a microfuge and carefully removing the supernatant.
12. Allow the pellet to air-dry (the pellet will dry faster at 37°C).
13. Dissolve the pellet in 50 µL of sterile distilled water. Denature the pellet for 5 min at 95°C and then transfer to 4°C.
14. The extracted HDV RNA is either immediately used for PCR testing or stored at –20°C for further evaluations.

3.2. Reverse Transcriptase

1. Make a mix of the following reagents per sample and interspersed negative control: 2.2 µL 5X RT buffer, 1.1µL 0.1 *M* DTT, 1.1 µL 10 m *M* dNTPs, 0.55 µL 10X hexanucleotide, 0.55 µL M-MuLV RT (*see* **Note 4**), 0.5 µL RNAsin, 3.89 µL water, 9.89 µL total volume.
2. Dispense 9 µL of RT mix to each sample tube.
3. Add 1 µL of extracted RNA and 1 µL of extracted negative control for each testing sample and mix by pipeting. Briefly centrifuge. For each set of samples, a positive control should also be included (serum with known HDV RNA concentration).
4. To obtain cDNA, put 0.5-mL tubes in thermal cycler (Applied Biosystems Geneamp PCR System 2400 or 9700) following the program: 15 min 37°C, 15 min 42°C, 5 min 95°C, and 5 min 4° C.

3.3. PCR I

1. PCR reaction mix (40 µL) containing 0.5 µ*M* (25 pmol) of HDV primers (**Table 1**) and 2.5 U of Hot StarTaq should be added to 10 µL of cDNA obtained from **Subheading 3.2.** For each testing sample, prepare a PCR reaction mixture as following: 5.0 µL 10X PCR buffer, 7.0 µL 25 m*M* $MgCl_2$, 10.0 µL (5X) Q-solution, 1.25µL 20 µ*M* Primer 8276, 1.25 µL 20 µ*M* Primer 5413, 0.5 µL (5 U/µL) Hot StarTaq, 15 µL water, 40.0 µL total volume.
2. Reactions will take place at the following thermal cycle conditions: 15 min 95°C for initial activation step; 2 min 95°C for denaturing; 35 cycles for denaturing, annealing, extension at 1 min 94°C, 1 min 55°C, and 1 min 72°C. Final extension: 5 min 72°C; hold at 4°C.

3.4. PCR Nested

1. Prepare a PCR nested mixture of 49 µL containing 200 µ*M* deoxynucleotide triphosphate, 0.5 µ*M* of each PCR primer (**Table 1**), and 2.5 U Taq polymerase as follows: 5 µL 10X PCR buffer, 7 µL 25 m*M* $MgCl_2$, 1 µL m*M* dNTPs, 10 µL 5X Q-solution, 1.25 µL 20 µ*M* Primer

5414, 1.25 μL 20 μ*M* Primer 5415, 0.5 μL (5 U/μL Hot StarTaq, 23 μL water, 49 μL total volume.
2. Add 1 μL of PCR I reaction to each single tube containing 49 μL of PCR nested mix (**step 1**) and cover with 50 μL of mineral oil.
3. PCR nested reaction will take place at the following thermal cycle conditions: 15 min 95°C for initial activation step, 2 min 95°C for denaturing, 35 cycles for denaturing, annealing, extension at: 1 min 94°C, 1 min 55°C, and 1 min 72°C. Final extension: 5 min 72°C.

3.5. Gel Electrophoresis Analysis

Amplicons of both PCR reactions can be analyzed by gel electrophoresis using 2% agarose and ethidium bromide staining.

1. Dissolve 3 g agarose (in microwave or by boiling) in 150 mL of TAE buffer. Allow to cool to 50°C and add 3 μL of ethidium bromide solution (10 mg/mL).
2. Pour melted agarose on two small gel trays prepared with appropriate combs and let cool. Add TAE running buffer.
3. Prepare 100-bp DNA ladder (10 μL) as marker.
4. Add 2 μL of blue dye to 10 μL of PCR product and mix by pipetting.
5. Load stained PCR product **(step 4)** and marker **(step 3)** to gel well.
6. Run gel until bromophenol blue migrates about three-fourths the length of the gel.
7. Photograph the gel on ultraviolet transluminator to record marker position and PCR results. Positive amplicon for PCR I should give a size fragment of 454 bp, whereas amplicon for PCR nested should be of 405 bp **(Fig. 5)**.

4. Notes

1. Aliquots of 5 mL master mix, including 2X lysis buffer, tRNA, and proteinase K, can be prepared in advance and stored at −20°C.
2. A precipitate inevitably forms in this solution with storage at room temperature. The buffer continues to work well despite the precipitate.
3. The extraction procedure for serum HDV RNA allows the simultaneous extraction of HBV DNA.
4. The enzymes required for PCR should be kept in ice during handling.

References

1. Gerin, J. L. (1994) The taxonomy of Hepatitis Delta Virus. In: Nishioka K., Suzuki H., Mishiro S., Oda T., eds., *Viral Hepatitis and Liver Disease*, Springer-Verlag, Tokyo, 63–64.
2. Smedile, A., Niro, G. A., Rizzetto, M. (1997) Hepatitis D virus. In: Richman, D. D., Whitley, R. J., Hayden, F. G. (eds.), *Clinical Virology*, Churchill Livingstone, New York.
3. Brach, A. D., Robertson, H. D. (1984) A replication cycle for viroids and other small infectious RNAs. *Science* **223**, 450–455.
4. Taylor, J. M. (1990) Hepatitis delta virus: cis and trans functions required for replication. *Cell* **61**, 371–373.
5. Casey, J. L., Bergman, K. F., Brown, T. L., Gerin, J. L. (1992) Structural requirements for RNA editing in hepatitis delta virus: evidence for a uridine-to-cytidine editing mechanism. *Proc. Natl. Acad. Sci. USA* **89**, 1749–1753.

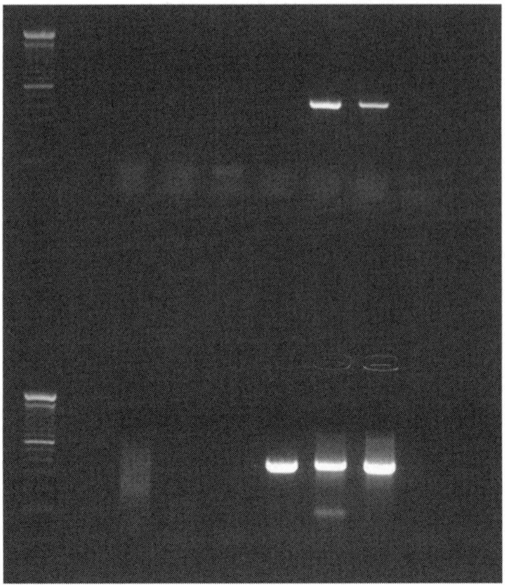

Fig. 5. Electrophoresis gel stained by ethidium bromide showing approx 470 (PCR I, *top*) and 406 (PCR nested, *bottom*) amplicon.

6. Casey, J. L., Gerin, J. L. (1995) Hepatitis delta virus RNA editing and genotype variations. In: Dinber-Gottlieb, G. (ed.) *The Unique Hepatitis Delta Virus*. Springer-Verlag, New York.
7. Denniston, K. J., Hoyer, B. H., Smedile, A., Wells, F. V., Nelson, J., Gerin, J. L. (1986) Cloned fragment of hepatitis delta RNA genome, sequence and diagnostic application. *Science* **232**, 873–875.
8. Smedile, A., Rizzetto, M., Denniston K., et al. (1986) Type D hepatitis: the clinical significance of hepatitis D virus RNA in serum as detected by a hybridization based-assay. *Hepatology* **6**, 1297–1302.
9. Smedile, A., Bergmann, K. F., Baroudi, B. M., et al. (1990) Riboprobe assay for HDV-RNA: a sensitive method for the detection of the HDV genome in clinical serum samples. *J. Med. Virol.* **30**, 20–24.
10. Ehrlich, H. (ed.) (1989) *PCR Technology: Principles and Applications for DNA Amplification*. Stockton Press, New York.
11. Smedile, A., Casey, J. L., Cote, P. J., et al. (1998) Hepatitis D viremia following orthotopic liver transplantation involves a typical HDV virion with hepatitis B surface antigen envelope. *Hepatology* **27**, 1723–1729.
12. Casey, J. L., Brown, T. L., Colan, E. J., et al. (1993) A genotype of hepatitis D virus that occurs in northern South America. *Proc. Natl. Acad. Sci. USA* **90**, 9016–9020.
13. Niro, G. A., Smedile, A., Andriulli, A., Rizzetto, M., Gerin, J. L., Casey, J. L. (1997) The predominance of hepatitis delta virus genotype I among chronically infected Italian patients. *Hepatology* **25**, 728–734.

14. Shakil, A. O., Hadziyannis, S., Hoofnagle, J. H., Di Bisceglie, A. M., Gerin, J. L., Casey, J. L. (1997) Geographic distribution and genetic variability of hepatitis delta virus genotype I. *Virology* **234**, 160–167.
15. Casey, J. L., Niro, G. A., Engle, R., et al. (1996) Hepatitis B virus/hepatitis D virus co-infection in outbreaks of acute hepatitis in the Peruvian Amazon basin: the role of HDV genotype III and HBV genotype F. *J. Infect. Dis.* **174**, 920–926.
16. Smedile, A., Rosina, F., Saracco, G., et al. (1991) Hepatitis B virus replication modulates pathogenesis of hepatitis D virus in chronic hepatitis D. *Hepatology* **13**, 413–416.
17. Rosina, F., Pintus, C., Meschievitz, C., et al. (1991) A randomized controlled trial of a 12-mo course of recombinant human interferon-a in chronic delta (type D) hepatitis: a multicenter study. *Hepatology* **13**, 1052–1056.
18. Cariani, E., Ravaggi, A., Puoti, M., Mantero, G., Alberti, A., Primi, D. (1992) Evaluation of hepatitis delta virus RNA levels during interferon therapy by analysis of polymerase chain reaction products with a nonradioisotopic hybridisation assay. *Hepatology* **15**, 685–689.
19. Cotrina, M., Buti, M., Jardi, R., et al. (1998) Hepatitis delta genotypes in chronic delta infections in the North East of Spain (Catalonia). *J. Hepatol.* **28**, 971–977.

11

Nonradioisotopic *In Situ* Hybridization for HDV RNA

Francesco Negro

1. Introduction

The procedure described here was reported to detect the genomic strand of the hepatitis virus (HDV) RNA *(1)* in formalin-fixed, paraffin-embedded liver sections (**Fig. 1**). The method used a 27-mer end-labeled with digoxigenin (DIG). Hybrids were detected by a specific antibody coupled to alkaline phosphatase. Earlier reports had described the detection of both genomic and antigenomic HDV RNA by radioactive ^{35}S-labeled RNA probes (**Fig. 2**) *(2)*. However, because the average number of genomic HDV RNA in each hepatocyte is very high (around 300,000 copies/cell) *(3)*, HDV is the ideal target to be detected by a nonradioactive *in situ* hybridization procedure, even using a short oligonucleotide probe, i.e., representing only approx 1.6% of the total length of the genome.

2. Materials

1. The oligonucleotide sequence is 5'-CCCCAGTGAATAAAGCGGGTTTCCACT-3', complementary to bases 936–962 of HDV RNA according to the proposed numbering *(4)*.
2. DIG-11-dUTP (Roche Molecular Biochemicals) is provided by the manufacturer as 1-m*M* solution in a kit for tailing 3' ends of oligonucleotides *(5)*; the same kit also contains the terminal deoxynucleotidyl transferase, 50 U/μL.
3. Poly-L-lysine-coated microscope slides.
4. Xylene and absolute ethanol and ethanol dilutions in water (Fluka Chemie AG).
5. Phosphate-buffered saline (PBS): 137 m*M* NaCl, 2.7 m*M* KCl, 4.3 m*M* Na_2HPO_4, 1.4 m*M* KH_2PO_4, pH 7.3.
6. Proteinase K, DNase- and RNase-free (Merck, Darmstadt).
7. PBS/0.1 *M* glycine.
8. Deionized formamide: Take 500 mL of formamide, add 50 g of resin (Bio-Rad AG 501-X8, 20–50 mesh), stir 30 min at room temperature, filter through Whatman 2, and store in 50-mL aliquots at –20° C, protecting from light.

From: *Methods in Molecular Medicine, vol. 95: Hepatitis B and D Protocols, volume 1*
Edited by: R. K. Hamatake and J. Y. N. Lau © Humana Press Inc., Totowa, NJ

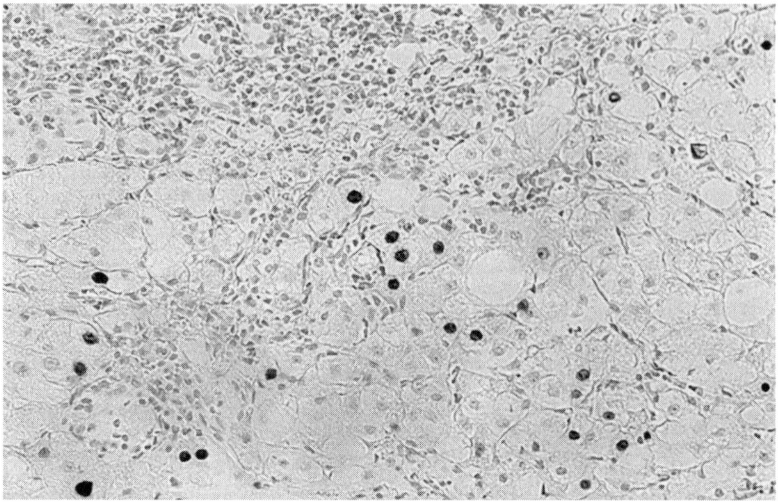

Fig. 1. Detection of genomic HDVRNA in nuclei of hepatocytes by nonradioisotopic *in situ* hybridization using a digoxigenin-labeled synthetic oligonucleotide. Counterstaining with methyl green. Original magnification ×40.

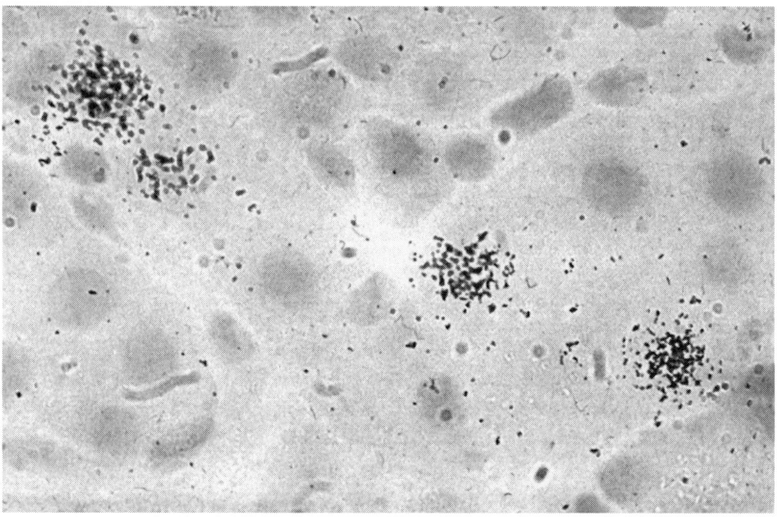

Fig. 2. Detection of genomic HDV RNA in nuclei of hepatocytes by *in situ* hybridization using ^{35}S-labeled RNA probes. Counterstaining with hematoxylin. Original magnification ×100.

9. 20X Standard saline citrate (SSC): 3 *M* NaCl, 0.3 *M* Na_3citrate, pH 7.0.
10. 50X Denhardt's solution: 5 g Ficoll 400, 5 g polyvinylpyrrolidone, 5 g bovine serum albumin (Pentax Fraction V, Miles Laboratories) in 500 mL H_2O; filter, sterilize, and store in aliquots at –20°C.

11. 10 mg/mL herring sperm DNA.
12. 10 mg/mL yeast tRNA.
13. TN buffer: 100 m*M* Tris-HCl, pH 7.5, 150 m*M* NaCl.
14. Normal sheep serum (Dakopatts).
15. Sheep anti-DIG-Fab fragments, conjugated to calf intestinal alkaline phosphatase (Roche Molecular Biochemicals).
16. TNM buffer: 100 m*M* Tris-HCl, pH 9.5, 100 m*M* NaCl, 50 m*M* $MgCl_2$.
17. Developing solution: Add 45 μL of nitroblue tetrazolium salt (100 mg/mL in dimethylformamide [Roche Molecular Biochemicals]), 35 μL of 5-bromo-4-chloro-3-indolyl-phosphate (50 mg/mL solution in dimethylformamide [Roche Molecular Biochemicals]), 0.024% tetramisole (Sigma) to 10 mL of TNM buffer; prepare immediately before use.
18. Stop buffer: 10 m*M* Tris-HCl, pH 8.0, 1 m*M* ethylenediaminetetraacetic acid (EDTA).
19. Methyl green.
20. Mounting medium (Entellan™, Merck).

3. Method

1. Label 25 pmol of the oligomer with DIG-11-dUTP following the manufacturer's instructions. Store at –20°C until use (up to 3 mo).
2. Deparaffinize tissue sections in xylene for 10 min twice.
3. Rehydrate to PBS through a standard series of ethanols (absolute, 5 min twice, then 95% for 5 min, and 70% for 5 min).
4. Digest in proteinase K, 0.15–0.5 mg/mL in PBS for 15 min at 37°C (*see* **Note 1**).
5. Block digestion in ice-cold PBS, 0.1 *M* glycine, 5 min twice.
6. Rinse in 2X SSC for 3 min.
7. Prehybridize for 1 h at room temperature in a mixture containing 50% formamide, 5X SSC, 1X Denhardt's solution, 0.5 mg/mL herring sperm DNA, 0.25 mg/mL yeast tRNA.
8. Tap excess prehybridization mixture and hybridize overnight at 37°C in a wet chamber with the same mixture as above containing the DIG-labeled probe diluted 1:100 (final concentration of 100 n*M*) (*see* **Note 2**).
9. Wash 1 h at room temperature in 2X SSC, then 1 h in 1X SSC, then 30 min at 42°C in 0.5X SSC, and finally 1 h at room temperature in 0.1X SSC. (Unless specified, all subsequent steps are to be performed at room temperature.)
10. Rinse briefly in TN buffer.
11. Incubate the sections with TN buffer containing 2% normal sheep serum and 1:100 AP-anti-DIG-Fab for 30 min.
12. Wash in TN buffer for 15 min twice.
13. Incubate for 2 min in TNM buffer.
14. Develop 10–40 min in the developing mixture, checking the intensity of the staining periodically with the microscope (*see* **Note 3**). **Do not allow the sections to dry at any time.**
15. Block with 10 m*M* Tris-HCl, pH 8.0, 1 m*M* EDTA for 5 min.
16. Countercolor with 1% methyl green.
17. Rinse in water, dehydrate (passage in 95% ethanol should be quick because it may destain the section), and mount.

4. Notes

1. The proteinase K concentration used to pretreat sections cannot be predetermined because it depends on the amount of crosslinks formed during the formalin fixation. The longer the tis-

sue has been kept in the fixative, the tighter the crosslinks will be, hence the higher the protease concentration needed to improve the accessibility of the probe to its target. Excessive digestion may result in loss of morphological details as well as poor retention of small tissue molecules (including the target RNA) during the various steps of the *in situ* hybridization protocol.

2. The protocol does not include a denaturation step of the sections before hybridization, because only a minority of the genomic HDV RNA is base-paired, most likely to its antigenomic counterpart *(2)*. Denaturation would be necessary if detection of antigenomic HDV RNA is desired; the antigenomic strand of HDV appears to be fully base-paired *(2)*.
3. The HDV RNA (both genomic and antigenomic strands) is exclusively localized in the hepatocyte nuclei. These nuclei may have a "sanded" appearance *(1)*. No other cell type seems to support HDV replication in vivo. Hepatocytes containing HDV RNA, as detected by *in situ* hybridization, also express the hepatitis D antigen (HDAg), in most cases although exceptions have been observed *(6)*. Occasionally, nuclei may only contain HDV RNA or HDAg. The expression of the HDAg alone may be consistent with the fact that HDVAg is an early viral antigen *(7)*. Conversely, the finding of HCV RNA in the absence of detectable levels of expression of HDAg is more difficult to explain, as a result of the known role of HDAg in activating the HDV replication *(8)*. Neither the expression of HDV RNA nor that of HDAg seems to be associated with morphological changes of hepatocytes, such as eosinophilic degeneration *(6)*.

References

1. Pacchioni, D., Negro, F., Chiaberge, E., Rizzetto, M., Bonino, F., and Bussolati, G. (1992) Detection of hepatitis delta virus RNA by a nonradioactive in situ hybridization procedure. *Hum. Pathol.* **23**, 557–561.
2. Gowans, E.J., Baroudy, B.M., Negro, F., Ponzetto, A., Purcell, R. H., and Gerin, J. L. (1988) Evidence for replication of hepatitis delta virus RNA in hepatocyte nuclei after in vivo infection. *Virology* **167**, 274–278.
3. Chen, P. J., Kalpana, G., Goldberg, J., et al. (1986) Structure and replication of the genome of the hepatitis delta virus. *Proc. Natl. Acad. Sci. USA* **83**, 8774–8778.
4. Schmitz, G. G., Walter, T., Seibl, R., and Kessler, C. (1991) Nonradioactive labeling of oligonucleotides in vitro with the hapten digoxigenin by tailing with terminal transferase. *Anal. Biochem.* **192**, 222–231.
5. Wang, K. S., Choo, Q. L., Weiner, A. J., et al. (1986) Structure, sequence and expression of the hepatitis delta (δ) viral genome. *Nature* **323**, 508–514.
6. Negro, F., Bonino, F., Di Bisceglie, A., Hoofnagle, J. H., and Gerin, J. L. (1989) Intrahepatic markers of hepatitis delta virus infection: a study by in situ hybridization. *Hepatology* **10**, 916–920.
7. Modahl, L. E., and Lai, M. M. (2000) The large delta antigen of hepatitis delta virus potently inhibits genomic but not antigenomic RNA synthesis: a mechanism enabling initiation of viral replication. *J. Virol.* **74**, 7375–7380.
8. Kuo, M. Y., Chao, M., and Taylor, J. (1989) Initiation of replication of the human hepatitis delta virus genome from cloned DNA: role of delta antigen. *J. Virol.* **63**, 1945–1950.

12

Detection and Characterization of Small and Large HDV Antigens

Thomas B. Macnaughton and Michael M. C. Lai

1. Introduction

Hepatitis delta virus antigen (HDV Ag) was discovered by Rizzetto and associates in 1977 following the detection of a novel nuclear antigen in the hepatocytes of some hepatitis B virus carriers *(1)*. HDV Ag is the nucleocapsid protein of a small RNA virus known as HDV. In infected liver tissue, HDV Ag is generally localized to the nucleoplasm of the nucleus but has also been detected in the cytoplasm in patients with acute HDV infection *(2)*. In cell cultures transfected with HDV cDNA, three different patterns of nuclear staining of HDV Ag have been reported: nucleolar, mixed nucleolar and nucleoplasmic, and exclusively nucleoplasmic *(3)*. Although the reason for these differences is unknown, we have noted that the nucleolar pattern is more commonly seen when only the HDV Ag gene is expressed *(4)*.

In Western blots of HDV-infected liver *(5)* and cell cultures containing replicating HDV RNA *(3)*, HDV Ag appears as two closely related species of approximate molecular masses of 24 kDa and 27 kDa. These two species are referred to as small and large hepatitis delta antigens (S-HDV Ag and L-HDV Ag, respectively). The L-HDV Ag species arises as the result of a specific RNA-editing event, in which the stop codon for S-HDV Ag is changed to a tryptophan, allowing translation to continue for a further 19 amino acids *(6)*. As a result of the temporal regulation of this editing event, L-HDV Ag appears only during the later stage of the HDV life cycle (**Fig. 1**). L-HDV Ag is essential for virus packaging *(7)* and thus is always found in the virus particle (in an approximately equimolar amount with S-HDV Ag).

2. Materials

2.1. Solutions

1. 4X lower buffer: Dissolve 90.85 g of Tris-HCl in 400 mL distilled water; add 10.0 mL of 20% sodium dodecyl sulfate (SDS) and adjust pH to 8.8 with HCl. Adjust volume to 500 mL with distilled water. Store at room temperature.

From: *Methods in Molecular Medicine, vol. 95: Hepatitis B and D Protocols, volume 1*
Edited by: R. K. Hamatake and J. Y. N. Lau © Humana Press Inc., Totowa, NJ

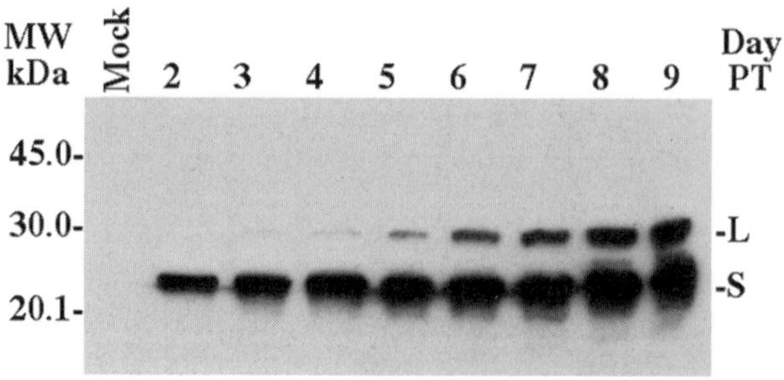

Fig. 1. Western blot examining the kinetics of S- and L-HDV Ag synthesis. HuH7 cells transfected with HDV RNA were harvested from d 2–9 post-transfection and analyzed for HDV Ag by Western blot. The primary antibody comprised a 1:200 dilution of a mixture of three monoclonal antibodies specific for both L- and S-HDV Ag *(8)*. The secondary antibody was a 1:5000 dilution of rabbit anti-mouse (Dako, cat. no.) conjugated to horseradish peroxidase. The "Mock" track is mock-transfected HuH7 cells, and the numbers on the left-hand side indicate the positions of three of the Rainbow Molecular weight markers (Amersham Pharmacia Biotech). The Western blot shows the typical kinetics of HDVAg appearance. S-HDV Ag (S) is detected at all time points, whereas L-HDV Ag (L) first appeared 3 to 4 days post-transfection and gradually became stronger with time.

2. 4X upper buffer: Dissolve 30.3 g of Tris-HCl in 400 mL distilled water; add 10.0 mL of 20% SDS and adjust pH to 6.8 with HCl. Adjust volume to 500 mL with distilled water. Store at room temperature.
3. 4X running buffer: Dissolve 12.0 g of Tris-HCl and 57.6 g of glycine in 900 mL distilled water. Add 20.0 mL 20% SDS and make up volume to 1 L with distilled water.
4. 2X sample buffer: Mix 1.0 mL of glycerol, 1.50 mL of 20% SDS, 1.25 mL of 4X upper buffer, 0.50 mL β-mercaptoethanol, and 5.75 mL distilled water. Add bromophenol blue powder to color (approx 0.01 mg). Store at 4°C for up to 3 mo. Stable for 1 yr or longer prior to addition of β-mercaptoethanol.
5. 10% ammonium persulfate in distilled water. Store at –20°C for up to 1 yr or at room temperature for up to 2 wk.
6. TEMED (Sigma, cat. no.T 7024). Store at room temperature.
7. 40% acrylamide (19:1, Amresco ultra pure cat. no. 0496). Store at room temperature.
8. 10X transfer buffer: Dissolve 30.3 g of Tris-HCl and 144 g glycine in distilled water to a final volume of 1 L. Store at room temperature. Mix 100 mL of the transfer buffer with 200 mL of methanol and 700 mL of distilled water before use.
9. Blocking buffer: Phosphate-buffered saline (PBS; 150 m*M* NaCl, 6 m*M* K_2HPO_4, 2 m*M* KH_2PO_4, pH 7.2) containing 0.05% Tween-20, 5% nonfat dried milk, and 2% bovine calf serum (optional).
10. 20% sucrose in PBS. Filter-sterilize; do not autoclave. Store at 4°C.
11. Antibodies: Commercial antibodies specific for HDV Ag are difficult to obtain. If no other sources are available, choose a high-titer serum from HDV-infected patients. Secondary antibodies for Western blotting need to be conjugated to horseradish peroxidase, whereas those for immunofluorescence need to be conjugated to fluorescein isothiocyanate (FITC) or rhodamine (*see* **Note 1**).

2.2. Equipment and Kits

1. Noninterfering Protein Assay kit (Geno Technology, cat. no. 786-005) for quantifying protein levels in samples containing SDS and β-mercaptoethanol.
2. Polyacrylamide gel electrophoresis equipment, 0.75–1-mm combs and spacers. We use a Hoefer Mighty Small II system for analysis of HDV Ag proteins (Amersham Pharmacia Biotech, cat. no. 80-6147-45).
3. Wet transfer apparatus. We use a Hoefer TE 22 Mini Tank (Amersham Pharmacia Biotech cat. no. 80-6204-26).
4. Hybond-C extra (Amersham Pharmacia Biotech, cat. no. RPN303E) protein transfer membrane.
5. Rocker platform. Any variable-speed model will do. We use The Belly Dancer (Stovall Life Science Inc).
6. Nonradioactive Western blotting detection system, ECL+plus (Amersham Pharmacia Biotech, cat. no. RPN2132).
7. Biomax MR scientific imaging film (Kodak, cat. no. 8701302) and X-ray cassettes to suit.
8. Falcon 4- or 8-chamber CultureSlides (Becton Dickinson), NJ, cat nos. 354104 and 354108, respectively) and cover glasses to suit (VWR Scientific, cat. no. 48393106).
9. ProLong Antifade Kit (Molecular Probes, OR, cat. no. P-7481).
10. Any microscope with ultraviolet viewing capabilities, preferably with filters for detection of both FITC and rhodamine.

2.3. Materials for Analysis

In our laboratory, the most common source material for HDV Ag analysis is a cell line transfected with HDV cDNA or HDV RNA. We have also used virus particles generated from HDV-transfected cells and from the serum of HDV-infected patients. In the latter case, it is important that the sera have not undergone too many freeze–thaw cycles.

3. Methods

3.1. Preparation of Samples for Analysis by Western Blot

3.1.1. Cultured Cells

The procedure given is for cells grown in 35-mm Petri dishes or 6-well-plate cultures. Scale up accordingly for larger cultures.

1. Trypsinize cells and transfer to 1.5-mL Eppendorf tubes. Pellet cells at low speed for 20 s and remove as much supernatant as possible with a micropipet. There is no need to wash the pellet.
2. Immediately add 100 μL of 2X sample buffer and vortex vigorously for 15 s. The solution will become very viscous at this stage. If a number of samples are to be processed, store them on ice prior to and after addition of the sample buffer.
3. After the sample buffer has been added to all samples, place them in a boiling water bath for 5 min and then quench on ice. Samples can be analyzed immediately or stored at –20°C for later use (*see* **Note 2**).
4. Where necessary, total protein concentrations of the samples can be determined using the noninterfering Protein Assay kit.

3.1.2. Virus Particles

1. Serum samples should first be diluted at least 1:3 with PBS. Culture fluids can be used as they are. Clarify samples by centrifugation in a bench-top centrifuge at 5,000*g* for 10 min.
2. Carefully layer the clarified sample over a 0.5-mL cushion of 20% sucrose (in PBS) in 4-mL polypropylene ultracentrifuge tubes suitable for use in a Beckman SW-60 (or equivalent) rotor. Ensure that the tubes are precisely balanced and filled to approx 2–3 mm from the top.
3. Centrifuge at 40,000 rpm in a Beckman SW-60 rotor for 4 h at 4°C; pour off supernatant and drain tubes upside down on paper towel for 5–10 min.
4. Carefully dry the inside of the tube with tissue paper without disturbing the pellet. Add 50 μL of 2X sample buffer, vortex briefly, cover the top of the tube with Parafilm, and place in a boiling water bath for 5 min. Quench on ice.

3.2. Western Blot Analysis for the Detection of L- and S-HDV Ag

1. Assemble apparatus and pour polyacrylamide gels according to the manufacturer's directions. For HDV Ag detection, we use 12.5% polyacrylamide gels prepared according to the following mixtures. For 20 mL of lower gel: 8.7 mL of distilled water, 5 mL of 4X lower buffer, 6.3 mL of 40% acrylamide solution, 80μL of 10% ammonium persulfate, and 10 μL of TEMED. For 10 mL of stacker gel: 6.5 mL of distilled water, 2.5 mL of 4X upper buffer, 0.9 mL of 40% acrylamide, 75 μL of 10% ammonium persulfate, and 20 μL of TEMED.
2. Load samples on the gel and electrophorese at 20 mA (for Mighty Small II system gels) until just after the bromophenol blue dye runs off the bottom of the gel. To serve as molecular weight markers and to monitor protein transfer from the gel, we also load a dye-linked protein marker mix (Rainbow molecular weight markers, Amersham Pharmaicia Biotech cat. ca. RPN756). For preprepared samples stored at –20°C, place them in a boiling water bath for 1–2 min prior to loading.
3. Remove gel from plates and excise stacker gel with a razor blade. Assemble gel in wet transfer apparatus and transfer to Hybond-C extra at 90 V for 60 min.
4. Remove the Hybond-C membrane containing the transferred proteins and let dry at room temperature. This step facilitates fixation of the proteins to the membrane. If necessary, the membrane can be stored at this stage for later processing.
5. Incubate membrane in blocking buffer for 2 h at room temperature or overnight at 4°C while shaking on a rocker platform.
6. Incubate with an HDV Ag-specific antibody diluted in PBS containing 0.05% Tween-20 and 5% nonfat dried milk for 2 h at room temperature. The degree of dilution depends on the quality of the antibody and will need to be determined empirically. In most cases, 1:500 to 1:1000 dilutions work well.
7. Wash membrane four times for 5 min each in PBS containing 0.05% Tween-20, then incubate with a secondary antibody conjugated with horseradish peroxidase and diluted in PBS containing 0.05% Tween-20 and 5% nonfat dried milk. Usual dilutions for the secondary antibody are 1:5000 or higher.
8. Wash membrane as described, and then visualize HDV Ag proteins using an ECL+plus non-radioactive Western blotting detection system and expose to Biomax MR scientific imaging film. We recommend a first exposure of approx 10 s. Use the results from this first exposure to determine the optimum exposure time. The ECL signal remains stable for 1–2 h. S- and L-HDV Ag should run somewhere in between the 20.1 kDa and 30.0 kDa Rainbow molecular weight markers **(Fig. 1)** (*see* **Note 3**).

3.3. Immunofluorescent Analysis for HDV Ag

1. Culture cells on Falcon 4- or 8-chamber "CultureSlides." For best results, cells should be subconfluent at the time of harvest for staining.
2. Pour off culture media, and carefully remove and discard upper chamber using the tool provided with the slides. Rinse slide briefly in PBS, and then fix cells by incubating in PBS containing 2% formalin at room temperature for 30 min. Permeabilize cells by transferring the slide to cold acetone (4°C) for 5 min. Best results are obtained if the staining step is performed immediately after fixation. However, if necessary, slides can be dried after the acetone step and stored at 4°C for later use.
3. Rehydrate cells in PBS for 5 min, shake off excess fluid, wipe edges of slide with tissue paper, and then apply the primary HDV Ag-specific antibody diluted in PBS. Use approx 25 μL or 50 μL of antibody per well of the 8- or 4-well chamber slides, respectively. The appropriate antibody dilution will depend on the quality of the antibody; however, 1:50 to 1:100 dilution will usually produce satisfactory results. Immediately cover slide with a cover slip, then place it in a humid chamber and incubate at 37°C for 60 min. Placing a wet sponge inside a plastic container that has a tightly fitting lid can make a simple humid chamber.
4. Remove the cover slip by dipping the slide in PBS, and then wash the slide in PBS twice for 5 min each.
5. Add appropriate secondary antibody conjugated with FITC or rhodamine. Usual dilution for this antibody is about 1:100. Cover with a cover slip and incubate in a humid chamber for 40 min at 37°C. **Important**: Before use, centrifuge diluted conjugate for 5 min at maximum speed in a microfuge to remove particulate FITC or rhodamine that has dissociated from the antibody.
6. Remove the cover slip and wash as in **step 4**. After last wash, remove excess fluid and mount using ProLong antifade reagent. Under the ultraviolet microscope, HDV Ag appears predominantly in the nucleus, although some of the antigen is occasionally detected in the cytoplasm. The nuclear distribution may vary among nucleolar, nucleoplasmic (excluding the nucleolus), or a combination of both. Some typical results are shown in **Fig. 2** (*see* **Note 4**).

4. Notes

1. The shelf-life of all antibodies can be extended considerably by mixing 50:50 with 100% glycerol and storing at –20°C.
2. Do not store trypsinized cultured cells at –20°C prior to boiling in a sample buffer because this will lead to partial degradation of HDV Ag. After boiling, samples can be stored at –20°C for more than 1 yr. However, repeated freeze–thaw cycles should be avoided. Always aliquot samples required for repeated assays.
3. If the HDV Ag signal from the Western blot is still weak after long exposure, rinse the membrane briefly in PBS containing 0.05% Tween-20 to remove the ECL+plus reagent and repeat **steps 6–8**. This step generally leads to about a 5–10-fold increase in the signal.
4. During the immunofluorescent staining procedure, it is imperative that the cells do not dry out; otherwise, very high background staining will be observed.

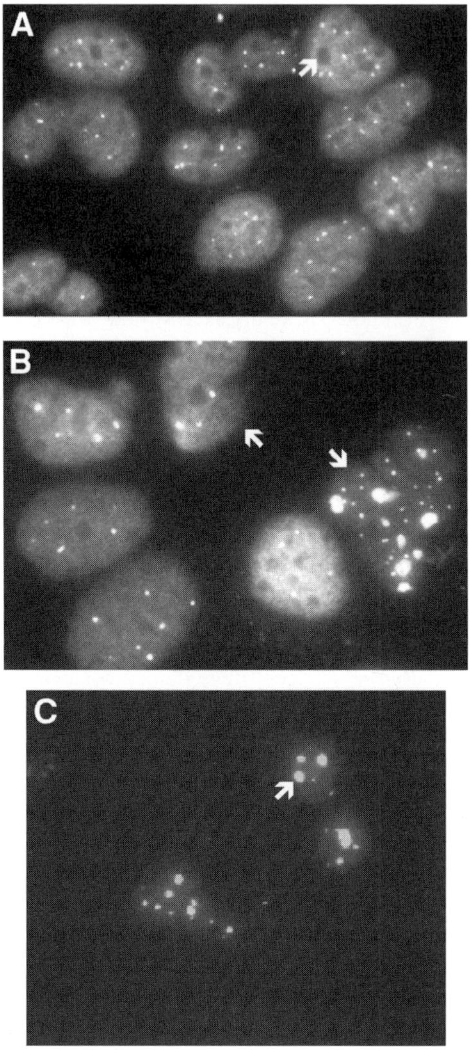

Fig.2. Immunofluorescence analysis for HDV Ag. HuH7 cells were transfected with either HDV-RNA (**Panels A** and **B**) or an expression plasmid for S-HDV Ag **(Panel C)** and stained for HDV Ag on d 4 post-transfection. The primary antibody was the same HDV Ag–specific monoclonal antibody mixture as used in **Fig. 1** but diluted 1:10. The secondary antibody was a 1:100 dilution of an FITC-conjugated goat anti-mouse antibody (Jackson ImmunoResearch Inc., cat no. 115-095-146). **(Panel A)** The typical nucleoplasmic HDV Ag distribution observed in cultured cells undergoing HDV-RNA replication. Note: the nucleolus (indicated by arrow) is usually negative. **(Panel B)** Here two different patterns of HDV Ag staining can be seen. Nucleolus negative and positive (left and right arrows, respectively). **(Panel C)** When the HDV Ag alone is expressed in the absence of HDV-RNA replication, the HDV Ag staining pattern is usually only nucleolar (indicated with arrow), excluding the nucleoplasm.

References

1. Rizzetto, M., Canese, M.G., Arico, S., et al. (1977) Immunofluorescence detection of a new antigen-antibody system (δ/anti-δ) associated to the hepatitis B virus in the liver and serum of HBsAg carriers. *Gut* **18**, 997–1003.
2. Rizzetto, M. (1983) The delta agent. *Hepatology* **3**, 729–737.
3. Macnaughton, T. B., Gowans, E. J., Jilbert, A. R., and Burrell, C. J. (1990). Hepatitis delta virus RNA, protein synthesis and associated cytotoxicity in a stably transfected cell line. *Virology* **177**, 692–698.
4. Macnaughton, T. B., Gowans, E. J., Reinboth, B., Jilbert, A. R., and. Burrell. C. J (1990) Stable expression of hepatitis delta virus antigen in a eukaryotic cell line. *J. Gen. Virol.* **71**, 1339–1345.
5. Bergmann, K. F. and Gerin, J. L. (1986) Antigens of hepatitis delta virus in the liver and serum of humans and animals. *J. Infect. Dis.* **154**, 702–706.
6. Luo, G., Chao, M., Hsieh, S.-Y. Sureau, C., Nishikura, K., and Taylor, J. (1990) A specific base transition occurs on replicating hepatitis delta virus RNA. *J. Virol.* **64**,1021–1027.
7. Chang, F.-L., Chen, P.-J., Tu, S.-J., Wang., C.-J., and Chen, D.-S. (1991) The large form of hepatitis delta antigen is crucial for the assembly of hepatitis delta virus. *Proc. Natl. Acad. Sci. USA* **88**, 8490–8494.
8. Hwang, S. B. and Lai, M. M. (1993) A unique conformation at the carboxyl terminus of the small hepatitis delta antigen revealed by a specific monoclonal antibody. *Virology* **193**, 924–931.

13

Immunohistochemical Detection of Hepatitis Delta Antigen

Karim Abid and Francesco Negro

1. Introduction

There is only one antigen specifically associated with the hepatitis delta virus (HDV) infection, i.e., the hepatitis delta antigen (HDAg) ***(1,2)***. HDAg is a phosphoprotein encoded by an open reading frame conserved among all HDV isolates. HDAg is a structural protein, because approx 200 subunits of HDAg bind via specific domains to genomic RNA, forming a core-like structure within an envelope provided by the co-infecting helper hepadnavirus ***(3)***. HDAg consists of two protein species of 24 kDa (195 amino acids) and 27 kDa (214 amino acids), referred to as small HDAg (S-HDAg) and large HDAg (L-HDAg), respectively. Those two proteins share the same primary structure, except for a unique 19-amino-acid sequence found at the C-terminus of L-HDAg, which possesses packaging activity. This additional sequence found in L-HDAg is synthesized via an RNA-editing process during HDV replication.

The stop codon UAG of the antigenomic RNA causes the translation of HDAg to terminate, thereby giving rise to S-HDAg. This stop codon is deaminated by cellular enzymes (ADAR1 and ADAR2) to UIC (where I stands for inosine) ***(4)***. Further base changes occur during the next replication cycle, resulting in the replacement of UAG by UGG, which directs the incorporation of tryptophan into the nascent HDAg. Translation of HDAg then proceeds until a new stop codon is reached, 19 amino acids downstream, thereby giving rise to L-HDAg. The S-HDAg and L-HDAg share many biochemical activities and functions, but they also play distinct roles, especially in replication and packaging. S-HDAg is required for genome replication, whereas L-HDAg is responsible for the packaging process. A complete discussion of all different functions of these two forms of HDAg is beyond the scope of this chapter.

Although antibodies specifically reacting with each of the two HDAg forms have been developed ***(5)***, most polyclonal antisera detect both of them. We report here the

From: *Methods in Molecular Medicine, vol. 95: Hepatitis B and D Protocols, volume 1*
Edited by: R. K. Hamatake and J. Y. N. Lau © Humana Press Inc., Totowa, NJ

procedure for detecting total HDAg in formalin-fixed, paraffin-embedded tissue sections using horseradish peroxidase (HRP)–conjugated anti-HD (*see* **Fig. 1**). HDAg can also be conveniently detected by immunofluorescence on frozen liver sections, fixed in various ways (*see* **Fig. 2**). However, we will focus on the former procedure. Because anti-HD antisera are difficult to obtain in the market, it is advised to purify total IgG from a HDV-infected patient and directly conjugate them to HRP. Protocols for conjugation of HRP to antibodies are available in most reference laboratory manuals ***(6)***.

The pattern of staining usually reported is nuclear. Some variations may occur, and their interpretation has been the object of debate. In vitro, the small form of HDAg seems exclusively nucleolar, whereas the large form seems to accumulate in the nucleoplasm ***(7)***. However, the pure nucleolar pattern is never seen in vivo, where, on the contrary, two patterns are most frequently reported: 1) an intense, nucleolar staining together with a weaker nucleoplasmic reactivity, and 2) a diffuse nucleoplasmic with negative nucleoli ***(8)***. Some doubts have been raised about the real nature of the intranuclear speckles containing HDAg: whether they are indeed nucleoli ***(9)*** or sites of accumulation of small HDAg involved in viral replication ***(10)*** remains an open issue. The genotype-specific detection of HDAg by immunohistochemistry is also possible ***(11)***, but its clinical relevance has not been universally recognized.

Although various other open reading frames are present on the genomic or the antigenomic strands of HDV, most of them are not found in all isolates and their products have not been detected in vivo, except indirectly, via detection of the corresponding antibodies in infected patients ***(12,13)***. The clinical and biological significance of these viral proteins has not been elucidated.

2. Materials

1. Poly-L-lysine-coated microscope slides.
2. Xylene and absolute ethanol and ethanol dilutions in water (Fluka Chemie AG, Buchs, Switzerland).
3. Phosphate-buffered saline (PBS): 137 m*M* NaCl, 2.7 m*M* KCl, 4.3 m*M* Na_2HPO_4, 1.4 m*M* KH_2PO_4, pH 7.3.
4. Proteinase K, DNase- and RNase-free (Merck, Darmstadt, Germany).
5. PBS/0.1 *M* glycine.
6. Quenching solution: 3% hydrogen peroxide (Fisher Scientific) in distilled water.
7. Primary antibody: To be prepared by conjugation with HRP ***(5)***.
8. Developing solution: Mix 250 µL of a 25 mg/mL solution (store at –20°C) of 3,3'-diaminobenzidine DAB (Fisher Scientific), 12.5 mL of 100 m*M* Tris-HCl, pH 7.6, and 125 µL of 3% hydrogen peroxide (to be prepared immediately before use).
9. Mayer's hematoxylin (Merck).
10. Mounting medium (Entellan™, Merck).

3. Method

1. Deparaffinize tissue sections in xylene for 10 min twice.
2. Rehydrate to PBS through a standard series of ethanols (absolute, 5 min twice, then 95% for 5 min and 70% for 5 min).
3. Digest in proteinase K, 0.15–0.5 mg/mL in PBS for 15 min at 37°C (*see* **Note 1**).

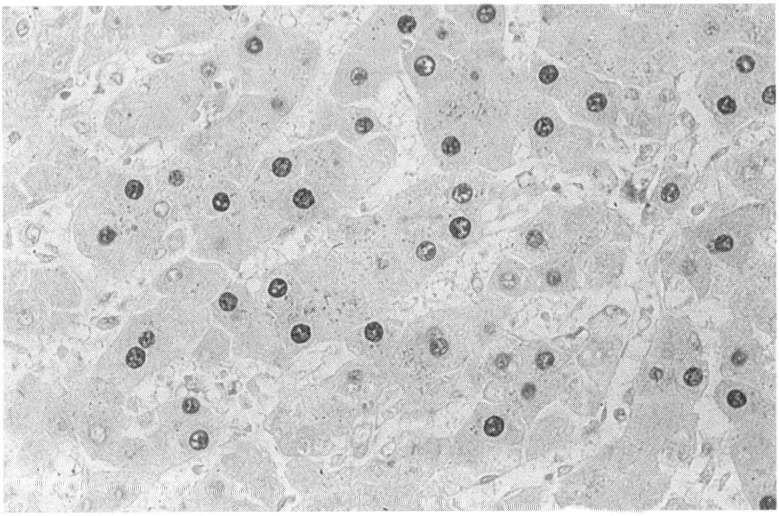

Fig. 1. Detection of HDAg in the nuclei of hepatocytes by immunohistochemistry using a HRP-labeled antiserum. Counterstaining with hematoxylin and eosin. Original magnification ×40.

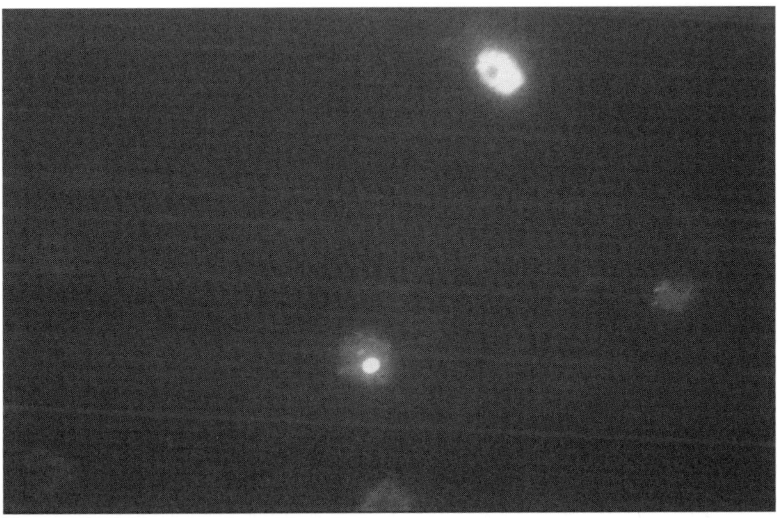

Fig. 2. Detection of HDAg in the nuclei of hepatocytes by direct immunofluorescence using fluorescein-labeled antiserum. Original magnification ×60.

4. Block digestion in ice-cold PBS, 0.1 *M* glycine, 5 min twice.
5. Wash in PBS for 5 min.
6. Block endogenous peroxides with the quenching solution for 5 min at room temperature.
7. Wash in PBS for 5 min.

8. Incubate with HRP-conjugated anti-HD IgG in PBS, 60 min at 37° C; the appropriate concentration will have to be optimized by titration.
9. Wash in PBS for 5 min twice.
10. Incubate in the developing solution by placing 50 μL on each section and covering with a cover slip; allow to develop for 2–5 min at room temperature (check under the microscope from time to time). Do not allow the sections to dry at any time.
11. Wash under running tap water for 10 min.
12. Counterstain for 1 min in Mayer's hematoxylin.
13. Rinse in running tap water for 30 s.
14. Dehydrate through a standard series of ethanols (70% for 5 min, 95% for 5 min, absolute for 5 min twice).
15. Pass in xylene (5 min twice) and mount in mounting medium (Entellan, Merck).

4. Notes

1. The proteinase K concentration used to pretreat sections cannot be predetermined because it depends on the amount of crosslinks formed during the formalin fixation. The longer the tissue has been kept in the fixative, the tighter the crosslinks will be, hence the higher the protease concentration needed to improve the accessibility of the antibody to its epitope. Excessive digestion may result in loss of morphological details as well as poor retention of small-tissue molecules during the various steps of the protocol.

References

1. Lazinski, D. W. and Taylor, J. M. (1994) Recent developments in hepatitis delta virus research. *Adv. Virus Res.* **43**, 187–231.
2. Lai, M. M. (1995) The molecular biology of hepatitis delta virus. *Annu. Rev. Biochem.* **64**, 259–286.
3. Gudima, S., Chang. J., Moraleda, G., Azvolinsky, A., and Taylor, J. (2002) Parameters of human hepatitis delta virus genome replication: the quantity, quality, and intracellular distribution of viral proteins and RNA. *J. Virol.* **76**, 3709–3719.
4. Polson, A. G., Bass, B. L., and Casey, J. L. (1996) RNA editing of hepatitis delta virus antigenome by dsRNA-adenosine deaminase. *Nature* **380**, 454–456.
5. Cullen, J. M., David, C., Wang, J. G., Becherer, P., and Lemon, S. M. (1995) Subcellular distribution of large and small hepatitis delta antigen in hepatocytes of hepatitis delta virus superinfected woodchucks. *Hepatology* **22**, 1090–1100.
6. Ausubel, F. M., Brent, R., Kingston, R. E., et al. (eds.) (1998) *Current Protocols in Molecular Biology.* John Wiley & Sons, New York.
7. Wu, J. C., Chen, C. L., Lee, S. D., Sheen, I. J., and Ting, L. P. (1992) Expression and localization of the small and large delta antigens during the replication cycle of hepatitis D virus. *Hepatology* **16**, 1120–1127.
8. Negro, F., Pacchioni, D., Bussolati, G., and Bonino, F. (1991) Hepatitis delta virus heterogeneity: a study by immunofluorescence. *J. Hepatol.* **13 (Suppl 4)**, S125–S129.
9. Lee, C. H., Chang, S. C., Chen, C. J., and Chang, M. F. (1998) The nucleolin binding activity of hepatitis delta antigen is associated with nucleolus targeting. *J. Biol. Chem.* **273**, 7650–7656.
10. Bichko, V. V. and Taylor, J. M. (1996) Redistribution of the delta antigens in cells replicating the genome of hepatitis delta virus. *J. Virol.* **70**, 8064–8070.

11. Hsu, S. C., Syu, W. J., Ting, L. T., and Wu, J. C. (2000) Immunohistochemical differentiation of hepatitis D virus genotypes. *Hepatology* **32**, 1111–1116.
12. Khudyakov, Y. E., Favorov, M. O., and Fields, H. A. (1993) A small open reading frame of the hepatitis delta virus antigenomic RNA encodes a protein that elicits antibodies in some infected patients. *Virus Res.* **27**, 13–24.
13. Bichko, V. V., Khudyakov, Y. E., and Taylor, J. M. (1996) A novel form of hepatitis delta antigen. *J. Virol.* **70**, 3248–3251.

II

Viral Genotypes and Variants

14

HBV Vaccine-Escape Variants

Ashraf A. Basuni and William F. Carman

1. Introduction

The classical method for typing and subtyping individual hepatitis B viruses (HBV) is serotyping. Although serotyping has generally been useful for determining antigenic distinctions among viruses, some limitations have been observed. For example, some viruses, such as measles and cytomegalovirus (CMV), do not have significant antigenic differences and cannot be divided into types and subtypes. In addition, serotyping does not usually have the ability to distinguish individual isolates within a serotype. Molecular methods can circumvent such limitations and allow comprehensive and precise characterization of individual viruses.

Viral genomes can have variable nucleotide sequences without influencing their essential characteristics at the protein and thus virion level. These nucleotide substitutions, which do not alter amino acids, are termed synonymous sites and have been used as the basis for genotype definition and classification of viruses. However, some regions of the viral genome are hypervariable, whereas others are stable and resistant to mutation. Therefore, in studies using less than the whole genome, one must choose a suitable region that has sufficient variability for analysis.

During the past 20 years, molecular applications that allow the study of this viral variability have been developed: polymerase chain reaction (PCR), nucleic acid probe technology, and restriction fragment length polymorphism (RFLP). PCR not only detects minute levels of virus but also allows detection of viruses that were previously difficult to culture or grow in animal models. In conjunction with direct sequencing, PCR is the ideal and definitive method for studying the genetic variability of viruses.

HBV is hepatotropic with a small, approx 3.2 kb in length, circular DNA that contains a single-stranded region of variable length in different molecules and replicates via an RNA intermediate *(1)*. Variation in HBV is greater than many other DNA viruses because of the use of a nonproofreading reverse transcriptase enzyme in the replication cycle. On the other hand, the overlapping protein-coding pattern of HBV puts a substantial constraint on its variability and leads to a lack of synonymous mutations in most

From: *Methods in Molecular Medicine, vol. 95: Hepatitis B and D Protocols, volume 1*
Edited by: R. K. Hamatake and J. Y. N. Lau © Humana Press Inc., Totowa, NJ

of the coding sequence. The rate of sequence change of HBV is therefore complicated and uncertain. Another factor compounding this difficulty is the type of predominating infection, perhaps a result of the differences in pathology and immune selection ***(2, 3)***.

HBV is estimated to undergo nucleotide substitution at a rate of $1.4–3.2 \times 10^{-5}$ per site per year ***(4)***. This rate is much closer to that of RNA viruses than to that of DNA viruses, which are relatively stable, with an estimated rate of nucleotide substitution of 10^{-9} per site per year. This relatively high rate of HBV mutation may contribute to its persistence by generating a pool of variants, some of which have altered, or inactive, viral epitopes and can escape immune surveillance. Mutations could lead to a diminished rate of replication, resulting in a low-titer immunologically negative HBV infection ***(5)***.

Two classes of HBV variants can be generally identified: class I variants, which occur naturally and have been selected over years, dependent on the genetic background of the host (e.g., subtype-defining determinants). In contrast, class II variants have been largely selected by human intervention. Vaccination, administration of immunoglobulin antibodies after liver transplantation, or during antiviral therapy all have been reported as inducing events ***(6–9)***.

Vaccine-escape mutants are the most highly covered variants in this particular literature. Viruses with mutations in the "a" determinant of hepatitis B surface antigen (HBsAg), the major B-cell epitope cluster in S protein (amino acids 124–147), have been found in several populations after launching vaccination ***(10–12)***. They probably have altered expression of HBsAg "a" determinant epitopes, which allows both infection in previously vaccinated individuals as well as a lack of detection by the conventional immunobased assays for HBV ***(13–15)***. Vaccine-escape viruses with mutations outside the "a" determinant have also been described in Japan ***(16)*** and Singapore ***(17)***. These variants express an altered binding affinity to antibodies ***(17)***. According to these results and previous observations, it has been suggested that this epitope could be extended up- and downstream to include the entire major hydrophilic region (MHR) (***18***; **Fig. 1**).

Identification of such mutations is of some importance because of the need to eliminate HBV, the hope that the use of alternate vaccines such as those with PreS may be more protective, and the requirement to develop novel assays with a better sensitivity for such variants. It may also be useful to characterize their functional activity and transmissibility.

The identification of these variants has been performed mainly by two molecular techniques: direct sequencing or RFLP analysis. Unlike PCR, RFLP is simple and less expensive and can detect variation across large genomic regions. RFLP was used earlier to relate HBV serotypes to certain restriction patterns ***(19)*** and recently for HBV genotyping ***(20,21)***. However, RFLP analysis detects only a small proportion of the total genetic variation. This fact probably limits its use in studying variation within a genotype or investigating and identifying transmission routes. In contrast, direct sequencing yields more complete information about variation at the sequenced site; however, its expense and technical requirements limit its application to small genomic regions (≤ 1000 bases).

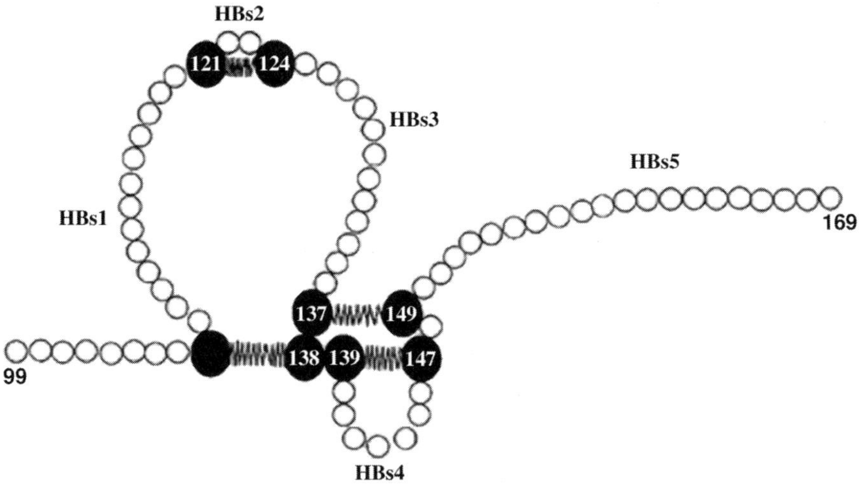

Fig. 1: Proposed model of major hydrophilic region (MHR). The five proposed antigenic regions are labeled HBsl through HBs5. Cysteine-to-cysteine disulfide bridges are also shown. (From ref. ***18***.)

Phylogenetically, HBV has been classified into seven genotypes, denoted A to G, often with a distinct geographic association ***(22–24)***. The molecular basis for the serological heterogeneity of HBsAg, which is encoded by the small surface (S) gene, has also been defined ***(25)***. HBV genotyping, based on limited sequencing within the S gene, is consistent with those based on sequencing of the full HBV genome ***(26)***. The validity of S gene sequencing analysis for HBV genotyping has been further confirmed in several studies ***(21, 27)***. Norder et al. ***(23)*** also devised a scheme that showed a substantial correlation between antigenic subtypes and genotypes, except for the heterogeneity of both *ayw1* and *adw2* subtypes. Extended studies in wider geographical contexts are likely to contribute to the finer mapping of both the regional strains and the relationship between genotypes and antigenic subtypes.

In recent years, powerful computerized tools for phylogenetic analysis of nucleotide and amino acid sequences have been produced, where the relationship between members of a given data set or evolutionary history of organisms and genes generated from sequence alignments can be presented in the form of "trees" or "networks." In a tree, each terminal node (branch end) represents a single sequence from the alignment, whereas internal nodes (where branches meet) represent hypothetical ancestral sequences. Based on a range of philosophical and mathematical approaches, a wide variety of tree-building techniques have been developed. Phylogenetic techniques either examine a sample of all possible tree topologies, looking for the best possible tree as defined by chosen criteria (searching methods; e.g., maximum parsimony [MP]), or they use an algorithm to generate a tree starting with a few members of the data set and adding the rest one at a time (clustering methods; e.g., neighbor joining [NJ]) ***(28)***.

On the other hand, networks have proven to be an effective way to represent ambiguity and try to explicitly place mutations on the branches of a tree. A network contains one or more cycles (a group of nodes for which it is possible to trace a path that starts and ends at the same node without visiting any other node more than once), whereas trees do not.

To date, two network models have been developed: reduced median (RM) and median joining (MJ). Briefly, RM networks display the principal character relationships present in the data and resolve likely parallel events while retaining character conflicts in the form of reticulations when ambiguity remains *(29)*. In MJ networks, larger sets of data can be analyzed and a faster speed can be achieved *(30)*. A network approach is particularly useful in studying intraspecific data, such as variation within human mitochondrial DNA (mtDNA) and virus genotypes, where alternative potential evolutionary paths can be displayed.

For detection and characterization of HBV S gene escape variants, several issues should be addressed. First, the sensitivity of the laboratory reagents and kits used for isolation of the virus should be determined. Second, the sensitivity and specificity of the PCR should be explored. Third, purification reagents that give the highest yield and the best quality of purified amplified PCR products should be chosen for optimal sequencing results. Finally, in addition to the database and geographically matched reference-virus sequences, a powerful computer with a good software package for phylogenetic analysis is essential for analyzing the acquired sequence data (**Fig. 2**).

2. Materials

2.1. Kits and Reagents

2.1.1. High Pure Viral Nucleic Acid Kit (Roche Diagnostics, Lewes, East Sussex, UK)

1. Binding buffer: 6 *M* guanidine HCl, 10 m*M* urea, 10 m*M* Tris-HCl, 20% Triton X-100 (v/v), pH 4.4.
2. Poly (A) carrier RNA: 0.2 mg/40 µL (after reconstitution).
3. Proteinase K: 20 mg/mL (after reconstitution).
4. Wash buffer: 20 m*M* NaCl, 2 m*M* Tris-HCl, pH 7.5.
5. Elution buffer: Nuclease-free redistilled H_2O.
6. High pure filter tubes: Polypropylene tubes have two layers of glass fiber fleece and can hold up to 700 µL of sample volume.
7. Collection tubes: 2 mL polypropylene tubes.

2.1.2. Reagents, Enzymes, and Buffers for PCR

1. 10X PCR buffer: 200 m*M* Tris-HCl, pH 8.4, 500 m*M* KCl.
2. 10X dNTPs: 100 m*M* of each dATP, dCTP, dGTP, dTTP.
3. TaqStart antibody, 1.1 µg/µL in storage buffer (50 m*M* KCl, 10 m*M* Tris-HCl, pH 7.0, 50% glycerol).
4. TaqStart dilution buffer: 50 m*M* KCl, 10 m*M* Tris-HCl, pH 7.0.
5. 10X TBE: 890 m*M* Tris, pH 8.0, 890 m*M* boric acid, 10 m*M* ethylenediaminetetraacetic acid (EDTA).
6. 10X agarose gel-loading buffer: 1X TBE, 1% sodium dodecyl sulfate (SDS), 50% sucrose, 1 mg/mL bromophenol blue.
7. *Taq* DNA polymerase, Roche Diagnostics, cat. no. 1956594.

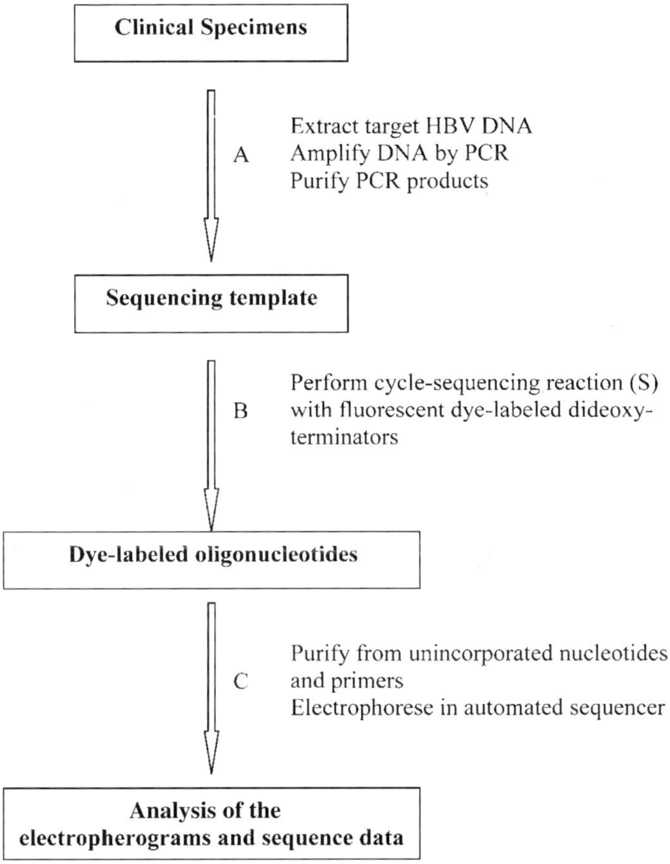

Fig. 2. Automated sequencing of PCR products. **(A)** The target HBV DNA is extracted and amplified, and the PCR products are purified from unincorporated nucleotides and primers. **(B)** The sequencing template is amplified in another PCR mixture containing the sequencing primer. Fluorescent dyes are coupled to dideoxynucleotides with a different color for each of the four bases and act as terminators of the growing oligonucleotides. The large array of oligonucleotides is then separated in a polyacrylamide gel, and the colors are detected as they pass a laser scan point. **(C)** The detection information is then fed into a computer for analysis and construction of the electropherogram, which is translated into linear sequences by commercially available software.

2.1.3. Geneclean Kit for DNA Purification (Bio 101; Vista, CA)

1. NaI, 125 mL of a 6 *M* sodium iodide solution.
2. TBE modifier, 15 mL of a proprietary mixture concentrated salts.
3. New concentrate: 14 mL of a concentrated solution of NaCl (prepared by adding to 280 mL distilled water and 310 mL ethanol).
4. GLASSMILK, 1.5 mL of specially prepared suspension of silica matrix.

2.2. Equipment

1. Water bath.
2. Vaccum centrifuge.
3. Ultraviolet transilluminator.
4. ThermalCycler (Perkin-Elmer Applied Biosystems, Cheshire, UK).
5. Automatic sequencer.

2.3. S Gene Primers

Name	Primer sequence (5' → 3')	Position	Type
S1	CCTGCTGGTGGCTCCAGTTC	56–75	Sense
S4*	GTATGTTGCCCGTTTGTCCTC	459–479	—
S6C	GCACACG †GAATTCCCGAGGACTGGGGACCCTG	129–146	—
S10*	TCCTATGGGAGTGGGCCTCAG	636–656	—
S2Na	CCACAATTCKTTGACATACTTTCCA (K=G/T)	1003–979	Antisense
S3*	AATGGCACTAGTAAACTGAGCC	690–669	—
S7D	GACACC ‡AAGCTTGGTTAGGGTTTAAATGTATACC	842–823	—
S8*	AGAAGATGAGGCATAGCAGC	434–415	—

* Primers used mainly for sequencing.
† *EcoR*1 restriction site (underlined).
‡ *Hind*III restriction site (underlined).
Nucleotide position numbering is according to Okamoto et al., 1988 ***(22)***.

3. Methods

3.1. HBV DNA Extraction

1. Two hundred microliters of working solution [binding buffer supplemented with poly(A) carrier RNA] and subsequently 40 μL of 20 mg/mL proteinase K are added to 200 μL sera in a sterile Eppendorf tube, mixed, and incubated for 10 min at 72°C (*see* **Note 1**).
2. After the incubation, 100 μL of isopropanol is added.
3. The filters and collection tubes are combined and the samples are pipetted into the upper reservoir followed by centrifugation for 1 min at 8000*g*. Discard the flowthrough.
4. The filter is washed twice with the wash buffer, and the flowthrough is discarded after each wash.
5. Finally, centrifuge for 10 s at full speed to remove all the residual wash buffer.
6. Collection tubes are discarded, and clean nuclease-free 1.5 mL tubes are used to collect the eluted DNA in 50 μL of elution buffer. To control for each experiment, HBV DNA positive standard at a reasonable titration [10–100 genomic equivalents/mL] and negative HBV sera should be extracted and amplified along with any specimens.

3.2. PCR

3.2.1. Preparation of Primers

The primers were designed with reference to alignments of the S gene of HBV and are provided in (**Subheading 2.3.**). Primers are high purity salt free (HPSF) grade and are synthesized by MWG-Biotech UK Ltd., Milton Keynes. Primers are diluted to 500 pmol/μL in sterile nuclease-free water, and aliquots are made and stored at −20°C. Primer concentrations are confirmed by measuring the optical density (OD) at 260 and 280 nm (where a 260/280 reading ratio should be around 1.8 to minimize any contamination). The PCR working dilutions are made up from these stock dilutions.

3.2.2. HBV DNA S Gene PCR

Hot start PCR is performed using a nested protocol and antibody to Taq polymerase to amplify the surface (S) gene of HBV.

1. Five microliters of extracted DNA (*see* **Note 2**) is amplified in 50 μL solution containing 1.25 U Taq polymerase, 2.5 U TaqStart antibody, 0.25 m*M* dNTPs, 2.5 m*M* $MgCl_2$, 10X PCR buffer, and 25 pmol of each primer (S1: sense 5'-CCTGCTGGTGGCTCCAGTTC-3' and S2Na: antisense 5'-CCACAATTCKTTGACATACTTTCCA-3'; where K=G or T).
2. Amplify for 5 cycles of 95°C for 1 min, 55°C for 1 min, and 72°C for 90 s followed by 35 cycles with the denaturation temperature reduced to 90°C.
3. One microliter of first-round PCR product is then reamplified in the same solution as above except for nested primers (S6C: sense and S7D: antisense, *see* **Subheading 2.3.**). Conditions used are 5 cycles of 95°C for 1 min, 55°C for 75 s, and 72°C for 90 s followed by 25 cycles with the denaturation temperature reduced to 90°C.

3.2.3. Agarose Gel Electrophoresis

Agarose gel electrophoresis is used to confirm the presence and correct size of amplified PCR products by visualizing the gel on an ultraviolet transilluminator.

1. Gels are prepared by adding 1 g agarose to 100 mL 1X TBE buffer.
2. The solution is boiled until dissolved and left to cool. Then, 50 μL ethidium bromide (1 mg/mL) is added before pouring the gel.
3. One microliter of agarose gel-loading buffer is added to each sample before loading, followed by running the gel at 80–90 V in 1X TBE buffer for 30 min.

3.3. DNA Sequencing and Phylogenetic Analysis

3.3.1. Purification of the PCR Product

1. After an adequate amount of the PCR product (20–30 μL) is run on the gel, DNA fragments of the expected size are located by visualizing the gel on an ultraviolet transilluminator.
2. The correct bands are excised and placed in 1.5-mL tubes with 4.5 vol of sodium iodide and 0.5 vol of TBE gel-modified buffer and incubated at 55°C for 10–15 min.
3. After complete melting of the gel, 5 μL of GLASSMILK is added to each tube.
4. The tubes are vortexed and incubated at room temperature for 10 min.
5. The tubes are spun for 30 s at 6000*g* in a bench-top microfuge, and the resulting pellet is washed twice with 0.5 mL ice cold NEW wash (containing 14 mL concentrate provided with the Geneclean kit, 280 mL distilled water, and 310 mL 100% ethanol).
6. The pellet is dried (*see* **Note 3**), and the DNA is eluted in 10 μL of dH_2O by incubation at 55°C for 5 min.
7. Finally, the supernatant is collected after spinning the suspension at 6000*g* rpm for 2 min (*see* **Note 4**).

3.3.2. Sequencing of the Amplified Products

1. After purification (*see* **Note 5**), sequencing of the S gene is performed directly from the purified PCR products according to the dideoxy method by means of a Taq Dye Deoxy Terminator cycle sequencing kit using an automated sequencer (ABI Prism, 377 DNA sequencer, Perkin Elmer, Applied Biosystem) according to the manufacturer's instructions.

2. The reaction mix is prepared by adding 4 μL of the terminator ready reaction mix to 1.6–3.2 pmol of the sequencing primer (*see* **Notes 6** and **7**) and 30–90 ng purified PCR product (*see* **Note 8**) in a total volume of 10 μL, the total volume to be adjusted by dH_2O.
3. Cycling program for 30 cycles of 96°C for 20 s, 50°C for 20 s, and 60°C for 4 min followed by holding at 4°C.
4. For each reaction, prepare a sterile well-labeled 1.5-mL microcentrifuge tube by adding 2 μL of 3 *M* sodium acetate, pH 4.6 (stop solution).
5. Transfer the sequencing reaction to the appropriately labeled tubes and then add 50 μL cold 95% ethanol.
6. Immediately centrifuge at 12,000*g* at 4°C for 15 min and carefully remove the supernatant with a micropipettor.
7. Rinse the pellet twice with 250 μL 70% cold ethanol; for each rinse, centrifuge immediately for a minimum of 2 min.
8. Remove all the supernatant after centrifugation and dry the pellet in a vacuum centrifuge.
9. Finally, resuspend the sample in a loading buffer (deionized formamide and 25 m*M* EDTA pH 8.0, containing 50 mg/mL blue dextran in a ratio of 5:1 formamide to EDTA/blue dextran) and transfer the resuspended samples to the appropriate wells.
10. The presence of different DNA populations in a sample, detected by the appearance of double bands in sequencing gel or double peaks in a sequencing chromatogram, can be confirmed by the following procedures: sequencing the complementary DNA strand (*see* **Note 9**) or the use of a second amplificate and/or another fresh sample. If two DNA populations are present in the sample, the number of base differences between DNA samples should be determined. The relative concentration of the DNA population can be roughly estimated by comparing the respective intensities of the double bands.

3.3.3. Molecular Analysis

1. The Sequence Navigator software program included in the ABI 373 software package (Applied Biosystem, Cheshire, UK) was used to edit and align the forward and reverse sequences to ensure reliability of the generated sequences and to resolve possible ambiguous nucleotides.
2. Sequences were then aligned, and a pairwise matrix of evolutionary distances of nucleotide sequences was generated using DNADIST (Kimura's two-parameters method), which is included in MacVector™ 7.0 package (Accelrys Ltd, Regent House Business Centre).
3. To confirm the reliability of the phylogenetic analysis, bootstrap resampling and reconstruction must be performed 1000, or at least 100, times. If more than 75% of trees constructed from the resampled data are essentially similar to the tree generated from the original set, the topology is considered stable.
4. The HBV genotype for each sequenced strain was then determined on the basis of this analysis, which showed co-clustering with reference genotype strains. Comparison with the published sequences in the European Molecular Biology Laboratory (EMBL), other international databases, and local regional sequences is essential to characterize and identify the genetic variability of isolated viral sequences (*see* **Note 10**).

4. Notes

1. Care must be taken during the incubation step to use proteinase K for digestion; otherwise, incomplete recovery of HBV DNA from some samples may occur.
2. To control for every PCR experiment, HBV DNA-positive and -negative sera should be included.

3. For complete removal of the residual washing buffer, sufficient air-drying is advisable.
4. Centrifuge the DNA solution and transfer it to a new reaction tube to remove any residual silica matrix before using for sequencing.
5. The gel-purification method is more precise as it allows identifying the right sized band visually; however, DNA purification directly from PCR products is easier and faster (High Pure PCR Product purification kit [Roche Diagnostics]).
6. PCR primer concentrations should be checked and confirmed by measuring the optical density (260/280 reading ratio) or by running various primer concentrations on the gel.
7. For maximum PCR sensitivity, test the determined primer concentration by performing PCR using different concentrations of the two primers in a chessboard format.
8. Optimal DNA quantity and high purity are essential for successful sequencing.
9. Sequencing on both strands is essential to resolve possible ambiguities during sequencing.
10. Choosing the correct reference sequence (with the same geographical region as the study samples) is mandatory, especially in cross-sectional studies, otherwise overestimation of mutations can occur.

References

1. Ganem, D. (1996) Hepadnaviridae and their viral replication. In: Fields B. N. (ed.) *Fields Virology*, Lippincott-Raven, Philadelphia, PA, 2703–2737.
2. Bozkaya, H., Akarca, U. S., Ayola, B., and Lok, A. S. (1997) High degree of conservation in the hepatitis B virus core gene during the immune tolerant phase in perinatally acquired chronic hepatitis B virus infection. *J. Hepatol.* **26**, 508–516.
3. Hannoun, C., Horal, P., and Lindh, M. (2000) Long-term mutation rates in the hepatitis B virus genome. *J. Gen. Virol.* **81**, 75–83.
4. Okamoto, H., Imai, M., Kametani, M., Nakamura, T., and Mayumi, M. (1987) Genomic heterogeneity of hepatitis B virus in a 54-year-old woman who contracted the infection through materno-fetal transmission. *Jpn. J. Exp. Med.* **57**, 231–236.
5. Preisler-Adams, S., Schlayer, H. J., Peters, T., Hettler, F., Gerok, W. and Rasenack, J. (1993) Sequence analysis of hepatitis B virus DNA in immunologically negative infection. *Arch. Virol.* **133**, 385–396.
6. Carman, W. F., Zanetti, A. R., Karayiannis, P., et al. (1990) Vaccine-induced escape mutant of hepatitis B virus. *Lancet* **336**, 325–329.
7. Hawkins, A. E., Gilson, R. J., Gilbert, N., et al. (1996) Hepatitis B virus surface mutations associated with infection after liver transplantation. *J. Hepatol.* **24**, 8–14.
8. Tipples, G. A., Ma, M. M., Fischer, K. P., Bain, V. G., Kneteman, N. M., and Tyrrell, D. L. (1996) Mutation in HBV RNA-dependent DNA polymerase confers resistance to lamivudine in vivo. *Hepatology* **24**, 714–717.
9. Protzer-Knolle, U., Naumann, U., Bartenschlager, R., et al. (1998) Hepatitis B virus with antigenically altered hepatitis B surface antigen is selected by high-dose hepatitis B immune globulin after liver transplantation. *Hepatology* **27**, 254–263.
10. Okamoto, H., Yano, K., Nozaki, Y., et al. (1992) Mutations within the S gene of hepatitis B virus transmitted from mothers to babies immunized with hepatitis B immune globulin and vaccine. *Pediatr. Res.* **32**, 264 to 268.
11. Oon, C. J., Lim, G. K., Ye, Z., et al. (1995) Molecular epidemiology of hepatitis B virus vaccine variants in Singapore. *Vaccine* **13**, 699–702.
12. Hsu, H. Y., Chang, M. H., Liaw, S. H., Ni, Y. H., and Chen, H. L. (1999) Changes of hepatitis B surface antigen variants in carrier children before and after universal vaccination in Taiwan. *Hepatology* **30**, 1312–1317.

13. Karthigesu, V. D., Allison, L. M., Fortuin, M., Mendy, M., Whittle, H. C. and Howard, C. R. (1994) A novel hepatitis B virus variant in the sera of immunized children. *J. Gen. Virol.* **75**, 443–448.
14. Carman, W. F., Van Deursen, F. J., Mimms, L. T., et al. (1997) The prevalence of surface antigen variants of hepatitis B virus in Papua New Guinea, South Africa, and Sardinia. *Hepatology* **26**, 1658–1666.
15. Coleman, P. F., Chen, Y. C., and Mushahwar, I. K. (1999) Immunoassay detection of hepatitis B surface antigen mutants. *J. Med. Virol.* **59**, 19–24.
16. Miyake, Y., Oda, T., Li, R., and Sugiyama, K. (1996) A comparison of amino acid sequences of hepatitis B virus S gene in 46 children presenting various clinical features for immunoprophylaxis. *Tohoku J. Exp. Med.* **180**, 233–247.
17. Oon C. J., Chen, W.N., Shiuan, K., and Lim, G. K. (1999) Identification of hepatitis B surface antigen variants with alterations outside the "a" determinant in immunized Singapore infants. *J. Infect. Dis.* **179**, 259–263.
18. Wallace, L.A., and Carman, W. F. (1997) Surface gene variation of HBV: scientific and medical relevance. *Viral Hepatitis Rev.* **3**, 5–16.
19. Shih, J. W., Cheung, L. C., Alter, H. J., Lee, L. M., and Gu, J. R. (1991) Strain analysis of hepatitis B virus on the basis of restriction endonuclease analysis of polymerase chain reaction products. *J. Clin. Microbiol.* **29**, 1640–1644.
20. Lindh, M., Andersson, A. S., and Gusdal, A. (1997) Genotypes, nt 1858 variants, and geographic origin of hepatitis B virus—large-scale analysis using a new genotyping method. *J. Infect. Dis.* **175**, 1285–1293.
21. Mizokami, M., Nakano, T., Orito, E., et al. (1999) Hepatitis B virus genotype assignment using restriction fragment length polymorphism patterns. *FEBS Lett.* **450**, 66–71.
22. Okamoto, H., Tsuda, F., Sakugawa, H., et al. (1988) Typing hepatitis B virus by homology in nucleotide sequence: comparison of surface antigen subtypes. *J. Gen. Virol.* **69**, 2575–2583.
23. Norder, H., Hammas, B., Lofdahl, S., Courouce, A. M., and Magnius, L. O. (1992) Comparison of the amino acid sequences of nine different serotypes of hepatitis B surface antigen and genomic classification of the corresponding hepatitis B virus strains. *J. Gen. Virol.* **73**, 1201–1208.
24. Stuyver, L., De Gendt, S., Van Geyt, C., et al. (2000) A new genotype of hepatitis B virus: complete genome and phylogenetic relatedness. *J. Gen. Virol.* **81**, 67–74.
25. Norder, H., Courouce, A. M., and Magnius, L. O. (1992) Molecular basis of hepatitis B virus serotype variations within the four major subtypes. *J. Gen. Virol.* **73**, 3141–3145.
26. Norder, H., Courouce, A. M., and Magnius, L. O. (1994) Complete genomes, phylogenetic relatedness, and structural proteins of six strains of the hepatitis B virus, four of which represent two new genotypes. *Virology* **198**, 489–503.
27. Arauz-Ruiz, P., Norder, H., Visona, K. A., and Magnius, L. O. (1997) Molecular epidemiology of hepatitis B virus in Central America reflected in the genetic variability of the small S gene. *J. Infect. Dis.* **176**, 851–858.
28. Page, R.D.M., and Holmes, E.C. (1998) Molecular Evolution A Phylogenetic Approach. Blackwell Science, London.
29. Bandelt, H. J., Forster, P., Sykes, B. C., and Richards, M. B. (1995) Mitochondrial portraits of human populations using median networks. *Genetics* **141**, 743–753.
30. Bandelt, H. J., Forster, P., and Rohl, A. (1999). Median-joining networks for inferring intraspecific phylogenies. *Mol. Biol. Evol.* **16**, 37–48.

15

HBV Genotyping and Analysis for Unique Mutations

Anna Ayres, Stephen Locarnini, and Angeline Bartholomeusz

1. Introduction

This chapter describes the methodology, analysis, and assessment of the significance of hepatitis B virus (HBV) mutations selected during antiviral therapy. Included in this description is the methodology for genotype classification. The major area of sequence-analysis methodology focuses on the reverse transcriptase region of the polymerase gene, in particular the catalytic domains A–E. This region coincides with the "a" determinant of the S gene in the overlapping reading frame. Other clinically significant HBV mutations, which are located in other genes and regulatory regions such as the basal core promoter and precore gene [(both of which are associated with loss or reduction in the production of hepatitis Be antigen (HBeAg)], may also be identified. Multiple mutations within a gene and the combination of mutations from other areas of the genome may act in a compensatory manner, altering the resistance pattern, replication phenotype, and pathogenesis profile of viral infection. Thus, the crosslinking of genomic data has potentially important implications for patient management.

There are currently seven major genotypes of HBV (A to G) that vary by greater than an 8% nucleotide divergence based on complete genomic sequence. Genotype identification can be determined by sequencing and phylogenetic analysis, by restriction fragment-length polymorphisms (RFLP), or by using different hybridization technologies ***(1–3)***. In this chapter, the genotype classification is performed by sequencing analysis. The HBV genotype may influence response to therapeutic agents, clinical outcome, and natural history ***(4,5)***. Differences in genomic length have caused problems in the nomenclature for different HBV mutants. These problems have been overcome by the development of new nomenclature that is independent of the HBV genotype ***(6)***.

Lamivudine is the first nucleoside analog approved for the treatment of HBV infection. The major limitation of lamivudine therapy is the emergence of viral mutants that are resistant to the drug. Antiviral resistance to lamivudine has been mapped to the YMDD motif in the reverse transcriptase domain of HBV polymerase. Based on the new nomenclature, the mutations in the reverse transcriptase (rt) most frequently selected during

From: *Methods in Molecular Medicine, vol. 95: Hepatitis B and D Protocols, volume 1*
Edited by: R. K. Hamatake and J. Y. N. Lau © Humana Press Inc., Totowa, NJ

Table 1
Accepted Domain-Specific Numbering System for HBV Polymerase, RT Domain

HBV	First Amino Acid RT Domain		Subdomain B LMV–Associated Mutation		Subdomain C LMV–Associated Mutation	
Genotype	Previously	Accepted	Previously	Accepted	Previously	Accepted
A	349	rt1	L528M	rtL180M	M552I/V	rtM204I/V
B/C/F	347	rt1	L526M	rtL180M	M550I/V	rtM204I/V
D	336	rt1	L515M	rtL180M	M539I/V	rtM204I/V
E/G	346	rt1	L525M	rtL180M	M549I/V	rtM204I/V

Modified from Stuyver et al. ***(6)***.

lamivudine therapy are designated rtM204I/V and rtL180M (**Table 1**). The process for the identification of these important mutations and/or other multiple mutations within the same gene or other genes that may act as compensatory mutations will be discussed.

2. Materials

2.1. Solutions

1. Sodium acetate (3 *M*) pH 5.2 (RMW = 82.03): Dissolve 24.6 g sodium acetate in 50 mL nuclease-free water. Stir until dissolved. Adjust pH to 5.2 with glacial acetic acid (>10 mL). Adjust volume to 100 mL with nuclease-free water. Sterilize by autoclaving. Store at room temperature (BDH, cat. no. 10236).
2. Nuclease-free water. Store at –20°C (Promega, cat. no. P1193).
3. Ethanol (analytical grade): Store at room temperature. Working concentration 70%, 95%. For 70%, add 7 mL of analytical grade ethanol to 3 mL of nuclease-free water. For 95%, add 9.5 mL of analytical grade ethanol to 0.5 mL of nuclease-free water (BDH).
4. Isopropanol (analytical grade): Store at ambient temperature (BDH).
5. Ethidium bromide: Dissolve a 10-mg tablet in 10 mL of water. Protect solution from exposure to light (Sigma, cat. no. 1239-45-8). *Potential teratogen, handle with extreme caution.*
6. Deoxynucleoside triphosphates (dNTP): Supplied at 100 m*M* each. Store at –20°C (Promega, cat. no. U1240). Stock solution, 20 m*M*: Add equal volumes of each of four dNTPS (100 m*M*) + equal volume of nuclease-free water.
7. DNA polymerase for polymerase chain reaction (PCR). *Thermus aquaticus* DNA polymerase; store at –20°C (Qiagen, cat. no. 201203).
8. ABI PRISM Dye Terminator Cycle Sequencing Ready Reaction Kit, version III (PE Applied Biosystems, cat. no. 402078).
9. 1-kb DNA ladder: For use as a marker in gel electrophoresis (MBI Fermentas, cat. no. SM0311). Store at –20°C.
10. Agarose: Analytical grade agarose (Promega, cat. no. V312A).
11. TE: 10 m*M* Tris-HCl, 1 m*M* ethylenediaminetetraacetic acid (EDTA) solution (pH 7.5).
12. TAE (gel-running buffer), 50X stock solution: Dissolve 242 g of Tris-base and 37.2 g EDTA into approx 700 mL of distilled water. Add 57.1 mL glacial acetic acid and make the solution up to 1 L using distilled water.

13. QIAamp DNA Mini Kit and QIA DNA Blood Mini Kit Handbook (Qiagen, cat. no. 51104 [50 X], cat. no. 51106 [250 X]).

2.2. Equipment

1. Micropipet tips (2–200 μL, Griener, cat. no. 739290, 200–1000 μL, Elkay, cat. no. 000-0000-025).
2. Sarstedt microtubes. These tubes come with screw caps and an O ring, which minimizes the amount of aerosols generated when opening specimens. Skirted Sarstedt microtubes, 1.5 mL, with cap (Disposable Products, cat. no. 72.692), unskirted Sarstedt microtubes, 1.5 mL, with cap (Bio-service, cat. no. EV-7161).
3. PCR Thermocycler tubes, 0.2-mL strip of eight tubes (Bio-service, tubes cat. no. EV-6361, caps, cat. no. EV-6411). For use with the PE2400 PCR machine.
4. 1.5-mL microfuge tubes (Elkay, cat. no. 000- MICRO-150).
5. Filtered pipet tips (Interpath, 2–20 μL, ART 20P cat. no. 2149, 40–200 μL; ART 200P, cat. no. 2069, 200–1000 μL; ART 1000, cat. no. 2079, 0.5–10 μL; ART 10F, cat. no. 2139F).
6. Perkin Elmer Gene Amp PCR Sysytem, PE2400.
7. Microcentrifuge.
8. Water bath/heat block.
9. Biological safety cabinet, class II.
10. Pipettors (*see* **Note 1**).

3 Methods

3.1. Extraction of HBV from Sera

All sera received are stored at –20°C as a minimum temperature, especially if the sample cannot be processed immediately. A temperature of –70°C is satisfactory for longer-term storage.

1. Safety: For safety of the user, all sera must be considered as potentially infectious. It is therefore advisable that all HBV DNA extractions from serum be performed in a laminar flow cabinet, Biosafety Level Class II.
2. Sample Contamination: The use of a laminar flow cabinet also greatly reduces the possibility of sample contamination. To minimize aerosols and contamination of gloves (thereby minimizing crosscontamination), vortex gently and centrifuge all solutions briefly before opening. Wherever possible, use screw-cap tubes rather than flip-top tubes. Filtered pipet tips should also be used to minimize contamination of pipets and therefore samples.

The QIAamp DNA MiniKit (Qiagen, CA) is used for the extraction of HBV DNA. The procedure is described by the manufacturer's specifications; however, the purified product is eluted in 50 μL instead of 200 μL. Other commercial kits are also suitable and will consistently provide the best source of material for further PCR and sequencing analysis.

3.2. PCR Amplification

3.2.1. HBV Oligonucleotide Primers for PCR Amplification and Sequencing of the HBV Genome

All primers for amplification and sequencing of the HBV genome are listed in **Table 2** and **Fig. 1**. All primers are purified by high-performance liquid chromatogra-

Table 2
HBV Primers[a]

Name	Position	Sequence (5' to 3')
204	204–223→	GTC GCA TGG AGA CCA CCG TGA
343	←343–364	ATC TCC TCC CCA ACT CCT CCC
344	344–361→	GGG AGG AGA TTA GGT TAA
540	←540–559	GGC AAA AAC GAG AGT AAC TC
1075	1075–1097→	AAG GTG GGA AAC TTT ACT GGG C
1408	1408–1430→	GCC TCA TTT TGT GGG TCA CCA TA
1437	←1437–1457	CAT GCT GTA GCT CTT GTT CC
1676	1676–1696→	TTG GGG TGG AGC CCT CAG GCT
1798	←1798–1819	CCA CTG CAT GGC CTG AGG ATG
2121	2121–2140→	TTG GCC AAA ATT CGC AGT C
2233	←2233–2255	GAA GAT GAG TAG CAG CAG G
2536	2536–2556→	CCC CAC TGT TTG GCT TTC AG
2628	2628–2648→	TTT TCT TTT GTC TTT GGG TAT
2798	←2798–2817	TCT CTG ACA TAC TTT CCA AT
3007	3007–3027→	GCT GAC GCA ACC CCA CTG G

[a]Numbering according to HPBADR1CG *(25)*.

phy (HPLC) to obtain more consistent results in both the PCR amplification and sequencing.

3.2.2. HBV–PCR Amplification Conditions for First- and Second-Round Amplification

PCR protocols have been optimized for the PE2400 PCR machine.

3.2.2.1. Controls

In every PCR run, several controls are included to monitor for contamination and to act as PCR reaction controls.

1. A HBV-negative serum control (antibody-negative donor) obtained from the Australian Red Cross Blood Service Victoria (ARCBS) is included in the extraction procedure. This agent acts as a control for sample crosscontamination during extractions.
2. A known second-round HBV PCR serum-positive control also obtained from the ARCBS is included for each PCR reaction This control monitors the sensitivity of each PCR amplification.
3. A reagent control that contains all reagents in the master mix is included, but nuclease-free water is used in place of the template DNA. This negative first-round PCR amplification is used as a template in the second round of amplification to determine whether (a) there is low-level contamination present and (b) there is PCR contamination during the second-round PCR amplification.

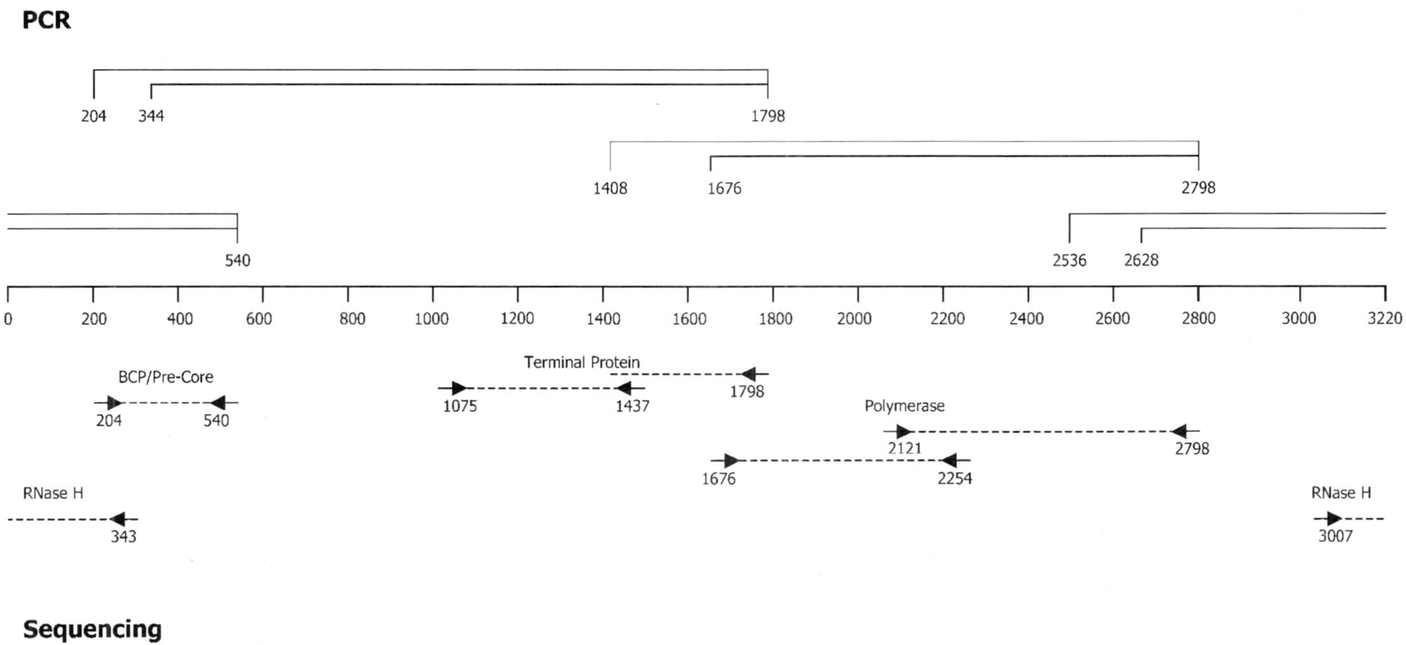

Fig. 1. Strategy for PCR amplification and sequencing of the HBV genome. The primers for first- and second-round PCR amplification and for sequencing the polymerase, S, and precore genes and the basal core promoter region are shown.

4. HBV DNA that has been cloned into a plasmid vector can be used as a template and acts as a positive PCR control.

3.2.2.2. PCR Protocol for the PE 2400 Series

DNA samples are taken through a first round of 40 cycles and then a subsequent second-round PCR of 25 cycles is performed if no product is produced in the first round. Use plugged pipet tips for all solution aliquoting. The PE2400 PCR machine uses strip tubes, so care must be taken when adding the different templates and removing the strip capping. As a rule, first-round products are removed from the strip tubes into 1.5-mL tubes because recapping the strip tubes could be a source of crosscontamination.

3.2.2.2.1. PCR Conditions for First-Round Amplification (PE2400)

1. For each amplification reaction, add the following components (*see* **Note 2**): 5.0 μL Template, 32.6 μL nuclease-free water, 5.0 μL 10X Qiagen amplification buffer, 6.0 μL 25 m*M* MgCl, 0.5 μL 20 m*M* dNTP, 0.3 μL 20 μ*M* Primer A, 0.3 μL 20 μ*M* Primer B, 0.3 μL DNA pol *Taq*.
2. First-round amplification is achieved by an initial cycle of denaturation at 94°C for 3 min, followed by 40 cycles of denaturation (94°C for 45 s), annealing (55°C for 45 s) and extension (72°C for 1.5 min). A final cycle of extension (72°C for 7 min) is employed for completion of the products.

3.2.2.2.2. PCR Conditions for Second-Round Amplification (PE2400)

1. For second-round PCR, add the following reagents for each amplification reaction (*see* **Note 2**): 2.0 μL Template, 35.6 μL nuclease-free water, 5.0 μL 10X Qiagen amplification buffer, 6.0 μL 25 m*M* MgCl, 0.5 μL 20 m*M* dNTP, 0.3 μL 20 m*M* Primer A, 0.3 μL 20 m*M* Primer B, 0.3 μL DNA pol *Taq*.
2. Second-round amplification is achieved by an initial cycle of denaturation at 94 °C for 3 min, followed by 25 cycles of denaturation (94°C for 45 s), annealing (55°C for 45 s), and extension (72°C for 1.5 min). A final cycle of extension (72°C for 7 min) is employed for completion of the products.

3.2.3. Analysis and Purification of PCR products

1. A 5-μL aliquot of each reaction is removed and analyzed on a 0.7% agarose gel.
2. The PCR products are purified using column purification kits. A number of these kits are available through several companies (e.g., Stratagene, Qiagen). We routinely use UltraClean columns (MO BIO) according to the manufacturer's specification.

3.3. DNA Sequencing

3.3.1. Sequencing Reactions

All automatic sequencing is carried out using the ABI Prism *Big Dye* Terminator Cycle Sequencing Ready Reaction Kit, Version III. The kit reagents include terminator ready reaction mix containing the following: A, C, G, T dye terminators, dNTPs, AmpliTaq DNA polymerase, thermally stable pyrophosphate, $MgCl_2$, Tris-HCl buffer, (pH 9.0), pGem-3Z double-stranded DNA control template, and 21M13 control primer (forward). The following sequencing reaction protocol has been optimized for the Perkin Elmer GeneAmp PCR Systems (PE-2400). Use 0.2-mL thin-walled PCR tubes.

1. Set up reactions as follows: 4.0 μL Terminator ready reaction mix, 30–90 ng template (purified PCR product), 1 μL primer (3 pmol), q.s. Deionized water, 15 μL total volume.
2. Spin briefly in microfuge for spin tubes.
3. Place tubes in thermal cycler PE2400 and set volume to 15 μL.
4. Sequencing is achieved by 25 cycles of denaturation (96°C for 10 s), annealing (50°C for 5 s), and extension (60°C for 4 min).

3.3.2. Purification of Extension Products Using Isopropanol Precipitation

1. For each sequencing reaction, label a 1.5-m*L* tube.
2. Add 6 μL 75% isopropanol and 1 μL 3 *M* sodium acetate to each reaction and incubate at room temperature for 15 min. Spin tubes at maximum speed for 20 min at room temperature.
3. Carefully remove the supernatant and discard.
4. Wash the pellet in 250 μL 75% isopropanol and spin again at maximum speed for 5 min.
5. Again, carefully remove the supernatant and discard.
6. Air-dry the pellet (do not over dry).

3.3.3. Electrophoresis of the Sequenced Products

Products can be separated by electrophoresis using one of a number of commercial automatic DNA sequencers. These protocols are designed for ABI Prism sequencers.

3.4. Analysis of Sequencing Data

1. The sequencing data are provided as a simple text document and as a chromatograph. The chromatograph provides the spectral analysis of dye/base relationships for each reaction. These sequence data should be saved and stored in a safe and secure environment.
2. For accuracy, sequencing is generated from each PCR product from both strands using at least two primers (reverse and forward). Any unspecified nucleotides, represented as N, in the chromatographs need to be resolved (if possible) by either examination of the peaks and peak heights or by comparing the sequencing results from the complementary strand. The two (or more) sequences generated from both strands can be used to form a consensus sequence, which is used in the final analysis.
3. In the analysis of patient samples undergoing antiviral therapy, it is not uncommon for sequencing to detect the presence of mixed viral populations with respect to important codons. An ambiguous nucleotide (N) in both strands at the same position indicates the presence of a mixed-virus population. The nucleotide is then given a code according to the IUPAC system. For example, where a mixture of an A and a T is detected, the IUPAC code assigned is W. The final consensus sequence is then imported into a DNA analysis program, such as Mac Vector (Oxford Scientific).
4. The integrity of the reading frame for each gene of interest should also be checked. Should the reading frame(s) be disrupted, the sequences used to generate the consensus must be rechecked against the chromatographs. For example, occasionally there are errors in the interpretation in the number of nucleotides when several of the same nucleotides occur in a row (GGGG may in fact be GGG, whereby the entire reading frame becomes disrupted from that point onward). Once this problem has been corrected, the consensus sequence is translated into the appropriate reading frame for analysis (e.g., hepatitis B surface antigen [HBsAg], polymerase).

3.4.1. Genotype Classification of HBV

The translated sequence for the specific gene(s) for each patient sample is compared with published reference sequence data. Norder et al. ***(3)*** have listed several representative HBV genotypes for comparison and deduced amino acid sequence data for the envelope genes and the precore/core genes. From these sequences, it is possible to determine the HBV genotype of each sample. Other genotype methods include PCR linked to RFLP *(1,7)*, PCR with specific primers *(2)*, commercial hybridization assay, and serological genotyping assay *(8,9)*.

3.4.2. Identification of Unique HBV Mutations

1. The HBV sequence from patient samples should be compared with the pretreatment sample in longitudinal samples.
2. In cross-sectional studies or studies where no additional samples are available, samples should be compared with a consensus sequence. Consensus sequences for the polymerase and HBsAg are shown in **Figs. 2** and **3.**
3. A number of programs are available to compare two or more sequences based on ClustalW. Either nucleotide or amino acid sequence can be compared using most sequence-comparison programs. However, the majority of mutations published are described relative to the deduced amino acid changes.
4. All mutations should be noted in both longitudinal and cross-sectional studies. However, the significance of the genotypic mutations can be made by comparison to either previously published in vitro phenotypic data or clinical data. In the next section, significant mutations that have been reported in the HBV genome are described.

3.4.3. Significant Mutations

3.4.3.1. Polymerase Mutations

The major polymerase mutations that have been reported to be selected during antiviral therapy with either lamivudine or famciclovir are presented in **Table 3.** Antiviral resistance to lamivudine has been mapped to the YMDD motif in the HBV polymerase gene. With the new nomenclature, the major mutations in the reverse transcriptase selected during lamivudine therapy are designated rtM204I/V and rtL180M **(Table 1)** *(6)*. The latter B-domain mutation is also selected during famciclovir treatment. To date, no polymerase mutations have been associated with adefovir or entecavir resistance. The conserved rt catalytic domains A–E coincide with the "a determinant" of the S gene in the overlapping reading frame. The changes to the S gene selected during antiviral therapy are also listed in **Table 3**.

3.4.3.2. Significant Mutations in the S Gene

Changes in the S gene that have been associated clinically with hepatitis B immune globulin (HBIG) breakthrough and vaccine failure are presented in **Table 4.** The major vaccine/HBIG escape mutant is within the "a" determinant located at codon sG145R *(10)*. The S gene encodes for a B-cell epitope at codons 124–148 and a T-cell epitope at codons 28–51 *(11)*. The majority of reported changes in the S gene are located in the "a" determinant. However, not all these changes are associated with vaccine/HBIG escape.

Mutations that have been tested in functional antigen–antibody binding studies to confirm this phenotype are listed in **Table 4**. Changes in the S gene may alter the overlapping polymerase gene *(12–14)*. Mutations selected in the S gene after nucleoside

75	76	77	78	79	80	81	82	83	84	85	86	87	88	89	90	91	92	93	94	95	96	97	98	99	100	101	102	103	104
421	422	423	424	425	426	427	428	429	430	431	432	433	434	435	436	437	438	439	440	441	442	443	444	445	446	447	448	449	450
								Domain A																					
S	N/D	L	S	W	L	S	L	D	V	S	A	A/G	F	Y	H	I/L	P	L	H	P	A	A/S	M	P	H	L	L	I/V	G
105	106	107	108	109	110	111	112	113	114	115	116	117	118	119	120	121	122	123	124	125	126	127	128	129	130	131	132	133	134
451	452	453	454	455	456	457	458	459	460	461	462	463	464	465	466	467	468	469	470	471	472	473	474	475	476	477	478	479	480
S	S/T/C	G	L/V	S/P/Q	R	Y	V	A	R	L/V	S	S/Y	N/T/D	S	R	N/I/Y	N/I/F/L/H/Y	N/D	N/H/Y	Q	H/Y/R	G/R	T/A	M/L	Q/P	N/D	L	H/R/N	D/N/S
135	136	137	138	139	140	141	142	143	144	145	146	147	148	149	150	151	152	153	154	155	156	157	158	159	160	161	162	163	164
481	482	483	484	485	486	487	488	489	490	491	492	493	494	495	496	497	498	499	500	501	502	503	504	505	506	507	508	509	510
																								Domain B					
S/Y	C	S	R	N/Q/H	L	Y/F	V/A	S	L	L/M	L	L	Y/F	K/Q	T/N	Y/F/L	G	W/R	K	L/V	H	L	Y	S	H	P	I	I/V	L/M
165	166	167	168	169	170	171	172	173	174	175	176	177	178	179	180	181	182	183	184	185	186	187	188	189	190	191	192	193	194
511	512	513	514	515	516	517	518	519	520	521	522	523	524	525	526	527	528	529	530	531	532	533	534	535	536	537	538	539	540
								Domain B																					
G	F	R	K	I	P	M	G/A	V/G/A	G	L	S	P	F	L	L	A	D	F	T	S	A	I/L	C	S/P/Q	V	V	R	R	A
195	196	197	198	199	200	201	202	203	204	205	206	207	208	209	210	211	212	213	214	215	216	217	218	219	220	221	222	223	224
541	542	543	544	545	546	547	548	549	550	551	552	553	554	555	556	557	558	559	560	561	562	563	564	565	566	567	568	569	570
								Domain C																					
F	P	H	C	L/V	A/G	F	S	Y	M	D	D	V/L/M	V	L	G	A	K/R	S/T	V	Q/H/R	H	L/R	E	S/A	L	Y/F	T/A	A/S	V/I
225	226	227	228	229	230	231	232	233	234	235	236	237	238	239	240	241	242	243	244	245	246	247	248	249	250	251	252	253	254
571	572	573	574	575	576	577	578	579	580	581	582	583	584	585	586	587	588	589	590	591	592	593	594	595	596	597	598	599	600
								Domain D																Domain E					
T	N/H	F	L	L	S	L/V	G	I	H	L	N	P/T	N/H/A/S/Q	K	T	K	R	W	G	Y	S/N	L	N/H	F	M	G	Y	V/I/R	I

Fig. 2. Consensus sequence of the deduced amino acid sequence for the HBV polymerase gene for the region spanning domains A–E. This consensus sequence encompasses all seven HBV genotypes.

1	2	3	4	5	6	7	8	9	10	11	12	13	14	15	16	17	18	19	20
M	E/D/G	N/S/K	I/T	T/A	S	G	F/L	L	G/R	P	L	L/R	V	L	Q	A	G/V	F/C	F
21	22	23	24	25	26	27	28	29	30	31	32	33	34	35	36	37	38	39	40
L/S/W	L	T	R/K	I	L/R	T/K	I	P	Q/K	S	L	D/H	S	W	W	T	S	L	N
41	42	43	44	45	46	47	48	49	50	51	52	53	54	55	56	57	58	59	60
F	L	G	G/E/A	S/A/V/T /L	P/T	V/R/T/K /G	C	L/P	G	Q/L/K	N	S/L	Q	S	P/Q	T/I	S	N/S	H
61	62	63	64	65	66	67	68	69	70	71	2	73	74	75	76	77	78	79	80
S/L	P	T/I	S/C	C	P	P	I/T	C	P/A	G	Y	R	W	M	C	L	R/Q	R	F
81	82	83	84	85	86	87	88	89	90	91	92	93	94	95	96	97	98	99	100
I	I	F	L	F/C	I	L	L	L	C	L	I	F	L	L	V	L	L	D	Y/C
101	102	103	104	105	106	107	108	109	110	111	112	113	114	115	116	117	118	119	120
Q	G	M	L	P/H/S	V	C	P	L	I/L	P	G/R	S/T	S/T	T	T	S	T/V/A	G/E/Q	P/S/A
121	122	123	124	125	126	127	128	129	130	131	132	133	134	135	136	137	138	139	140
C	K/R	T	C	T/M	T/I/S/A	P/T/A/I/ L	A/V	Q	G	N/T	S	M/K/L	F/Y/I	P	S/Y	C/S	C	C	T/I/S
141	142	143	144	145	146	147	148	149	150	151	152	153	154	155	156	157	158	159	160
K	P	T/S	D/A	G	N	C	T	C	I	P	I	P	S	S/T	W	A	F/L	A/G/V	K/R/T
161	162	163	164	165	166	167	168	169	170	171	172	173	174	175	176	177	178	179	180
Y/F	L	W	E	W/G	A/G	S	V/A	R	F/L	S	W	L	S/N	L	L	V/A	P/Q	F	V
181	182	183	184	185	186	187	188	189	190	191	192	193	194	195	196	197	198	199	200
Q	W/C/S	F/C	V/D/A	G/E	L	S/F	P	T/I	V	W	L/P	S/L	A/V	I	W	M/I	M/I	W	Y/F
201	202	203	204	205	206	207	208	209	210	211	212	213	214	215	216	217	218	219	220
W	G/E	P	S/N/K	L/Q	Y/F/H/D	S/G/N/D /T	I	V/L	S/N	P	F	I/M/L	P	L	L	P	I	F	F/C
221	22	223	224	225	226														
C/Y	L	W/R	V/A	Y/I/S	I														

Fig. 3. Consensus sequence of the deduced amino acid sequence for the HBV S gene. This consensus sequence encompasses all seven HBV genotypes.

analog therapy are listed in **Table 3**. There is the potential that some changes selected during antiviral therapy may alter the antigenicity of the S gene. The polymerase mutations at rtV173L plus rtL180M and rtM204V selected during lamivudine treatment result in changes to the S gene at codons sE164D and sI195M. In antigen–antibody binding studies, this S-gene mutant had reduced binding affinities compared with wild-type virus. Virus encoding these mutations may have the ability to behave as a vaccine/HBIG escape.

3.4.3.3. Mutations in the Basal Core Promoter and Precore Gene

The major mutations in the basal core promoter (BCP) and the precore gene are associated with a reduction ***(15,16)*** or loss in HBeAg synthesis ***(17)*** (**Table 5**). The major BCP mutations at nucleotides 1762 and 1764 have been detected in patients with fulminant hepatitis. However, they are also detected in patients with chronic hepatitis B. Buckwold et al. ***(18)*** have examined the effect of these mutations in the production of HBeAg in vitro. Patients with HBV encoding mutations within the BCP may still be HBeAg positive.

The A1764T, G1764A BCP mutations also cause changes in the overlapping reading frame of the X gene at codons 130 and 131.

The region that encodes the N terminus of the precore gene also encodes for the epsilon RNA, utilized both for the encapsidation signal and priming of DNA synthesis. The base pairing within the epsilon can affect the stability of the stem and loop, and a number of mutations may be selected to increase stability ***(17)***. The precore mutation G1896A results in a stop codon and therefore a loss of HBeAg expression. This nucleotide forms a base pair with nucleotide 1858, which in genotypes B, C, D, E, and G exists as a T. However, in genotypes A and F, nucleotide 1858 is a C, and the precore stop mutation at 1896 is not selected.

Three other nucleotide mutations (at positions 1817, 1874, and 1897) also cause truncation in HBeAg, and a number of changes that affect the initiation codon at 1814, 1815, and 1816 have been reported ***(19)***. HBeAg may still be detected in patients with HBV encoding the precore mutation as a result the presence of wild-type virus. During lamivudine treatment, there have been reports of phenotypic reversion of HBeAg status in patients with HBV encoding either the G1896A precore mutations or the BCP mutations at 1762/1764, because of the preferential selection of wild-type virus ***(20)***.

3.4.3.4. Compensatory Mutations

Multiple mutations within the same gene and/or in different genes should be examined for the effect on viral replication and/or antiviral sensitivity. Fulminant hepatitis B has been reported after nucleoside analog treatment alone, during combination with HBIG, and when no therapeutic selection pressure has been applied. In the case of the polymerase gene, the lamivudine resistance mutations were reported to be associated with a low replication yield phenotype relative to wild-type virus ***(21)***. Additional compensatory mutations may restore or enhance the replication yield phenotype and are associated with an increase in the HBV viral load and an exacerbation of disease. For

Table 3
Polymerase Mutations Selected During Antiviral Therapy of HBV

Antiviral Agent	Mutation[a]	Mutation Relative Genotype B,C,F[b]	Polymerase Domain	S Gene Changes	In Vitro Phenotypic Analysis	Comments	References
Lamivudine	L80V	L426V	A	No change	Not reported	Detected in association with M204I/V in HBV genotype C	***22***
Lamivudine	L80I	L426I	A	No change	Not reported	Detected in association with M204I/V in HBV genotype C	***22***
Lamivudine	L82M	L428M	A	No change	Not reported	Detected in association with M204I/V in HBV genotype C	***22,26***
Famciclovir	T128N	T474n	A-B Intermotif	P120T	Not reported	Possible compensatory mutation with M204I/V	***27***
Lamivudine	F166L	F512L	B	A157D	Drug sensitivity unknown Reduced replication	Detected with M204I	***28,29***
Lamivudine Famciclovir	V173L	V519L	B	E164D	No effect on 3TC-TP sensitivity (enzyme–based assay)	Detected with L180M M204V Associated with both lamivudine and	***26,30–32***

						famciclovir resistance	
Famciclovir	P177L	P523L	B	No change	2.4-fold reduction in PCV–TP sensitivity	Detected in association with V173L+L180M	***33***
Lamivudine	L179P	L525P	B	Not reported	Not reported	Transient minority species	***34***
Lamivudine Famciclovir	***L180M***	***L526M***	B	No change	3–18-fold reduction in 3TC sensitivity (cell–based assays) 2.6-fold reduction in 3TC-TP sensitivity (enzyme–based assay) Little effect on replication	Detected in association with M204V Associated with famciclovir breakthrough Possible compensatory mutation for M550V replication deficiency	***26,28, 30–32***
Lamivudine	A181T	A527T	B	Stop	Complete resistance to 3TC (cell–based assay) Reduced replication efficiency	Selected during prolonged 3TC therapy Associated with famciclovir breakthrough	***34***
Lamivudine	T184S	T530S	B/C Intermotif	L175F	2.2-fold reduction in 3TC-TP sensitivity (enzyme–based assay.		***26,30,32***

(continued)

Table 3 *(continued)*
Polymerase Mutations Selected During Antiviral Therapy of HBV

Antiviral Agent	Mutation[a]	Mutation Relative Genotype B,C,F[b]	Polymerase Domain	S Gene Changes	In Vitro Phenotypic Analysis	Comments	References
Lamivudine	A200V	A546V	B/C Intermotif	L192F	No effect on 3TC sensitivity (cell–based assay) No effect on replication efficiency	Possible compensatory mutation for M550I replication deficiency	***30,31,35***
Lamivudine	***M204I***	***M550I***	C	W196S, or W196L, or Stop	Complete resistance to 3TC (cell–based assays) Reduced replication efficiency	Mutation at YMDD locus	***26,28 30–32 36–38***
Lamivudine	***M204V***	***M550V***	C	I195M	Complete resistance to 3TC (with L526M mutation, cell–based assays) Reduced replication efficiency	Detected in association with L180M Mutation at YMDD locus	***26, 28, 30–32, 36–38***

Lamivudine Famciclovir	V207I	V553I	C	M198I +W199S	Associated with famciclovir resistance 6.2-fold reduction in PCV-TP (enzyme–based assay) No effect on replication efficiency	Possible compensatory mutation for M550I replication deficiency	***27,38,39***
Lamivudine	S213T	S559T	C/D Intermotif	No change	Not reported	—	***26,30,32***
Lamivudine Famciclovir	S219A	S565A	C/D Intermotif	S210R	Not reported	—	***35***
Lamivudine	I224S	I570S	C/D Intermotif	Not reported	Not reported	Minority species	***31***
Lamivudine	L229M	L575M	C/D Intermotif	F220L	Not reported	Detected with L180M + M204V	***40***
Famciclovir	N248T	N594T	E	After end of HBsAg	Not reported	Minority species	***41***
Adefovir	None detected	None detected	—	—	—	None detected	—

[a] Numbering of amino acid residues in the polymerase are relative to methionine in the YMDD motif as 204 ***(6)***.
[b] Numbering of amino acid residues in the polymerase are relative to methionine in the YMDD motif as 550 ***(42)***.

Table 4
Significant Changes in the S Gene

Changes in the S gene	Selection pressure	Comments	References
G145R*G145A+ G145K also detected	Vaccine/HBIG/naturally occurring	Reported in vaccinated children and their mothers as well as after HBIG treatment in the liver transplant setting. In vitro phenotype testing antigen/antibody binding studies were performed. In conjuction other multiple mutations associated with fulminant hepatitis	***10, 12, 14, 24, 43–47***
K141E	Vaccine/HBIG	Detected in vaccinated children in Gambia. In vitro phenotype testing antigen/antibody binding studies were performed	***48–50***
D144A D144G	Vaccine/naturally occurring	D144A—May not affect antigenicity D144G—In vitro phenotype testing antigen/antibody	***14, 43, 51, 52***

		binding studies were performed with reduced binding to polyclonal HBIG	
T131I	Vaccine/HBIG	In vitro phenotype testing antigen/antibody binding studies were performed	***50***
T114R	HBIG	—	***53***
T118A	HBIG	—	***53***
Insertion 1 or 2 AA at codons 122 or 124	Vaccine/naturally occurring	Associated with fulminant hepatitis	***12, 50, 54–56***
T123N	HBIG	—	***53***
T/I126S T/I126N	Vaccine/HBIG	In vitro phenotype testing antigen/antibody binding studies were performed	***53, 57***
P120T/E P120S	HBIG Naturally occurring	—	***14, 53, 58***
P142S	Vaccine/HBIG	—	***12, 53***
G130R	HBIG	—	***53***
N131S	HBIG	—	***53***

Table 5
Significant Mutations in the Basal Core Promoter and Precore Gene

Regulatory Region or Gene	Mutation	Deduced Amino Acid Change	Comments	References
BCP (1742–1805)	A1762T/G	—	Reduction in HBeAg antigen expression. HNF4 binding site altered Associated with fulminant hepatitis. In vitro HBeAg expression experiments performed	***15,16,18,59–62***
BCP	G1764A/T	—	Reduction in HBeAg antigen expression. HNF4 binding site altered Associated with fulminant hepatitis. In vitro HBeAg expression experiments performed.	***15,16***
BCP	T1753A/C		HNF4 binding site altered. Potential marker for advanced liver disease in association with G1613A and C1653T within enhancer II.	***63,64***
BCP	Deletions 5–21 bp	—	A number of deletions have been described, most commonly 8bp. The majority of deletions affect the second TA-rich region that can bind TATA-binding.	Reviewed in ***65***

			protein, resulting in a reduction in HBeAg expression	
BCP	Insertions	—	Creation of new HNF binding sites reported Associated with fulminant hepatitis	***66***
Precore	A1814T/C	M1L	Disruption of start codon, loss of HBeAg	***17***
Precore	T1815C/A/G	M1T/K/R	Disruption of start codon, loss of HBeAg	Reviewed in ***19***
Precore	G1816A/T	M1I	Disruption of start codon, loss of HBeAg	Reviewed in ***19***
Precore	C1817A	Q2Stop	Stop at codon 2 results in truncation and loss of HBsAg	Reviewed in ***19***
Precore	C1856T	P15S	Involved with base pairing with codon 1898	***17***
Precore	C1857T	P15L	Involved with base pairing with codon 1897	***17***
Precore	T1858C	No change	Involved with base pairing with codon 1896; C1858 already present in genotypes A and F as well as some strains of genotype C prevents selection of G1896C precore stop mutant	***17***
Precore	A1874T	K20Stop	Stop at codon 20 results in truncation and loss of HBsAg	Reviewed in ***19***

(continued)

Table 5 *(continued)*
Significant Mutations in the Basal Core Promoter and Precore Gene

Regulatory Region or Gene	Mutation	Deduced Amino Acid Change	Comments	References
Precore	G1896A	W28Stop	Stop at codon 28 results in truncation and loss of HBsAg	***17***
Precore	G1897A	W28Stop	Stop at codon 28 results in truncation and loss of HBsAg	***17***
Precore	G1898A	G29S	Involved with base pairing with codon 1856	***17***
Precore	G1899A	G29D	Involved with base pairing with codon 1855	***17***
Precore	Insertions	1838/39 1899/1900	Frame-shift mutation resulting in abrogation of HBeAg synthesis	Reviewed in ***19***
Precore	Deletions	1839	Frame-shift mutation resulting in abrogation of HBeAg synthesis	Reviewed in ***19***

example, the mutation rtL80V within the polymerase (domain A), in addition to the lamivudine resistance mutation at rtM204I, was detected in HBV isolated from a patient during a severe flare of hepatitis *(22)*. The patient's HBV-DNA levels were higher than pretreatment levels.

In another study, the vaccine-escape mutations that concomitantly encode changes in the polymerase gene at sP120T (and rtT128N) or sG145R (rtR/W143Q), in conjunction with the lamivudine-resistance mutations, replicated to a greater extent in the presence of lamivudine than in its absence *(23)*. Recently, Chen et al. (*67*) have shown that HBV mutants that encode both the precore mutation at G1896A and the lamivudine-resistance mutations had a replication fitness phenotype similar to that of the wild-type virus. Mutations detected within a gene or genes should be considered within the context of the entire genetic framework. Kalinina et al. *(24)* highlight the need for functional analysis to determine the significance of multiple mutations.

4. Notes

1. We strongly recommend the use of separate pipets and solutions for the extraction of HBV DNA from serum samples, the preparation of all reagents used in the PCR-amplification reactions (before the addition of a template), and the addition of a template into PCR reactions, especially for second-round amplification. (At least the set of pipets reserved for HBV DNA extraction could also be used for the addition of a template.)
2. Where possible, master mixes and reagents for master mixtures (e.g., dNTPs, buffers, and primers) for PCR reactions should be prepared in a designated clean area. In this way preparation of PCR reactions greatly reduces the risk of contamination from external sources.

References

1. Mizokami, M., Nakano, T., Orito, E., et al. (1999) Hepatitis B virus genotype assignment using restriction fragment length polymorphism patterns. *FEBS Lett,* **450**, 66–71.
2. Naito, H., Hayashi, S. and Abe, K. (2001) Rapid and specific genotyping system for hepatitis B virus corresponding to six major genotypes by PCR using type-specific primers. *J. Clin. Microbiol.* **39**, 362–364.
3. Norder, H., Courouce, A. M., and Magnius, L. O. (1994) Complete genomes, phylogenetic relatedness, and structûral proteins of six strains of the hepatitis B virus, four of which represent two new genotypes. *Virology* **198**, 489–503.
4. Kao, J. H., Wu, N. H., Chen, P. J., Lai, M. Y., and Chen, D. S. (2000) Hepatitis B genotypes and the response to interferon therapy. *J. Hepatol.* **33**, 998–1002.
5. Orito, E., Mizokami, M., Sakugawa, H., et al. (2001) A case-control study for clinical and molecular biological differences between hepatitis B viruses of genotypes B and C. Japan HBV Genotype Research Group. *Hepatology* **33**, 218–223.
6. Stuyver, L. J., Locarnini, S. A., Lok, A., et al. (2001) Nomenclature for antiviral-resistant human hepatitis B virus mutations in the polymerase region. *Hepatology* **33**, 751–77.
7. Lindh, M., Andersson, A. S., and Gusdal, A. (1997) Genotypes, nt 1858 variants, and geographic origin of hepatitis B virus—large-scale analysis using a new genotyping method. *J. Infect. Dis.* **175**, 1285–1293.
8. Usuda, S., Okamoto, H., Iwanari, H., et al. (1999) Serological detection of hepatitis B virus genotypes by ELISA with monoclonal antibodies to type-specific epitopes in the preS2-region product. *J. Virol. Methods* **80**, 97–112.

9. Usuda, S., Okamoto, H., Tanaka, T., et al. (2000) Differentiation of hepatitis B virus genotypes D and E by ELISA using monoclonal antibodies to epitopes on the preS2-region product. *J. Virol. Methods* **87**, 81–89.
10. Carman, W. F., Zanetti, A. R., Karayiannis, P., et al. (1990) Vaccine-induced escape mutant of hepatitis B virus. *Lancet* **336**, 325–329.
11. Tai, P. C., Banik, D., Lin, G. I., et al. (1997) Novel and frequent mutations of hepatitis B virus coincide with a major histocompatibility complex class I-restricted T-cell epitope of the surface antigen. *J. Virol.* **71**, 4852–4856.
12. Ghany, M. G., Ayola, B., Villamil, F. G., et al. (1998) Hepatitis B virus S mutants in liver transplant recipients who were reinfected despite hepatitis B immune globulin prophylaxis [see comments]. *Hepatology* **27**, 213–222.
13. Locarnini, S. (1998) Hepatitis B virus surface and polymerase gene variants: potential virological and clinical significance. *Hepatology* **27**, 294–297.
14. Protzer-Knolle, U., Naumann, U., Bartenschlager, R., et al. (1998) Hepatitis B virus with antigenically altered hepatitis B surface antigen is selected by high-dose hepatitis B immune globulin after liver transplantation. *Hepatology* **27**, 254–263.
15. Okamoto, H., Tsuda, F., Akahane, Y., et al. (1994) Hepatitis B virus with mutations in the core promoter for an e antigen-negative phenotype in carriers with antibody to e antigen. *J. Virol.* **68**, 8102–8110.
16. Sato, S., Suzuki, K., Akahane, Y., et al. (1995) Hepatitis B virus strains with mutations in the core promoter in patients with fulminant hepatitis. *Ann. Intern. Med.* **122**, 241–248.
17. Lok, A. S., Akarca, U., and Greene, S. (1994) Mutations in the pre-core region of hepatitis B virus serve to enhance the stability of the secondary structure of the pre-genome encapsidation signal. *Proc. Natl. Acad. Sci. U S A* **91**, 4077–4081.
18. Buckwold, V. E., Xu, Z., Chen, M., Yen, T. S., and Ou, J. H. (1996) Effects of a naturally occurring mutation in the hepatitis B virus basal core promoter on precore gene expression and viral replication. *J. Virol.* **70**, 5845–5851.
19. Gunther, S., Fischer, L., Pult, I., Sterneck, M., and Will, H. (1999) Naturally occurring variants of hepatitis B virus. *Adv. Virus Res.* **52**, 25–137.
20. Cho, S. W., Hahm, K. B., and Kim, J. H. (2000) Reversion from precore/core promoter mutants to wild-type hepatitis B virus during the course of lamivudine therapy. *Hepatology* **32**, 1163–1169.
21. Melegari, M., Scaglioni, P., and Wands, J. (1998) Hepatitis B virus mutants associated with 3TC and famciclovir administration are replication defective. *Hepatology* **27**, 628–633.
22. Ogata, N., Fujii, K., Takigawa, S., Nomoto, M., Ichida, T., and Asakura, H. (1999) Novel patterns of amino acid mutations in the hepatitis B virus polymerase in association with resistance to lamivudine therapy in japanese patients with chronic hepatitis B. *J. Med. Virol.* **59**, 270–276.
23. Bock, T., Torresi, J., Tillmann, H., Locarnini, S., Manns, M., and Trautwein, C. (1999) Replication and fitness of hepatitis B virus polymerase mutants after antiviral treatment following liver transplantation. *Hepatology* **30**, 79A.
24. Kalinina, T., Riu, A., Fischer, L., Will, H., and Sterneck, M. (2001) A dominant hepatitis B virus population defective in virus secretion because of several S-gene mutations from a patient with fulminant hepatitis. *Hepatology* **34,** 385–394.
25. Gan, R. B., Chu, M. J., Shen, L. P., Qian, S. W., and Li, Z. P. (1987) The complete nucleotide sequence of the cloned DNA of hepatitis B virus subtype adr in pADR-1. Sci. Sin. [B] **30**, 507–521.

26. Allen, M. I., Deslauriers, M., Andrews, C. W., et al. (1998) Identification and characterization of mutations in hepatitis B virus resistant to lamivudine. Lamivudine Clinical Investigation Group. *Hepatology* **27**, 1670–1677.
27. Tillmann, H. L., Trautwein, C., Bock, T., et al. (1999) Mutational analysis of hepatitis B virus on sequential therapy with famciclovir and lamivudine in patients with hepatitis B virus reinfection occurring under HBIg immunoglobulin after liver transplantation. *Hepatology* **30**, 244–256.
28. Ling, R., Mutimer, D., Ahmed, M., et al. (1996) Selection of mutations in the hepatitis B virus polymerase during therapy of transplant recipients with lamivudine. *Hepatology* **24**, 711–713.
29. Peters, M. G., Singer, G., Howard, T., et al. (1999) Fulminant hepatic failure resulting from lamivudine-resistant hepatitis B virus in a renal transplant recipient: durable response after orthotopic liver transplantation on adefovir dipivoxil and hepatitis B immune globulin. *Transplantation* **68**, 1912–1914.
30. Bartholomew, M., Jansen, R., Jeffers, L., et al. (1997) Hepatitis B virus resistance to lamivudine given for recurrent infection after orthotopic liver transplantation. *Lancet* **349**, 20–22
31. Chayama, K., Suzuki, Y., Kobayashi, M., et al. (1998) Emergence and takeover of YMDD motif mutant hepatitis B virus during long-term lamivudine therapy and re-takeover by wild type after cessation of therapy. *Hepatology* **27**, 1711–1716.
32. De Man, R., Bartholomeuz, A., Shaw, T., et al. (1997) The occurrence of sequential viral mutations in a liver transplant recipient reinfected with hepatitis B: primary famciclovir resistance followed by a lethal hepatitis hudring acquired lamivudine resistance. *Hepatol.* **26 (Suppl 1)**, 77.
33. Aye, T. T., Bartholomeusz, A., Shaw, T., et al. (1997) Hepatitis B virus polymerase mutations during antiviral therapy in a patient following liver transplantation. *J. Hepatol.* **26**, 1148–1153.
34. Yeh, C. T., Chien, R. N., Chu, C. M., and Liaw, Y. F. (2000) Clearance of the original hapatitis B virus YMDD-motif mutants wit emergence of distinct lamivudine-resistant mutants during prolonged lamivudine therapy. *Hepatology* **31**, 1318–1326.
35. Cane, P. A., Mutimer, D., Ratcliffe, D., et al. (1999) Analysis of hepatitis B virus quasispecies changes during emergence and reversion of lamivudine resistance in liver transplantation. *Antiviral Ther.* **4**, 7–14.
36. Honkoop, P., Niesters, H. G., de Man, R. A., Osterhaus, A. D., and Schalm, S. W. (1997) Lamivudine resistance in immunocompetent chronic hepatitis B. Incidence and patterns. *J. Hepatol.* **26**, 1393–1395.
37. Seta, T., Yokosuka, O., Imazeki, F., Tagawa, M., and Saisho, H. (2000) Emergence of YMDD motif mutants of hepatitis B virus during lamivudine treatment of immunocompetent type B hepatitis patients. *J. Med. Virol.* **60**, 8–16.
38. Tipples, A., Ma, M. M., Fischer, K. P., Bain, V. G., Kneteman, N. M., and Tyrrell, D. L. (1996) Mutation in HBV RNA-dependent DNA polymerase confers resistance to lamivudine in vivo. *Hepatology* **24**, 714–717.
39. Pichoud, C., Seigneres, B., Wang, Z., Trepo, C., and Zoulim, F. (1999) Transient selection of a hepatitis B virus polymerase gene mutant associated with a decreased replication capacity and famciclovir resistance. *Hepatology* **29**, 230–237.
40. Allen, M. I., Deslauriers, M., Andrews, C. W. et al. (1998) Identification and characterisation of mutations in hepatitis B virus resistant to lamivudine. Lamivudine Clinical Investigation Group. *Hepatology* **27**, 1670–1677.

41. Seigneres, B., Pichoud, C., Ahmed, S. S., Hantz, O., Trepo, C., and Zoulim, F. (2000) Evolution of hepatitis B virus polymerase gene sequence during famciclovir therapy for chronic hepatitis B [in process citation]. *J. Infect. Dis.* **181**, 1221–1233.
42. Bartholomeusz, A., Schinazi, R., and Locarnini, S. (1998) Significance of mutations in the hepatitis B virus polymerase selected by nucleoside analogues and implications for controlling chronic disease. *Viral Hepatitis Rev.* **4**, 167–187.
43. Cariani, E., Ravaggi, A., Tanzi, E., et al. (1995) Emergence of hepatitis B virus S gene mutant in a liver transplant recipient. *J. Med. Virol.* **47**, 410–415.
44. Carman, W. F., Trautwein, C., van Deursen, F. J., et al. (1996) Hepatitis B virus envelope variation after transplantation with and without hepatitis B immune globulin prophylaxis. *Hepatology* **24**, 489–493.
45. Fujii, H., Moriyama, K., Sakamoto, N., et al. (1992) Gly145 to ARG substitution in HBs antigen of immune escape mutant of hepatitis B virus. *Biochem. Biophys. Res. Commun.* **184**, 1152–1157.
46. Oon, C. J., Lim, G. K., Ye, Z., et al. (1995) Molecular epidemiology of hepatitis B virus vaccine variants in Singapore. *Vaccine* **13**, 699–702.
47. Waters, J. A., Kennedy, M., Voet, P., et al. (1992) Loss of the common "a" determinant of hepatitis B surface antigen by a vaccine-induced escape mutant. *J. Clin. Invest.* **90**, 2543--2547.
48. Howard, C. R. (1995) The structure of hepatitis B envelope and molecular variants of hepatitis B virus. *J. Viral. Hepat.* **2**, 165–170.
49. Karthigesu, V. D., Allison, L. M., Fortuin, M., Mendy, M., Whittle, H. C., and Howard, C. R. (1994) A novel hepatitis B virus variant in the sera of immunized children. *J. Gen. Virol.* **75**, 443–448.
50. Seddigh-Tonekaboni, S., Waters, J. A., Jeffers, S., et al. (2000) Effect of variation in the common "a" determinant on the antigenicity of hepatitis B surface antigen. *J. Med. Virol.* **60**, 113–121.
51. Chen, W. N., Oon, C. J., and Koh, S. (2000) Horizontal transmission of a hepatitis B virus surface antigen mutant [letter]. *J. Clin. Microbiol.* **38**, 938–939.
52. Lee, P. I., Chang, L. Y., Lee, C. Y., Huang, L. M., and Chang, M. H. (1997) Detection of hepatitis B surface gene mutation in carrier children with or without immunoprophylaxis at birth. *J. Infect. Dis.* **176**, 427–430.
53. Carman, W. F. (1997). The clinical significance of surface antigen variants of hepatitis B virus. *J. Viral. Hepat.* **4**, 11–20.
54. Carman, W. F., Korula, J., Wallace, L., MacPhee, R., Mimms, L., and Decker, R. (1995) Fulminant reactivation of hepatitis B due to envelope protein mutant that escaped detection by monoclonal HBsAg ELISA [see comments]. *Lancet* **345**, 1406–1407.
55. Hou, J., Karayiannis, P., Waters, J., Luo, K., Liang, C., and Thomas, H. C. (1995) A unique insertion in the S gene of surface antigen—negative hepatitis B virus Chinese carriers. *Hepatology* **21**, 273–278.
56. Yamamoto, K., Horikita, M., Tsuda, F., et al. (1994) Naturally occurring escape mutants of hepatitis B virus with various mutations in the S gene in carriers seropositive for antibody to hepatitis B surface antigen. *J. Virol.* **68**, 2671–2676.
57. Okamoto, H., Yano, K., Nozaki, Y., et al. (1992) Mutations within the S gene of hepatitis B virus transmitted from mothers to babies immunized with hepatitis B immune globulin and vaccine. *Pediatr. Res.* **32**, 264–268.
58. Tillmann, H. L., Trautwein, C., Bock, T., et al. (1999) Mutational pattern of hepatitis B virus on sequential therapy with famciclovir and lamivudine in patients with hepatitis B virus

reinfection occurring under HBIg immunoglobulin after liver transplantation. *Hepatology* **30**, 244–256.

59. Hasegawa, K., Huang, J., Rogers, S. A., Blum, H. E., and Liang, T. J. (1994) Enhanced replication of a hepatitis B virus mutant associated with an epidemic of fulminant hepatitis. *J. Virol.* **68**, 1651–1659.
60. Laskus, T., Rakela, J., Nowicki, M. J., and Persing, D. H. (1995) Hepatitis B virus core promoter sequence analysis in fulminant and chronic hepatitis B. *Gastroenterology* **109**, 1618–1623.
61. McMillan, J. S., Bowden, D. S., Angus, P. W., McCaughan, G. W., and Locarnini, S. A. (1996). Mutations in the hepatitis B virus precore/core gene promoter in patients with severe recurrent disease following liver transplantation. *Hepatology* **24**, 1371–1378.
62. Sterneck, M., Gunther, S., Santantonio, T., et al. (1996) Hepatitis B virus genomes of patients with fulminant hepatitis do not share a specific mutation. *Hepatology* **24**, 300–306.
63. Takahashi, K., Akahane, Y., Hino, K., Ohta, Y., and Mishiro, S. (1998) Hepatitis B virus genomic sequence in the circulation of hepatocellular carcinoma patients: comparative analysis of 40 full-length isolates. *Arch. Virol.* **143**, 2313–2326.
64. Takahashi, K., Ohta, Y., Kanai, K., et al. (1999) Clinical implications of mutations C-to-T1653 and T-to-C/A/G1753 of hepatitis B virus genotype C genome in chronic liver disease. *Arch. Virol.* **144**, 1299–1308.
65. Kramvis, A., and Kew, M. C. (1999) The core promoter of hepatitis B virus. *J. Viral. Hepat.* **6**, 415–427.
66. Pult, I., Chouard, T., Wieland, S., Klemenz, R., Yaniv, M., and Blum, H. E. (1997) A hepatitis B virus mutant with a new hepatocyte nuclear factor 1 binding site emerging in transplant-transmitted fulminant hepatitis B. *Hepatology* **25**, 1507–1515.
67. Chen RY, Edwards R, Shaw T, et al. (2003) Effect of the G1896A precore mutation on drug sensitivity and replication yield of lamivudine-resistant HBV in vitro. *Hepatology* **37**(1), 27–35.

16

A One-Filter–Three-Probe Assay for Defective Interference (DI) Effects of Naturally Occurring Core Internal Deletion (CID) Variants of Human Hepatitis B Virus

Chiaho Shih and Ta-Tung Thomas Yuan

1. Introduction

"Incomplete particles" were discovered during successive undiluted passages of the influenza viruses *(1)*. In general, these incomplete particles contain a less than full-length genome and are replication-defective. They can be rescued by, and interfere with, the replication of homologous helper viruses. Another important characteristic of incomplete particles is their ability to enrich their proportion in the total viral yield in cells infected with wild-type and incomplete viruses *(2–4)*. Based on these properties, Huang and Baltimore defined these biologically active incomplete particles as defective interfering (DI) particles and the replication-competent homologous helper viruses as standard viruses *(5)*.

DI particles are widespread among many DNA and RNA viruses in bacteria, plants, and animals. In tissue culture, DI viruses are capable of establishing persistent viral infections *(3)*. In animal models, some DI viruses have been shown to modulate the disease course by attenuating the virulence of standard viruses *(6,7)*. Co-infection with DI RNA of tomato bushy stunt virus (TBSV) can modify the disease course induced by the wild-type TBSV infection *(8)*. In humans, it has been proposed that DI particles might be responsible for the chronic recurrence of viral diseases. Perturbation of the balance between DI and standard viruses could trigger an episode of disease manifestation *(5)*.

Despite the extensive research of DI viruses, the molecular basis leading to a DI phenotype is often unclear. Most DI studies have demonstrated a correlation between a genomic deletion and the DI phenotype. There is no formal proof, beyond correlation, that a deletion is indeed the cause, entirely or in part, for the DI phenotype *(2)*. To date, most, if not all, DI particles were discovered in laboratory settings. Although human DI viruses have been found to occur during serial passages at high multiplicity of infection in tissue culture, it remains unclear whether or not DI particles also exist in natural infections *(2–4)*.

From: *Methods in Molecular Medicine, vol. 95: Hepatitis B and D Protocols, volume 1*
Edited by: R. K. Hamatake and J. Y. N. Lau © Humana Press Inc., Totowa, NJ

Hepatitis B virus (HBV) is one of the most common infectious agents in humans. Chronic active hepatitis B often leads to the development of cirrhosis and liver cancer ***(9,10)***. Although it is generally believed that liver damage caused by HBV infection is the result of immune-mediated injury ***(11,12)***, the molecular and cellular mechanisms of pathogenesis and chronicity of HBV infection remain to be elucidated. HBV core antigen (HBcAg or nucleocapsid protein) has been shown to be a major target of T-cell immunity ***(11–15)***.

Recently, a naturally occurring core antigen internal deletion (CID) was found to be geographically ubiquitous and highly prevalent in *chronic* HBV carriers ***(16–19)***. These deletions of CID mutants could be in-frame or out-of-frame ***(20)***, variable in size, and mapped to the central portion of HBcAg. Interestingly, CID mutants have never been found in patients with *acute* hepatitis ***(21,22)***. The significance of the correlation between HBV CID mutation and chronicity of infection, if any, is obscured by the fact that HBV variants in chronic carriers often contain a number of mutations, in addition to the CID mutation. Although the biological significance of CID mutations remains unclear, the deletions coincide with a potent and protective T-cell epitope ***(11,23–26)***, suggesting an immune escape nature of this mutation.

Previous approaches to identifying DI particles have mainly relied on the plaque assay in tissue culture or passage in animal models. At present, there is neither a plaque assay nor a reliable in vitro infection system for HBV ***(27)***. Another major difficulty in the conventional research of DI virus is in the complete separation of DI particles from the standard viruses. Although DI particles of vesicular stomatitis virus (VSV) can be separated from their standard viruses ***(28–30)***, this is more an exception than a rule for other viruses. In addition, the DI population could be rather heterogeneous in an individual animal in some viral systems ***(31)***. This finding also contributes to the variability of DI particles from preparation to preparation.

To circumvent these classic problems, we developed a new approach for the study of DI virus. Using a novel combination of methods, including gene cloning, co-transfection, and the "one-filter–three-probe" quantitative Southern assay **(Fig. 3)**, we demonstrated that the DI mutation most likely occurred in natural human infections ***(32,33)***.

1.1. HBV CID Mutants Are Replication Defective but Rescuable by Wild-Type Core Protein in trans

The functional definitions of a DI virus include its being replication defective, being rescuable by standard helper virus, and interfering with the production of standard virus and relative enrichment of DI particles. We have characterized two different CID mutants (DEL85 and DEL109) isolated from two different patients using two different hepatoma cell lines (Huh7 and HepG2) ***(32,33)***. To determine whether the CID mutants are capable of replication, either DEL85 or DEL109 alone was transfected into a human hepatoma cell line Huh7 (only DEL85 is exemplified here). DEL85 contains an internal deletion in the core gene from nucleotides 88 to 135 **(Fig. 1)**. Core particle-associated HBV DNA was then assayed for viral replication.

As demonstrated by Southern blot analysis **(Fig. 2A)**, DEL85 was replication-defective. The deficiency in its DNA synthesis is the result of the defect in RNA encap-

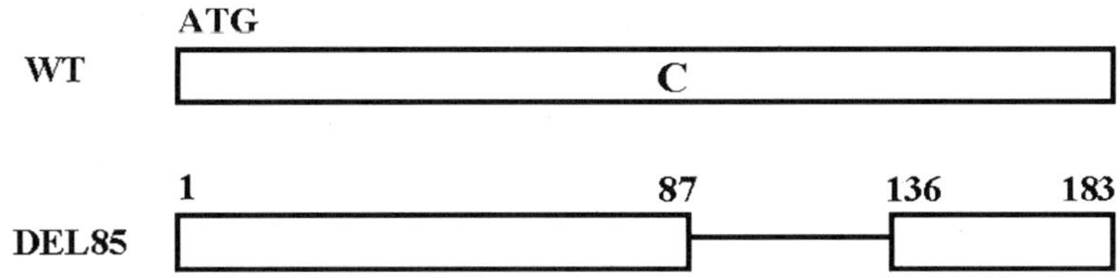

Fig. 1. This diagram illustrates the deletion regions of HBV core antigen of CID variant (DEL85) identified from a patient with hepatoma T85. This deletion region does not overlap with any other HBV genes, including X, P (polymerase), and preS/S (envelope). DEL85 deleted HBV core amino acids 88–135.

sidation, because no encapsidated pregenomic RNA from the CID mutant can be detected by primer extension analysis *(33)*. The fact that these replication-defective CID mutants can be detected by polymerase chain reaction (PCR) suggests that they may survive in the presence of other replicating HBV. We tested this possibility by co-transfecting CID mutants with a wild-type HBcAg expression vector (pSVC). The replication of DEL85 mutant was rescued to a level similar to that of the wild type **(Fig. 2B)**. These rescued CID mutants were also secreted into the medium *(33)*. The sedimentation profile of these rescued and secreted CID viral particles on gradient centrifugation appeared to be indistinguishable from that of the wild type in the Dane particle fraction *(33)*. The presence of the core gene deletions in the HBV CID genome in the secreted Dane particle fractions was confirmed by PCR amplification (data not shown).

1.2. Interference and Enrichment

In addition to the replication defect and rescuability **(Fig. 3)**, another major feature of DI particles is their characteristic behavior of interference and enrichment *(30)*. Since there is neither a plaque assay nor a reliable in vitro infection system for HBV, we used co-transfection and the "one-filter–three-probe" Southern assay **(Fig. 1)** to characterize the interference and enrichment effects of HBV CID mutants. As shown in **Fig. 3C** (top panel), Southern blot analysis using the full-length HBV DNA as a probe revealed that when increasing amounts of CID mutants were co-transfected with a fixed amount of wild-type HBV, the replication activity of the total HBV population did not change dramatically (approx 70–90% level of the signals compared with the wild type alone). Because the full-length HBV probe cannot differentiate between wild-type and CID mutants, the respective proportion of the CID mutant and wild-type viruses in the total viral yield is unclear. To measure the proportional yield of wild-type virus from this co-transfected culture, we stripped the full-length HBV probe from the filter (**Fig. 2C** [top panel]) and reprobed it with a wild-type–specific DNA fragment representing part of the deleted region of the HBcAg gene **(Fig. 3A)**, which should not hybridize with the CID mutant DNA.

Surprisingly, in contrast to the results shown in **Fig. 3C** (top panel), an equal amount of CID mutant DNA (DEL85) reduced the wild-type DNA replication by approximately

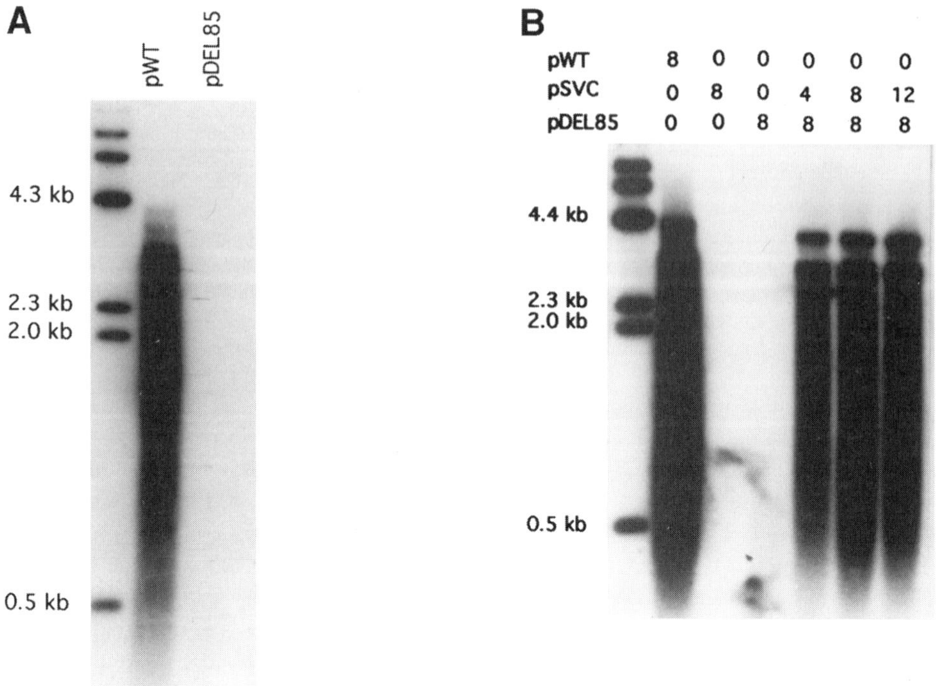

Fig. 2. **(A)** HBV CID variants are replication-defective upon transfection into the human hepatoma cell line, Huh7 cells. Five days after transfection with wild-type HBV (pWT) **(38)** or DEL85, viral DNAs of intracellular core particles were harvested and subjected to Southern blot analysis using the 3.1-kb full-length vector-free HBV DNA probe. No detectable replication of mutant DEL85 was observed. **(B)** The replication-defective CID mutants can be rescued by transcomplementation with wild-type HBV core. Various doses of a wild-type HBcAg expression vector (pSVC) were co-transfected with a constant amount of pDEL85. Viral DNAs of intracellular core particles were analyzed by Southern blot using the 3.1-kb full-length HBV probe.

sevenfold (**Fig. 3C**, middle panel). To demonstrate directly that the signals of HBV replication in the co-transfection experiment **(Fig. 3C**, top panel) were largely the result of the replication of CID mutants, we reprobed the same filter a third time with a probe specific for CID mutants **(Fig. 3B)**. The results were consistent with the prediction **(Fig. 3C**, bottom panel). Taken together, the results in **Fig. 3** suggest that the CID mutant can replicate at the expense of the wild-type HBV and become the predominant component of the viral progeny.

To determine whether the DI-like behavior of HBV CID mutants is idiosyncratic to the Huh7 cell line, we repeated the same experiment using another replication-permissive human hepatoblastoma cell line, HepG2. The DI effect of DEL85 appears to be even stronger in HepG2 (16-fold reduction in wild-type replication) than in Huh7 *(32)*. This DI-like phenomenon, including interference of wild-type and enrichment of

CID mutants, was also evident when extracellular HBV particles were examined using the full-length HBV probe and wild-type–specific probe *(32)*. The interference effect varied from 3- to 16-fold in a single cycle in vitro, depending on the specific DI virus, the host cell lines, the specificity of probes, and the relative dose of DI and helper viruses used in the assay. Theoretically, this effect could expand exponentially during sequential cycles of infection.

1.3. The Long-Sought DI Virus in Nature

DI viruses in previous studies were always generated by either brief or continuous passages in tissue culture, chicken eggs, or animal models under a laboratory setting *(3,4,31,34)*. Physically defective genomes of viruses have been found in clinical specimens. However, a direct *functional* proof that the same defective viruses are indeed "replication defective," "interfering," or able to "enrich" themselves has not been provided *(35,36)*. Structurally "defective" viruses do not necessarily "interfere" functionally, which is often assumed rather than proven to fulfill the standard definition of DI particles *(5)*. Indeed, the preS1 or preS2 envelope deletion variants of human hepatitis B virus is not defective interfering *(20)*. The demonstration here of the CID mutants of HBV in human chronic carriers is the first example of DI-like particles in the Hepadnaviridae family, which replicates the DNA genome through an RNA intermediate *(37)*. More important, to the best of our knowledge, this is the first report of DI particles found in natural infections *(3,4,31)*. This novel combination of gene cloning, co-transfection, and the "one-filter–three-probe" Southern assay should be useful for identifying DI-like particles in other viruses, which neither form plaque nor have an established in vitro infection system.

2. Materials

2.1. Solutions and Buffers

1. 1 *M* Tris-HCl, pH 7.5 and pH 7.4.
2. 5 *M* NaCl.
3. 0.5 *M* ethylenediaminetetraacetic acid (EDTA).
4. 10 mg/mL proteinase K.
5. 10% sodium dodecyl sulfate (SDS).
6. 70% and 100% ethanol.
7. Nonidet P-40.
8. 25% sucrose.
9. 1 *M* $CaCl_2$.
10. 1 *M* $MgCl_2$.
11. 26% polyethylene glycol (molecular weight 8000).
12. Phenol.
13. Chloroform.
14. α-^{32}P-dCTP. (deoxycytidine 5'-triphosphate; 3000 Ci/mmol).
15. dATP, TTP, dCTP, dGTP.
16. Sephadex G 50.
17. 20X standard saline citrate (SSC): 3 *M* NaCl and 0.3 *M* sodium citrate.
18. 50X Denhardt's solution: 1% (w/v) Ficoll 400, 1% (w/v) polyvinylpyrrolidone, and 1% (w/v) bovine serum albumin.

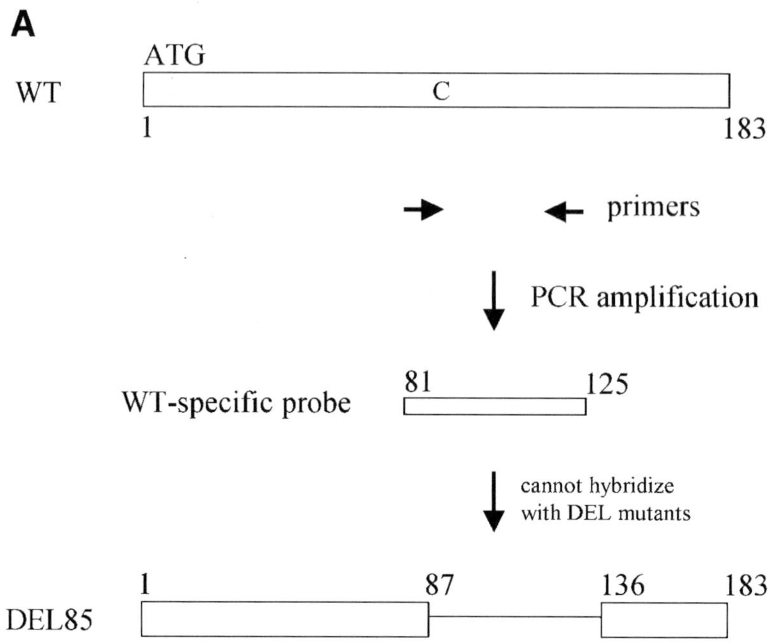

Fig.3. A defective–interfering phenomenon of HBV CID variants was observed in human hepatoma cell lines, Huh7 cells. **(A)** The wild-type–specific DNA fragment of 135 nt (from nt 2141 to 2275) was synthesized by PCR using pSV2ANeoHBV as the DNA template (**Subheading 3.4.2.**). The wild-type–specific probe can only hybridize with the wild-type virus but not with DEL85, which lacks the central core gene. **(B)** The DEL85-specific DNA probe is 181 nt in length (from nt 2041 to nt 2365 with a deletion of 144 nt) and synthesized by PCR using pDEL85 as a DNA template (**Subheading 3.4.3.**). The DEL85 probe can only anneal to the DEL85 DNA genome but not the wild-type virus at the hybridization temperature. **(C)** Seven micrograms of pWT were co-transfected with increasing amounts of pDEL85. HBV core particle–associated DNA was analyzed by Southern blot using the 3.1-kb full-length HBV fragment (top panel). Arrows indicate replicative intermediates of relaxed-circular (RC) and single-stranded (SS) DNAs. After the 3.1-kb full-length HBV probe was removed from the nitrocellulose filter used in the top panel, the same filter was reprobed with a radiolabeled wild-type–specific DNA fragment (middle panel). The relative intensity of replicative intermediates was measured by densitometer image analysis. After the wild-type–specific probe was removed, the nitrocellulose filter reused in the middle panel was reprobed with DEL85-specific fragments (bottom panel).

B

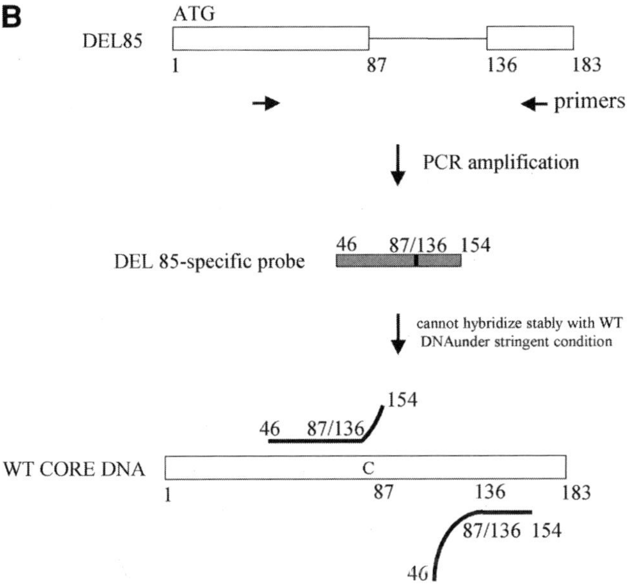

C

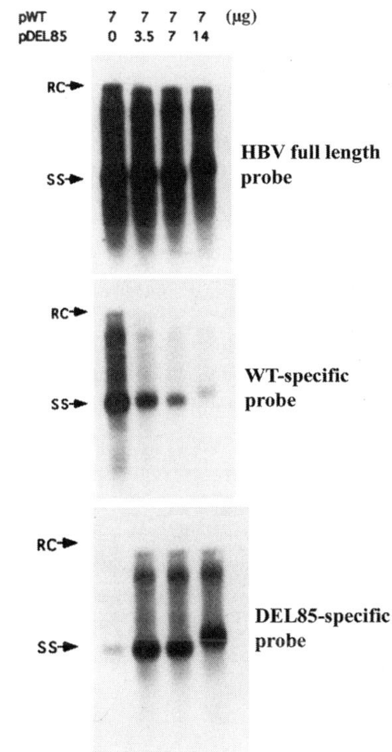

Fig. 3. *(continued)*

2.2. Cell Lines, Media, and Primary Tissues

The human hepatoma cell lines Huh7 and HepG2, which have been shown to be permissive for HBV replication, were used for DNA transfection. All cell lines were maintained in Dulbecco's modified Eagle's medium (DMEM) with 10% fetal bovine serum at 37°C in the presence of 5.5% CO_2. Primary hepatoma samples were obtained from the National Taiwan University Hospital *(17)*.

3. Methods

3.1. Plasmid Constructs (pDEL85)

1. To construct pDEL85, DNA fragments from nt 1636 to 2688 containing the HBV-deleted core gene were PCR amplified from total DNA of an HBV-replicating hepatoma T85 *(17)* and were used to replace both copies of the wild-type counterpart in the HBV tandem dimer plasmid *(38)*.
2. The two oligonucleotide primers used in PCR amplification for T85 follow. One primer is a 30-mer (5'-A AGG GCA AAT ATT TGG TAA GGT TAG GAT AG-3') containing HBV minus-strand DNA sequences from nt 2659 to 2688 with a *Ssp*I cleavage site (underlined). The other primer is a 27-mer (5'-AGA AAT ATT GCC CAA GGT CTT ACA TAA-3') containing HBV plus strand DNA sequences from nt 1636 to 1659 with a *Ssp*I cleavage site (underlined).
3. Use 1 μg of tumor DNA and 100 ng of each primer in a 10-μL PCR reaction, consisting of a denaturing step at 94°C (20 s) followed by a 40-cycle amplification at 94°C (1 s), 47°C (1 s), and 72°C (40 s).
4. Subclone the amplified target sequence (0.9 kb) into the pGEM-T vector (Promega Co.) and screen the recombinant by DNA sequencing.
5. Digest the DNA fragments containing CID mutations with *Ssp*I and gel purify the *Ssp*I fragment; use it to replace the normal counterpart of the wild-type HBV genome carried on a pUC12–HBV plasmid.
6. Ligate the 3.1-kb *EcoR*I fragment containing the CID mutation with the *EcoR*I cleaved pUC12–HBV CID monomer. The resulting tandem dimer plasmids, pDEL85, were then confirmed by restriction enzyme digestion and DNA sequencing.

3.2. Preparation of Intracellular Core Particles

1. Plasmid DNA was prepared by the polyethylene glycol (PEG) precipitation method without the use of a Qiagen column or CsCl gradient centrifugation. Briefly, the bacteria pellet from 100-mL bacteria culture was collected through centrifugation and resuspended in 6 mL solution I (50 m*M* glucose/25 m*M* Tris-HCl, pH 8.0/10 m*M* EDTA), followed by lysis on ice for 5 min using 12-mL solution II (0.2 *N* NaOH/1% SDS). The lysed bacteria solution was mixed with 6 mL solution III (3 *M* potassium acetate/11.5% glacial acetic acid) and vortexed briefly. The supernatant was collected after centrifugation for 15 min at 3,500 rpm in the Beckman SW41 rotor. DNA was precipitated by 0.6 volume of isopropanol at room temperature for 10 min. Following centrifugation, the DNA pellet was resuspended in 250 μL of TE. One hundred microliters of ammonium acetate (10 *M*) was added to the solution and incubated on ice for 10 min. The supernatant was collected after centrifugation and then precipitated by 2 vol of alcohol (100%). The DNA pellet was dissolved in 100 μL TE and incubated with 5 μL of RNase (2 mg/mL) for 1 h at 37°C. DNA was precipitated again by adding 50 μL PEG (30%)/NaCl (1.5 *M*) on ice for 30 min. After centrifugation, the DNA pellet was

resuspended in 100 μL of 10% proteinase K buffer and treated with 10 μL of proteinase K (10 mg/mL) at 50°C for 30 min. Finally, DNA was purified by phenol/chloroform extraction and ethanol precipitation.

2. Approximately 2×10^6 to 3×10^6 Huh7 cells were seeded in each 10-cm-diameter dish 12–16 h before the calcium phosphate transfection. In each transfection, 7 μg of wild-type HBV plasmid DNA was mixed with various amounts of DEL85 plasmid DNA, and the total amount of donor DNA was kept constant (35 μg of DNA per $2\text{–}3 \times 10^6$ cells per 10-cm dish per transfection). Carrier DNA of Huh7 origin was used to adjust the final amount of donor DNA to 35 μg total. Donor DNA was removed at approx 6 h posttransfection, and cells were fed with fresh DMEM containing 10% fetal bovine serum.
3. At 5 d posttransfection, lyse the cells from one 10-cm dish (6×10^6 cells) at 37°C (15 min) in 1 mL of buffer containing 10 m*M* Tris-HCl (pH 7.5), 1 m*M* EDTA, 50 m*M* NaCl, 0.25% Nonidet P-40, and 8% sucrose.
4. Spin the lysate in a microcentrifuge for 2 min, and transfer the supernatant to another tube.
5. Add 30 U of micrococcal nuclease and 1 U of DNase I to the supernatant (adjusted to 8 m*M* $CaCl_2$ and 6 m*M* $MgCl_2$), and incubate at 37°C for 15 min.
6. Precipitate the crude core particles by adding 330 μL of 26% PEG (molecular weight 8000) in 1.5 *M* NaCl and 60 m*M* EDTA.
7. After incubation for 1 h at 4°C, pellet the crude core particle by spinning in a microcentrifuge for 4 min.

3.3. Preparation of Core-Associated DNA

1. Resuspend the core pellet in 100 μL of buffer containing 10 m*M* Tris-HCl (pH 7.5), 8 m*M* $CaCl_2$, and 6 m*M* $MgCl_2$.
2. Add 30 U of micrococcal nuclease and 1 U of DNase I and incubate for 15 min at 37°C.
3. Lyse the core particles by adding 300 μL of lysis buffer containing 25 m*M* Tris-HCl (pH 7.5), 10 m*M* EDTA, and 1% SDS in the presence of proteinase K, at a final concentration of 400 μg/mL. Incubate at 50°C for 1 h.
4. Phenol/chloroform and then ethanol precipitate DNA.

3.4. DNA Probes for Southern Blot Analyses

3.4.1. Full-Length HBV Probe

1. Excise and purify the full-length 3.1-kb HBV DNA fragment from pSV2ANeoHBV by *Eco*RI digestion.
2. Label approx 25 ng of the 3.1-kb DNA fragment using a random primed DNA labeling kit (Boehringer Co.) and α-^{32}P-dCTP (3000 Ci/mmol).
3. Purify the labeled probe by passing through a Sephadex G 50 column.

3.4.2. Wild-Type–Specific DNA Probe

1. Synthesize the wild-type–specific DNA fragment of 135 nt (from nt 2141 to 2275) by PCR using pSV2ANeoHBV as the DNA template.
2. The oligonucleotides used to amplify the wild-type–specific fragment are both 21-mers (5'-TCT AGA GAC CTA GTA GTC AGT-3' and 5'-CCA CAC TCC GAA AGA CAC CAA-3').
3. Label the wild-type–specific DNA fragment with α-^{32}P-dCTP by PCR in a reaction mixture containing 1 ng DNA template, 200 μ*M* dATP, TTP, and dGTP, 10 μ*M* dCTP, 150 μCi ^{32}P-dCTP (3000 Ci/mmol, 2 μ*M*), 100 ng of each primer, 2.5 U *Taq* polymerase, 4 m*M* $MgCl_2$, and 10X PCR buffer (200 m*M* Tris-HCl, pH 8.3, 500 m*M* KCl).

4. The PCR procedure consisted of a denaturing step at 94°C (20 s) followed by a 40-cycle amplification step at 94°C (1 s), 55°C (1 s), and 72°C (40 s) (*see* **Note 1**).

3.4.3. DEL85-Specific DNA Probe

1. Synthesize the DEL85-specific DNA probe of 181 nt in length (from nt 2041 to nt 2365 with a deletion of 144 nt) by PCR using pDEL85 as a DNA template.
2. The oligonucleotides used to amplify the DEL85-specific DNA fragment follow: 5'-GGA CCT GCC TCG TCG TCT AAC AAC AGT AGT-3' and 5'-CAT TGT TCA CCT CAC CAT ACA-3'.
3. The PCR conditions used to synthesize α-^{32}P-labeled probe were the same as described above (**Subheading 3.4.2.**) (*see* **Note 1**).

3.5. Hybridization Procedure with DNA Probes (*see* Notes 2 and 3)

1. The standard Southern blot procedure was performed following the manufacturer's recommendation (Schleicher & Schuell). Briefly, DNA agarose gels were denatured by soaking in 3 *M* NaCl/0.5 *N* NaOH for 30 min, followed by neutralization with 0.5 *M* Tris-HCl (pH 7.0) 1.5 *M* NaCl for 30 min. Denatured single-stranded DNAs were transferred to nitrocellulose membranes (Schleicher & Schuell) by capillary transfer overnight in 10X SSC (made from the 20X stock solution). Agarose debris on nitrocellulose membrane was removed by washing in 2X SSC for 5–10 min. The nucleic acids on the membrane were immobilized by baking at 80°C for 2 h.
2. The baked nitrocellulose membrane was prehybridized at 42°C for at least 1 h in the plastic bag of hybridization buffer, containing 6X SSC, 5X Denhardt's solution (made from 50X stock solution), 100 μg/mL salmon sperm DNA, 50% (v/v) formamide, and 1% SDS.
3. The boiled radiolabeled probe was added to the plastic bag at a concentration of approx 5–20 ng/mL or $1–5 \times 10^6$ cpm/mL. Plastic bags were resealed after removing most of the air bubbles.
4. Hybridization was at 42°C for 16 h.
5. The blotted nitrocellulose membrane was washed twice with 2X SSC/0.1% SDS at room temperature for 5 min each time. Membranes were further washed twice for 15 min each with 0.1X SSC/1% SDS at room temperature. Finally, the membranes were washed twice for 30 min each time with 0.1X SSC/1% SDS at 65°C.
6. To reuse the membrane filter, old probes can be removed by heating the membrane in a boiling solution of 0.1X SSC/0.5% SDS. The solution was removed from the heat source and the membranes incubated for another 15 min. The removal of probes can be monitored using a Geiger counter. The same procedure can be repeated until the background level of radioactivity is not detectable (*see* **Note 4**).

4. Notes

1. Because we synthesized the wild-type–specific and DEL85-specific probes by using PCR to incorporate α-^{32}P-dCTP, extra precautionary measures should be exercised for the use of highly radioactive materials in the PCR machine. It is also important to examine the specificity of the synthesized probes. The control experimental set should always include transfections of pWT and pSVC + pDEL85. The wild-type–specific probe should only detect the replicative wild-type virus but not the rescued DEL85 genome. The DEL85-specific probe should only detect the rescued DEL85 genome but not the wild-type virus.
2. When the "one-filter–three-probe" Southern assay was first developed, we applied three probes sequentially to the filter in the order of HBV full-length, wild-type–specific, and DEL85-specific probes. We later realized that the background noise can be reduced if the full-length probe is used as the last probe.

3. In addition to the "one-filter–three-probe" quantitative Southern assay, one can measure the relative abundance between wild-type HBV and CID variants in serum or liver samples via quantitative PCR assay, as detailed elsewhere *(32)*.
4. The degree of interference and enrichment depends on a number of parameters, including the virus strains, host cell lines, and the relative proportion between the standard virus and the DI virus. Different CID deletions could have a different effect on defective interference. Of note, the same CID deletion as DEL85 has been found in a British patient *(39)*, a patient from Hong Kong *(40)*, and a Korean patient *(32)*.

References

1. von Magnus, P. (1947) Studies on interference in experimental influenza. I. biological observations. *Ark. Kemi. Mineral. Geol.* **24,** 1.
2. Dimmock, N.J. (1996) Antiviral activity of defective interfering influenza virus in vivo. In: Myint, S., and Taylor-Robinson, D. (eds.), *Viral and Other Infections of the Human Respiratory Tract*, pp. 421–445.
3. Holland J.J. (1987) Defective interfering rhabdoviruses. In: Wagner, R. (ed), *The Rhabdoviruses,* Plenum Publishing, New York, p. 297.
4. Roux, L., Simon, A. E., and Holland J. J. (1991) Effects of defective interfering viruses on viral replication and pathogenesis in vitro and in vivo. *Adv. Virus Res.* **40,** 181–211.
5. Huang, A. S., and Baltimore, D. (1970) Defective viral particles and viral disease processes. *Nature* **226,** 325–327.
6. Doyle, M., and Holland, J. J. (1973) Prophylaxis and immunization in mice by use of virus-free defective T particles to protect against intracerebral infection by vesicular stomatitis virus. *Proc. Natl. Acad. Sci. USA* **70,** 2105–2108.
7. Spandidos, D. A., and Graham, A. F. (1976) Generation of defective virus after infection of newborn rats with reovirus. *J. Virol.* **20,** 234–247.
8. Hillman, B. I., Carrington, J. C., and Morris, T. J. (1987) A defective interfering RNA that contains a mosaic of a plant virus genome. *Cell* **51,** 427–433.
9. Shih, C., Tai, P-C, Whitehead, W., Hosono, S., Lee, C.-S. and Yang, C.-S. (1996) Hepatitis B and C viruses and liver cancer. In: Bertino, J.R. (eds), *Encyclopedia of Cancer.* Academic Press, New York, pp. 824–834.
10. Tiollais, P., Pourcel, C., and Dejean, A. (1985) The hepatitis B virus. *Nature* 317, 489–495.
11. Chisari, F. V., and C. Ferrari. (1995) Hepatitis B virus immunopathogenesis. *Annu. Rev. Immunol.* **13,** 29–60.
12. Milich, D. R. (1991) Immune response to hepatitis B virus proteins: relevance of the murine model. *Semin. Liver Dis.* **11,** 93–112.
13. Ferrari, C., Bertoletti, A., Pena, A., et al. (1991) Identification of immunodominant T cell epitopes of the hepatitis B virus nucleocapsid antigen. *J. Clin. Invest.* **88,** 214–222.
14. Mondelli, M., Vergani, G. M., Alberti, A., et al. (1982) Specificity of T lymphocyte cytotoxicity to autologous hepatocytes in chronic hepatitis B virus infection: evidence that T cells are directed against HBV core antigen expressed on hepatocytes. *J. of Immunol.* **129,** 2773–2778.
15. Tsai, S. L., Chen, P. J., Lai, M. Y., et al. (1992) Acute exacerbations of chronic type B hepatitis are accompanied by increased T cell responses to hepatitis B core and e antigens. *J. Clin. Invest.* **89,** 87–96.
16. Ackrill, A. M., Naoumov, N. V., Eddleston, A. L. W. F., and Williams, R. (1993) Specific deletions in the hepatitis B virus core open reading frame in patients with chronic active hepatitis B. *J. Med. Virol.* **41,** 165–169.

17. Hosono, S., Tai, P.-C., Wang, W., et al. (1995) Core antigen mutations of human hepatitis B virus in hepatomas accumulate in MHC class II-restricted T cell epitopes. *Virology* **212,** 151–162.
18. Okamoto, H., Tsuda, F., and Mayumi, M. (1987) Defective mutants of hepatitis B virus in the circulation of symptom-free carriers. *Jpn. J. Exp. Med.* **57,** 217–221.
19. Wakita, T., Kakumu, S., Shibata, M., et al. (1991) Detection of pre-C and core region mutants of hepatitis B virus in chronic hepatitis B virus carriers. *J. Clin. Invest.* **88,** 1793–1801.
20. Sahu, G. K., Tai P. C., Banerjee S., et al. (2002) Out-of-frame vs. in-frame core internal deletion (CID) variants of human and woodchuck hepatitis B viruses. *Virology* **292**, 35–43.
21. Aye, T. T., Uchida, T., Becker, S. O., et al. (1994) Variations of hepatitis B virus precore/core gene sequence in acute and fulminant hepatitis B. *Dig. Dis. Sci.* **39,** 1281–1287.
22. Ehata, T., Omata, M., Chuang, W-L., et al. (1993) Mutations in core nucleotide sequence of hepatitis B virus correlate with fulminant and severe hepatitis. *J. Clin. Invest.* **91,** 1206–1213.
23. Jung, M. C., Diepolder, H. M., Spengler, U., et al. (1995) Activation of a heterologous hepatitis B (HB) core and e antigen-specific CD4+ T-cell population during seroconversion to anti-HBe and anti-HBs in hepatitis B virus infection. *J. Virol.* **69,** 3358–3368.
24. Menne, S., Maschke, J., Tolle, T. K., Lu, M., and Roggendorf, M. (1997) Characterization of T cell response to woodchuck hepatitis core protein and protection of woodchucks from infection by immunization with peptides containing a T cell epitope. *J. Virol.* **71,** 65–74.
25. Milich, D. R., McLachlan, A., Moriarty, A., and Thornton, G. B. (1987) Immune response to hepatitis B virus core antigen (HBcAg): localization of T cell recognition sites within HBcAg/HBeAg. *J. Immunol.* **139,** 1223–1231.
26. Tsai, S. L., Chen, M. H., Yeh, C. T., et al. (1996) Purification and characterization of a naturally processed hepatitis B virus peptide recognized by CD8+ cytotoxic T lymphocytes. *J. Clin. Invest.* **97,** 577–584.
27. Gripon, P., Diot, C., and Guguen-Guillouzo, C. (1993) Reproducible high level infection of cultured adult human hepatocytes by hepatitis B virus: effect of polyethylene glycol on adsorption and penetration. *Virology* **192,** 534–540.
28. Crick, J., Cartwright, B., and Brown, F. (1966) Interfering components of vesicular stomatitis virus. *Nature* **211,** 1204–1205.
29. Hackett, A. J., Schaffer, F. L., and Madin, S. H. (1967) The separation of infectious and autointerfering particles in vesicular stomatitis virus preparations. *Virology* **31,** 114–119.
30. Huang, A. S., Greenwalt, J. W., and Wagner, R. R. (1966) Defective T particles of vesicular stomatitis virus. I. preparation, morphology, and some biologic properties. *Virology* **30,** 161–172.
31. Barrett, A. D. T. and Dimmock, N. J. (1986) Defective interfering viruses and infections of animals. *Curr. Top. Microbiol. Immunol.* **128,** 55–84.
32. Yuan, T.-T., Lin, M. H., Chen, D. S., and Shih, C. (1998) A defective interference-like phenomenon of human hepatitis B virus in chronic carriers. *J. Virol.* **72,** 578–584.
33. Yuan, T.-T., Lin, M. H., Qiu, S. M., and Shih, C. (1998) Functional characterization of naturally-occurring variants of human hepatitis B virus containing the core internal deletion mutation. *J. Virol.* **72,** 2168–2176.
34. Bean, W. J., Kawaoka, Y., Wood, J. M., Pearson, J. E., and Webster, R. G. (1985) Characterization of virulent and avirulent A/chicken/Pennsylvania/83 influenza A viruses: potential role of defective interfering RNAs in nature. *J. Virol.* **54,** 151–160.
35. Pedley, S., Hundley, F., Chrystie, I., McCrae, M. A., and Desselberger, U. (1984) The genomes of rotaviruses isolated from chronically infected immunodeficient children. *J. Gen. Virol.* **65,** 1141–1150.

36. Siegl, G., Nuesch, J. P. F., and Chastonay, J. de. (1990) Defective interfering particles of hepatitis A virus in cell cultures and clinical specimens. In: Brinton, M. A. and Heinz, F. X. (ed.), *New Aspects of Positive-Strand RNA Viruses*. American Society of Microbiology, Washington DC, pp. 102–107.
37. Summers, J. and Mason, W. S. (1982) Replication of the genome of a hepatitis B-like virus by reverse transcription of an RNA intermediate. *Cell* **29,** 403–415.
38. Shih, C., Li, L. S., Roychoudhury, S., and Ho, M. H. (1989) In vitro propagation of human hepatitis B virus in a rat hepatoma cell line. *Proc. Natl. Acad. Sci. USA* **86,** 6223–6327.
39. Marinos, G., Torre, F., Gunther, S., et al. (1996) Hepatitis B virus variants with core gene deletions in the evolution of chronic hepatitis B infection. *Gastroenterology* **111**, 183–192.
40. Akarca, U. S. and Lok, A. S. F. (1995) Naturally occurring core-gene-defective hepatitis B viruses. *J. Gen. Virol.* **76**, 1821–1826.

17

Detection of Hypermodified Middle-Envelope (M) Proteins Secreted from Naturally Occurring HBV Variants Containing a preS2 Internal Deletion

Chiaho Shih and Pei-Ching Tai

1. Introduction

Human hepatitis B virus (HBV) produces three structurally related envelope proteins (also called surface antigens) from a single open reading frame (ORF) **(Fig. 1)**. This ORF contains three in-frame translational initiation AUG codons, dividing it into three regions: preS1, preS2, and S *(1,2)*. The three envelope proteins are referred to in the literature as large (L) (p39/gp42), middle (M) (gp33/gp36), and small (S, major surface antigen) (p24/gp27) envelope proteins. These proteins are co-carboxy-terminal proteins with different amino terminal extensions.

Naturally occurring deletions in the preS2 region have been found in serum and liver samples from HBV carriers *(3–11)*. There are two major types of HBV preS2 variants found in patients with end-stage liver disease: one produces internally truncated M envelope proteins as a result of a preS2 internal deletion and the other does *not* produce any M protein as a result of ablation of its AUG. Furthermore, the prevalence rate of preS2 variants with a preS2 internal deletion seemed to be correlated with different stages of chronic HBV infection *(12)*. In accordance with this result, we detected preS2 deletion variants only in patients with chronic cirrhosis and hepatocellular carcinoma (HCC) but not in carriers without cirrhosis and HCC *(11)* (*see* **Note 1**).

The HBV preS2 internal deletion results in a truncated middle-envelope protein (M). To understand the roles of these preS2 internal deletion variants in the pathogenesis of HBV, we have characterized two mutant M envelope proteins from two HCC patients. In this chapter, we describe in further technical detail the detection of the secreted M envelope proteins containing a preS2 internal deletion by sodium dodecyl sulfate-polyacrylamide gel electrophoresis (SDS–PAGE) and Western blot analysis **(Fig. 2)**. These secreted mutant M proteins exhibited significantly increased size heterogeneity and molecular weights compared with the full-length wild-type M protein in transient transfection using a human hepatoma Huh7 cell line **(Fig. 2A)**.

From: *Methods in Molecular Medicine, vol. 95: Hepatitis B and D Protocols, volume 1*
Edited by: R. K. Hamatake and J. Y. N. Lau © Humana Press Inc., Totowa, NJ

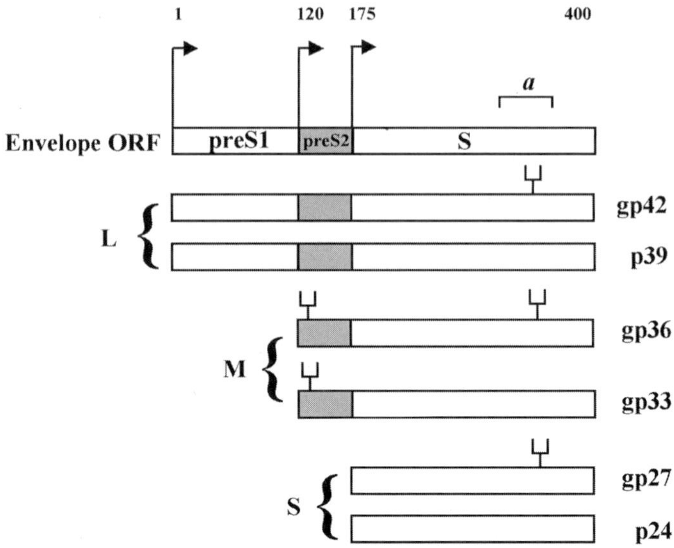

Fig. 1. Cartoon illustration of three related large (L), middle (M), and small (S) HBV envelope proteins. The top box represents the entire envelope open reading frame divided into preS1, preS2, and S domains. Amino acids methionine at positions 1, 120, and 175 indicate the respective translational initiation sites for L, M, and S envelope proteins. Position 400 is the common termination site for all three envelope proteins. The letter "*a*" indicates the group *a* determinant, which is located between amino acids 298 and 322 and shared by all three envelope proteins. The symbol Ψ represents N–linked complex glycans at asparagine (Asn) 123 and 320.

The same phenomenon can also be extended to stable transfection using a rat hepatoma cell line 7777 **(Fig. 3)**. We dubbed this paradoxical phenomenon "hypermodification" (*see* **Note 2**).

2. Materials

2.1. Plasmids

1. pSV2ANeoHBV2X (HBV wild-type tandem dimer DNA, subtype *ayw*): An HBV-containing plasmid, pcp10, was provided by Dr. P. Tiollais ***(13)***. After digestion of this plasmid DNA with *Eco*RI, the resulting 3.1-kb HBV DNA fragment was purified and ligated with an *Eco*RI-digested pSV2ANeo vector DNA (6.2 kb). The 9.3-kb pSV2ANeo–HBV monomer was then linearized by partial digestion with *Eco*RI. Tandem dimerization was performed by ligating the 3.1-kb HBV DNA fragment with the linearized 9.3-kb pSV2ANeo–HBV monomer at *Eco*RI site. The wild-type tandem dimer was screened by digestion with *Xho*I, which should give the 3.1-kb HBV DNA.
2. pΔ32 and pΔ79: These two plasmids are tandem dimer replicons of HBV preS2 internal deletion variants. To construct pΔ32 and pΔ79, a DNA fragment from nt 3213 to 990 encoding HBV M and S was polymerase chain reaction (PCR) amplified from total DNA of liver samples T32 and N79 ***(14)***, respectively. Both T32 and N79 carried actively replicating HBV

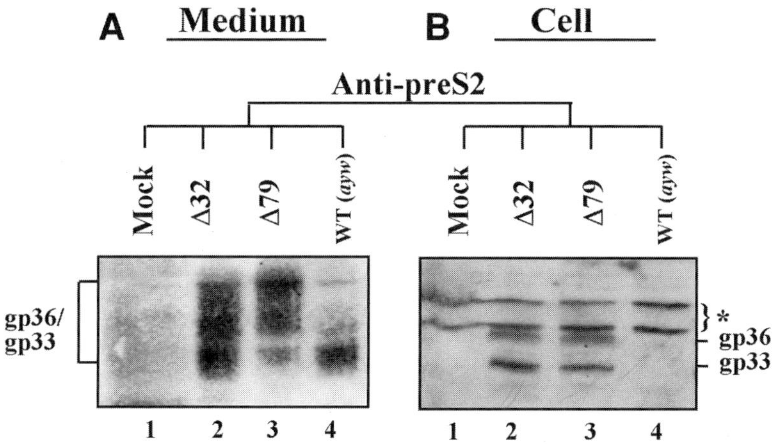

Fig. 2. **(A)** The secreted mutant M proteins (Δ32 and Δ79) exhibited significantly increased size heterogeneity and molecular weights compared with the full-length wild-type M protein in HBV replicon transfected human hepatoma Huh7 cell lines (lanes 2 and 3 vs 4). **(B)** The intracellular mutant M proteins were accumulated to a higher steady-state level than the wild-type control (lanes 2 and 3 vs 4). The wild-type preS2 protein (lane 4) is too faint to be visible in this figure. The conditioned medium and cell lysates were collected 6 d after transfection and analyzed by SDS-PAGE and Western blot analysis using an anti-preS2 specific antibody (Q19/10). The asterisk denotes the background of cellular proteins that crossreact nonspecifically with Q19/10. Mock indicates the negative control cells without transfection.

variants with an internal deletion in their preS2 region. Although Δ79 contains a 15-amino-acid deletion located between residues 127 and 141 in the preS2 region, Δ32 carries an 11-amino-acid deletion between residues 131 and 141 (*see* **Note 3**).

The preS2 internal deletions identical to Δ32 and Δ79 have also been found in samples of chronic carriers ***(15,16)***. The sense primer used in PCR amplification was derived from nt 3213 to 12 (5'- ATG CAG TGG AAT TCC ACA ACA-3'). This oligonucleotide starts with the ATG initiation codon of the preS2 ORF, and the *Eco*RI site (underlined) is at the fourth and fifth codon of the middle envelope protein. Consequently, the parental wild-type HBV and its derived mutants pΔ32 and pΔ79 have identical transcriptional regulatory elements and translational initiation context of their M envelope proteins. The antisense primer was from nt 988 to 972 (5'- ACT TTC CAA TCA ATA GG-3'). The PCR-amplified product of 0.8-kb was gel purified after digestion with *Eco*RI and *Acc*I. The DNA fragments from T32 and N79 were then used to replace the wild-type monomeric HBV counterpart in pSV2ANeoHBV1X before tandem dimerization at the *Eco*RI site.

3. pECEM-*adr* and pECEM-*ayw*: These two plasmids are HBV M envelope protein expression vectors that produce full-length wild-type M protein of subtypes *adr* and *ayw* origins (*see* **Note 4**). The HBV M envelope protein expression vector (P30) of subtype *adw2* was kindly provided by Dr. J. H. Ou ***(17)***. Plasmid P30 was used as a backbone to construct pECEM-*adr* and pECEM-*ayw*. The DNA fragments containing the preS2/S gene from nt 3213 to 1840 were amplified by PCR using wild-type HBV of *adr* and *ayw* origins as templates ***(13,18)***. The sense primer used in PCR amplification was derived from nt 3213 to 12

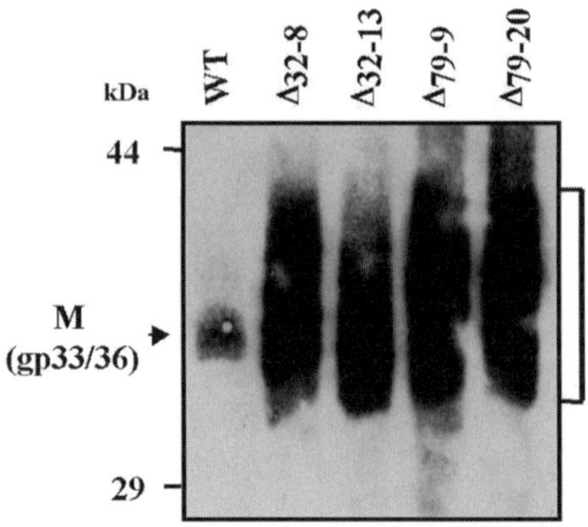

Fig. 3. Hypermodification of the secreted mutant M protein was also found in several rat Morris hepatoma cell lines stably transfected with HBV preS2 deletion variants. The immunoblot procedures were as detailed in the text and **Fig. 2.**

(5'- ATG CAG TGG AAT TCC ACA ACA-3'), and the antisense primer was from nt 1840 to 1811 (5'- TAGC GAA TTC TTA GGC AGA GGT GAA AAA GTT GCA TGG TGC-3'). Both primers contained an *Eco*RI cleavage site (underlined). The standard PCR condition was followed with an annealing temperature at 55°C ***(19)***. The 1.8-kb *Eco*RI HBV fragment containing the preS2/S sequence from either *adr* or *ayw* was used to replace the *adw2* counterpart in plasmid P30. All constructs were confirmed by restriction enzyme digestion and DNA sequencing.

2.2. Cell Culture

All cell lines were maintained in Dulbecco's modified Eagle's medium (DMEM) (Cellgro) with 10% fetal bovine serum (Hyclone) at 37°C in the presence of 5.5% CO_2 (*see* **Note 5**).

1. Human hepatoma cell line, Huh7: This human hepatoma cell line has been shown to be permissive for HBV replication ***(20)***.
2. Rat hepatoma cell line, 7777: This rat hepatoma cell line has been found to be competent to support HBV replication and maturation ***(21)***.

2.3. Solutions

1. TNE buffer: 40 m*M* Tris-HCl, pH 7.5, 150 m*M* NaCl, 1 m*M* ethylenediaminetetraacetic acid (EDTA), pH 8.0. Mix 4 mL of 1 *M* Tris-HCl, pH 7.5, 3 mL of 5 *M* NaCl, and 0.2 mL of 0.5 *M* EDTA, pH 8.0, to a final volume of 100 mL. The solution can be stably stored at room temperature.
2. 2X protein loading buffer: 0.125 *M* Tris-HCl, pH 6.8, 2% sodium dodecyl sulfate (SDS), 5% β-mercaptoethanol, 20% glycerol, and 0.1% bromophenol blue. Mix 2.5 mL of 0.5 *M* Tris-HCl, pH 6.8, 2 mL of 10% SDS, 0.5 mL of β-mercaptoethanol, 2 mL of glycerol, and 0.01 g of bromophenol blue in 3 mL of distilled H_2O. The solution can be stably stored at room temperature.

3. Phosphate-buffered saline (PBS): Dissolve 8 g of NaCl, 0.2 g of KCl, 1.44 g of Na_2HPO_4, and 0.24 g of KH_2PO_4 in 800 mL of distilled H_2O. PBS does not need to be sterilized for the purpose of Western blot analysis. The solution can be stably stored at room temperature.
4. 10X protein denaturing buffer: 5% SDS and 10% β-mercaptoethanol.
5. 10X G7 buffer: 0.5 *M* sodium phosphate, pH 7.5 at 25°C, and 10% NP-40 were provided with peptide: N-glycosidase F (PNGase F) (New England BioLabs). These reagents are stored at –20 °C.
6. Mouse monoclonal antibody to preS2 (Q19/10): A monoclonal antibody that reacts with all HBV genotypes and binds specifically to gp36 and gp33 of N-glycosylated M proteins *(22)*. It was kindly provided by Dr. W. H. Gerlich. Q19/10 detects the amino terminal glycopeptide region of M protein.
7. Mouse monoclonal antibody to HBs (H166): This monoclonal anti-HBs antibody is a generous gift from Dr. D. L. Peterson *(23)*. It reacts with all HBsAg subtypes and binds to all three envelope proteins (L, M, and S).

3. Methods

3.1. Transfections

Transient and stable transfections were performed by following the standard protocols *(21,24)* and are not detailed in this chapter.

3.2. Sample Preparation of the Secreted Mutant HBV Middle Envelope (M) Protein from the Cell Culture Medium

1. Collect cell medium from the transfected culture and centrifuge at 2000 rpm in an IEC Centra-8 centrifuge for 20 min to clear cellular debris (*see* **Note 6**).
2. Layer the clarified medium onto a 20% sucrose cushion in TNE buffer and ultracentrifuge at 26,000 rpm in a Beckman SW28 rotor at 4°C for 16 h.
3. Discard the supernatant and resuspend the subviral particle pellet in 100 μL of TNE buffer.
4. Add equal volume of 2X protein loading buffer into the 100 μL of TNE buffer.
5. The secreted M proteins can be stored at –20°C before SDS–PAGE and Western blot analysis.

3.3. Sample Preparation from the Cell Lysates

1. Harvest 6×10^6 cells from a 10-cm dish 6 d after transfection (cells should already reach confluence).
2. Rinse cells twice with PBS.
3. Collect cells in 200 μL of 2X protein loading buffer.
4. The cell lysates can be stored at –20°C before SDS–PAGE and Western blot analysis.

3.4. PNGase F Treatment

1. Denature the extracellular protein samples (resuspended in TNE buffer) in 1X protein denaturing buffer at 100°C for 10 min.
2. Add 1/10 volume of 10X G7 buffer and 10% NP-40.
3. Add 50–250 U of PNGase F (enzyme can be diluted in 10X G7 buffer) and allow incubation at 37°C for at least 5 h.

3.5. Detection of Hypermodification of the Secreted Mutant HBV Middle Envelope (M) Proteins by SDS–PAGE and Western Blot Analysis

1. To denature proteins, heat the sample at 100°C for 5 min. Resuspend the sample by pipetting up and down several times. Spin briefly to collect all samples to the bottom of the microcentrifuge tube and leave on ice.
2. Load 60 μL of protein samples into each well of a 12.5% full-sized SDS–PAGE gel and run at a constant current at 30 mA for at least 4 h (*see* **Note 7**).
3. Transfer protein samples from gel to nitrocellulose membrane by electric transfer at a constant 80 V for 1 h.
4. Block nitrocellulose membrane with 100 mL of 1% nonfat dry milk and 0.2% Tween-20 in PBS for 30 min at room temperature.
5. Wash nitrocellulose membrane three times with 100 mL of PBS containing 0.05% Tween-80 for 10 min per wash.
6. Apply the primary antibody (prepared in PBS containing 3% bovine serum albumin) to nitrocellulose membrane in a plastic bag and incubate overnight at 4°C (*see* **Note 8**).
7. After overnight incubation, wash membrane three times as in **step 5**.
8. Dilute the secondary antibody conjugated to horseradish peroxidase or alkaline phosphatase 1000-fold in 10 mL of PBS containing 5% nonfat dry milk, apply to nitrocellulose membrane in a plastic bag, and incubate for 2 h at room temperature.
9. Wash nitrocellulose membrane three more times as in **step 5**.
10. Detect signals by the ECL chemiluminescence kit (Amersham Pharmacia Biotech) or a Sigma *Fast* BCIP/NBT (5-bromo-4-chloro-3-indolyl phosphate/nitroblue tetrazolium) substrate.

4. Notes

1. There are two major types of HBV preS2 variants found in patients with end-stage liver disease: one produces internally truncated M envelope proteins as a result of a preS2 internal deletion and the other does *not* produce any M protein as a result of its AUG ablation. Hypermodification was observed in the secreted mutant M protein with a preS2 internal deletion.
2. Hypermodification is defined by the paradoxical increased-size heterogeneity and molecular weight of the secreted mutant M envelope proteins, relative to the secreted wild-type M protein control. It should be pointed out that hypermodification does not refer to the mobility up-shift of the secreted M protein when compared with its intracellular counterpart **(Fig. 2A,B)**. Nor does it refer to any subtype difference in the secreted wild-type M protein. For example, as shown in **Fig. 4**, the M protein of subtype *adw2* (genotype A) exhibited two distinct bands in contrast to the smearing pattern of other subtypes (*adr* [genotype C] and *ayw* [genotype D]). Hypermodification is a mutant-specific phenotype.
3. As shown in **Fig. 2**, variations in hypermodification were observed in two mutant M envelope proteins: Δ79 appeared to have a slower migration than Δ32. This phenotypic difference could be the result of their difference in the exact location and/or size of deletions (Δ79 has a deletion of 15 amino acids in the preS2 region, where as Δ32 has a deletion of 11 amino acids).
4. Because of its low level of expression, the intracellular wild-type M envelope protein is more difficult to detect by Western blot analysis **(Fig. 2B)** when produced in the replicon system than when produced by a protein expression vector.
5. Consistent with our current knowledge, the extent of protein modification could be dependent on the host-cell types and species origins. For example, hypermodification appears to be more pronounced in the rat cell line (Morris 7777, Fig. 3) than in the human hepatoma cell

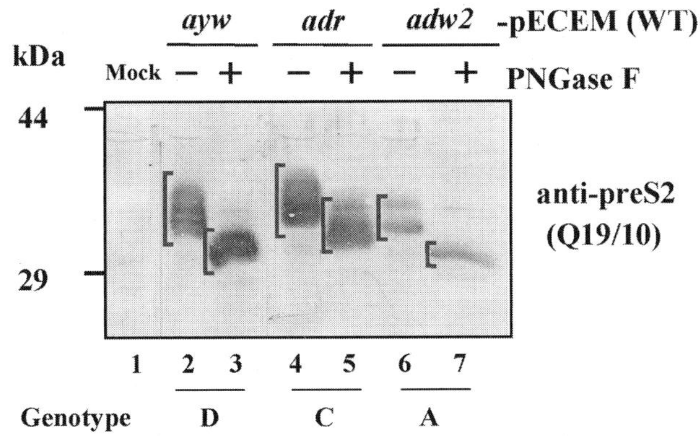

Fig. 4. Different subtypes or genotypes of wild-type HBV displayed different levels of O-linked glycosylation at the preS2 region of the secreted M envelope proteins. After removal of N-glycosylation by PNGase F, the smearing pattern persisted for both subtypes *ayw* (genotype D) and *adr* (genotype C), suggesting that they are O-glycosylated **(25)**. Subtype *adw2* (genotype A) did not have a similar up-shift pattern of mobility, before or after PNGase F treatment (lanes 6 and 7), indicating the lack of O-glycosylation in genotype A. The immunoblot procedures were as detailed in the text and **Fig. 2.**

line (Huh7, **Fig. 2A**).

6. According to our experience, preclearing the cell medium at 2000 rpm for 20 min before ultracentrifugation will decrease the background noise on Western blot results.
7. Better detection of hypermodification can be achieved by using the full-sized SDS–PAGE gel and by a longer period of electrophoresis.
8. Two reusable monoclonal antibodies were used in this chapter: Q19/10 and H166. H166 can be stored at –20°C, although repeated freezing and thawing should be avoided for Q19/10. Both of them can be reused several times.

References

1. Ganem, D. (1996) Hepadnaviridae and their replication. In: Fields, B. N., Knipe, D. M., and Howley, P. M. (eds.), *Virology*, 3rd ed., Lippincott-Raven Publishers, Philadelphia, PA, pp. 2703–2737.
2. Gerlich, W. H., Lu, X., and Heermann, K. H. (1993) Studies on the attachment and penetration of hepatitis B virus. *J. Hepatol.* **17(Suppl 3),** S10–S14.
3. Gerken, G., Kremsdorf, D., Capel, F., et al. (1991) Hepatitis B defective virus with rearrangements in the preS gene during chronic HBV infection. *Virology* **183**, 555–565.
4. Raimondo, G., Campo, S., Smedile, V., et al. (1991) Hepatitis B virus variant, with a deletion in the preS2 and two translational stop codons in the precore regions, in a patient with hepatocellular carcinoma. *J. Hepatol.* ***13*(Suppl 4),** S74–S77.
5. Santantonio, T., Jung, M. C., Schneider, R., et al. (1992) Hepatitis B virus genomes that cannot synthesize pre-S2 proteins occur frequently and as dominant virus populations in chronic carriers in Italy. *Virology* **188**, 948–952.
6. Yamamoto, K., Horikita, M., Tsuda, F., et al. (1994) Naturally occurring escape mutants of

hepatitis B virus with various mutations in the S gene in carriers seropositive for antibody to hepatitis B surface antigen. *J. Virol.* **68**, 2671–2676.
7. Kidd-Ljunggren, K., Ekdahl, K., Oberg, M., Kurathong, S., and Lolekha, S. (1995) Hepatitis B virus strains in Thailand: genomic variants in chronic carriers. *J. Med. Virol.* **47**, 454–461.
8. Pollicino, T., Campo, S., and Raimondo, G. (1995) PreS and core gene heterogeneity in hepatitis B virus (HBV) genomes isolated from patients with long-lasting HBV chronic infection. *Virology* **208**, 672–677.
9. Preikschat, P., Meisel, H., Will, H., and Gunther, S. (1999) Hepatitis B virus genomes from long term immunosuppressed carriers are modified by specific mutations in several regions. *J. Gen. Virol.* **10**, 2685–2691.
10. Gunther, S., Fischer, L., Pult, I., Sterneck, M., Piwon, N., and Will, H. (1999) Naturally occurring variants of hepatitis B virus. *Adv. Virus Res.* **52**, 25–137.
11. Tai, P.-C., Suk, F.-M., Gerlich, W. H., Neurath, A. R., and Shih, C. (2002) Hypermodification and immune escape of an internally deleted middle-envelope (M) protein of frequent and predominant hepatitis B virus variants. *Virology* **292**, 44–58.
12. Fan, Y.-F., Lu, C.-C., Chen, M.-C., et al. (2001) Prevalence and significance of hepatitis B virus (HBV) preS mutants in serum and liver at different replicative stages of chronic HBV infection. *Hepatology* **33**, 277–286.
13. Dubois, M. F., Pourcel, C., Rousset, S., Chang, C., and Tiollais, P. (1980) Excretion of hepatitis B surface antigen particles from mouse cells transformed with cloned viral DNA. *Proc. Natl. Acad. Sci. USA* **77**, 4549–4553.
14. Hosono, S., Tai, P. C., Wang, W., et al. (1995) Core antigen mutations of human hepatitis B virus in hepatomas accumulate in MHC class II-restricted T cell epitopes. *Virology* **212**, 151–162.
15. Kohno, H., Inoue, T., Tsuda F., Okamoto, H., and Akahane, Y. (1996) Mutations in the envelope gene of hepatitis B virus variants co-occurring with antibody to surface antigen in sera from patients with chronic hepatitis B. *J. Gen. Virol.* **77**, 1825–1831.
16. Takahashi, K., Akahane, Y., Hino, K., Ohta, Y., and Mishiro, S. (1998) Hepatitis B virus genomic sequence in the circulation of hepatocellular carcinoma patients, comparative analysis of 40 full-length isolates. *Arch. Virol.* **143**, 2313–2326.
17. Ou, J. H., and Rutter, W. J. (1987) Regulation of secretion of the hepatitis B virus major surface antigen by the preS-1 protein. *J. Virol.* **61**, 782–786.
18. Kobayashi, M., and Koike, K. (1984) Complete nucleotide sequence of hepatitis B virus DNA of subtype adr and its conserved gene organization. *Gene* **30**, 227–232.
19. Tai, P. C., Banik, D., Lin, G. I., (1997) Novel and frequent mutations of hepatitis B virus coincide with a major histocompatibility complex class I-restricted T-cell epitope of the surface antigen. *J. Virol.* **71**, 4852–4856.
20. Nakabayashi, H., Taketa, K., Miyano, K., Yamane, T., and Sato, J. (1982) Growth of human hepatoma cell lines with differentiated functions in chemically defined medium. *Cancer Res.* **42**, 3858–3863.
21. Shih, C., Li, L. S., Roychoudhury, S., and Ho, M. H. (1989) In vitro propagation of human hepatitis B virus in a rat hepatoma cell line. *Proc. Natl. Acad. Sci. USA* **86**, 6223–6327.
22. Heermann, K. H., Kruse, F., Seifer, M., and Gerlich, W. H. (1987) Immunogenicity of the gene S and pre-S domains in hepatitis B virions and HBsAg filaments. *Intervirology* **28**, 14–25.
23. Peterson, D. L., Paul, D. A., Lam, J., Tribby, I. I., and Achord, D. T. (1984) Antigenic struc-

ture of hepatitis B surface antigen, identification of the "d" subtype determinant by chemical modification and use of monoclonal antibodies. *J. Immunol.* **132**, 920–927.

24. Roychoudhury, S., Faruqi, A. F., and Shih, C. (1991) Pregenomic RNA encapsidation analysis of eleven missense and nonsense polymerase mutants of hepatitis B virus. *J. Virol.* **65**, 3617–3624.
25. Schmitt, S., Dieter, G., Alving, K., et al. (1999) Analysis of the pre-S2 *N*- and *O*-linked glycans of the M surface protein from human hepatitis B virus. *J. Biol. Chem.* **274**, 11,945–11,957.

18

Hepatitis B Viral Genotyping with the Research INNO-LiPA HBV Genotyping Line Probe Assay

Sija De Gendt, Fred Shapiro, Jelena Juras, Els Van Assche, Geert Maertens, and Erwin Sablon

1. Introduction

Hepatitis B continues to remain one of mankind's major infectious scourges, causing considerable morbidity and mortality. It has been estimated that no less than one-third of all individuals alive today have been infected at some time with the hepatitis B virus (HBV). Of the estimated 350 million people (6% of the world's population) who fail to resolve the disease and become chronic HBV carriers, up to one-third will inevitably develop progressive, life-threatening liver disease. However, the impact of HBV-related disease is not geographically uniform. Prevalence rates vary from less than 2% in Western Europe and North America, to 2–7% in Southern and Eastern Europe, and to more than 8% in Asia, Africa, and the Western Pacific *(1)*.

For such a small DNA virus (only 3200 nucleotides), HBV is characterized by a surprising degree of variability. Indeed, evidence of its serological heterogeneity emerged soon after its discovery by means of monoclonal antibodies directed against the surface antigen of the virus (HBsAg). These HBsAg subdeterminants consist of a common group-reactive "a" antigen, shared by all HBsAg isolates, and the mutually exclusive subtype-specific pairs "d" or "y" and "w" or "r." Together with other more recently characterized specificities, they make up the nine different serological subtypes: ayw1, ayw2, ayw3, ayw4, ayr, adw2, adw4, adrq+, and adrq– *(2)*.

In recent years, it has become evident that considerable molecular variation occurs throughout the HBV genome. This variation results from the fact that the infective HBV genome does not replicate directly from a DNA template using the replicative machinery of its host but relies instead on reverse transcription from an RNA intermediate that is prone to mutation. Given that a better understanding of HBV variation at the molecular level could provide useful information about the prevalence and clinical outcome of HBV infection in different regions of the world, a genetic classification

From: *Methods in Molecular Medicine, vol. 95: Hepatitis B and D Protocols, volume 1*
Edited by: R. K. Hamatake and J. Y. N. Lau © Humana Press Inc., Totowa, NJ

system based on the nucleotide sequencing of complete HBV genomes has been established.

With this system, up to seven genomic groups (designated A through G), showing an intergroup divergence of 8% or more with reference to the complete nucleotide sequence, have now been described *(3–5)*. These different genotypes show a distinct geographic distribution. Genotypes A and D are pandemic; genotypes B and C predominate in Asia; genotype E is uniquely African; genotype F is found among native Americans and Polynesians; and the recently discovered genotype G has been localized so far in the United States and in Europe. In addition to the geographical localization and delimitation of the genotypes and their correlation with HBV serotypes, such a genetic classification can be used epidemiologically to trace routes of HBV infection *(6)* and to help reconstruct the phylogenetic history of HBV *(7)*. Several recent studies have pointed to possible differences in clinical characteristics associated with different genotypes *(8,9)*. Preliminary investigations have also indicated that the outcome of HBV treatment may be influenced by genotype *(10,11)*.

To help investigate the possible influence of viral genotype on the pathogenesis, epidemiology, and clinical outcome of HBV infection, a genetic typing system targeting the HBsAg region of the HBV genome was developed *(12)*. This line probe assay (INNO-LiPA HBV Genotyping, Innogenetics, Ghent, Belgium) is based on the reverse hybridization principle and makes use of a series of immobilized oligonucleotide probes that are able to discriminate between nucleic acid fragments (*see* **Note 1**). In the LiPA system, these probes are attached as parallel lines on nitrocellulose membrane strips in a layout permitting easy identification of the viral genotypes (*see* **Note 2**). The LiPA principle is illustrated in **Fig. 1**.

An advantage of using the carboxy-terminal HBsAg coding open reading frame for genotyping is that the overlapping reading frame for the HBV polymerase covers the clinically significant drug-resistance (DR) motifs that reduce the susceptibility of the virus strains to antiviral drugs such as lamivudine. Consequently, the same amplified fragment can also be used to detect these mutations by methods such as the commercially available INNO-LiPA HBV DR assay.

In conclusion, the INNO-LiPA HBV Genotyping line probe assay is a rapid, accurate, and convenient system for HBV genotyping that is being used by researchers, epidemiologists, and clinicians alike. The results generated by means of this assay will undoubtedly increase our understanding of chronic hepatitis B viral disease.

1.1. Test Principle

In the HBsAg region between nucleotide positions 328 and 619, eight separate regions were recognized as containing sufficient variability for the design of a hepatitis B genotyping reverse hybridization LiPA. In this research version of the INNO-LiPA HBV Genotyping assay, a total of 15 genotype-specific probes were designed in these eight target regions (*see* **Note 3**). Three specific probes were designed for genotype A, two each for genotypes B, C, D, E, and F, and one for the newly discovered genotype G. However, genotype G amplicons will, next to the genotype G-specific probe, always display an additional reactivity with one specific genotype A probe (*see* **Note 4**). In

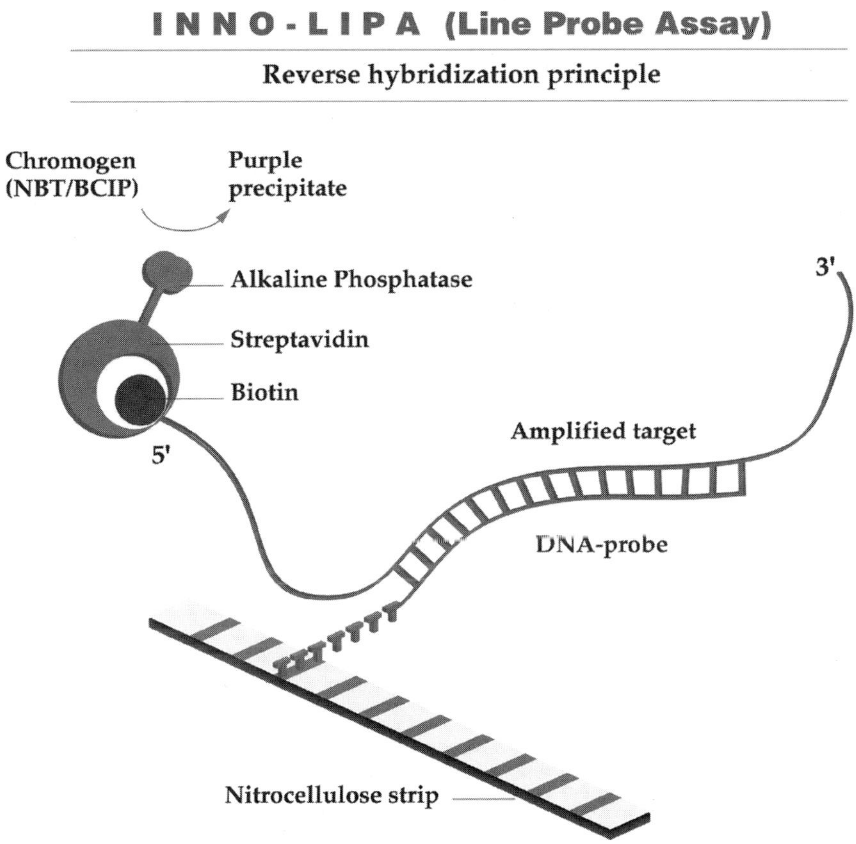

Fig. 1. Principle of the INNO-LIPA HBV Genotyping.

addition to these genotype-specific probes, the INNO-LiPA HBV Genotyping strip contains one marker line and two control lines. These two latter lines consist of a conjugate control line to check for the color development reaction and an amplification control line containing universal HBV probes to control for the presence of amplified material.

The test principle **(Fig. 1)** can be explained briefly as follows: oligonucleotide probes are immobilized as parallel lines on a nitrocellulose membrane strip. Biotin-labeled viral amplicons obtained from amplification of the HBsAg region from patients with hepatitis B will hybridize only to a probe (or line) giving a perfect match with the sequence of the isolate, allowing stringent discrimination of the HBV genotype(s) present in the sample. The presence of probe amplicon-biotin hybrids is subsequently revealed by adding streptavidin-labeled alkaline phosphatase, which binds to the biotin. In a final step, incubation with a chromogen results in a purple-brown precipitate at the site of hybridization.

2. Materials

2.1. Nucleic-Acid Isolation

1. High Pure PCR[1] Template Preparation kit provided by Roche Diagnostics (cat. no. 1 796 828).
2. Disposable gloves.
3. Disposable sterile pipet tips (preferably cotton-plugged).
4. Sterile microtubes.
5. Microtube racks.
6. Microtube centrifuge.
7. Pipets adjustable to deliver 1 to 20 μL, 20 to 200 μL, and 200 to 1000 μL.
8. Autoclaved distilled water.
9. Ethanol p.a.
10. Isopropanol p.a.

2.2. INNO-LiPA HBV Genotyping Amplification Procedure

2.2.1. Materials Not Included in the INNO-LiPA HBV DR Amplification Kit (P-1084)

1. DNA thermal cycler and equipment.
2. dNTPs (25 m*M*).
3. 10X Taq2000™ amplification buffer provided by Stratagene (cat. no. 600196).
4. Taq2000 DNA polymerase provided by Stratagene (cat. no. 600196).
5. Disposable gloves.
6. Disposable sterile pipet tips (preferably cotton-plugged).
7. Sterile microtubes.
8. Microtube racks.
9. Microtube centrifuge.
10. Pipets adjustable to deliver 1 to 20 μL, 20 to 200 μL, and 200 to 1000 μL.
11. Autoclaved distilled water.

2.2.2. Materials Included in the INNO-LiPA HBV DR Amplification Kit (P-1084) (see **Note 5**)

1. One green-capped tube containing 0.06 mL nested primers (NP; containing biotinylated primers).
2. One red-capped tube containing 0.06 mL outer primers (OP; containing biotinylated primers).

2.3. INNO-LiPA HBV Genotyping Hybridization Procedure

2.3.1. Materials Not Included in the INNO-LiPA HBV Genotyping hybridization Kit

1. Water bath with shaking platform (80 rpm; with inclined lid; temperature adjustable to 50°C ± 0.5°C).
2. Aspiration apparatus.

[1]The polymerase chain reaction (PCR) and methods are covered by patents and patent applications owned by F. Hoffmann—La Roche AG. No authorization, implicit license, or explicit license to practice PCR or any method using PCR is conveyed by purchase of this product. Information on licenses to practice PCR and methods using PCR may be obtained by contacting F. Hoffmann—La Roche AG, CH—4002 Basel, Switzerland.

3. Calibrated thermometer.
4. Distilled or deionized water.
5. Disposable gloves.
6. Disposable sterile pipet tips (preferably cotton-plugged).
7. Tweezers for strip handling.
8. Graduated cylinders (10, 25, 50, and 100 mL).
9. Orbital, reciprocal, or rocking platform shaker.

   Recommendations for an orbital shaker:

   - The diameter of the circular motion should be equal or superior to 13 mm.
   - Recommended speed for a 13-mm circular motion is 160 rpm.

   For a reciprocal shaker:

   - Recommended speed for the to-and-fro motion is 80 movements per min.

   For a rocking platform shaker:

   - The shaking angle should not exceed 13° to avoid spilling of liquid.
   - Recommended speed is 50 rpm.

10. Adjustable pipets to deliver 1–20 μL, 20–200 μL, and 200–1000 μL.
11. Dispensing multipipet (Eppendorf, optional).
12. Timer, 2 h (± 1 min).
13. Vortex mixer or equivalent.

2.3.2. Materials Included in the INNO-LiPA HBV Genotyping Hybridization Kit (see ***Note 6****)*

1. One plastic tube containing 20 INNO-LiPA HBV Genotyping strips marked with a red marker line (*see* **Note 7**).
2. One vial containing 0.8 mL of 100X concentrated conjugate (C), to be diluted 100-fold in conjugate diluent (CD) before use.
3. One vial containing 80 mL of CD.
4. One vial containing 1.0 mL of denaturation solution (DS) (*see* **Note 8**).
5. One vial containing 80 mL of hybridization solution (HS).
6. One vial containing 60 mL of concentrated rinse solution (RS), to be diluted fivefold (one part RS + four parts H_2O) in distilled water before use.
7. One vial containing 0.8 mL of 100X concentrated 5-bromo, 4-chloro, 3-indolyl phosphate/4-nitroblue tetrazolium (BCIP/NBT) substrate solution (S) to be diluted 100-fold in substrate buffer (SB) before use (*see* **Note 9**).
8. One vial containing 180 mL of SB.
9. One vial containing 200 mL of stringent wash (SW) solution.
10. Three incubation trays containing eight troughs each.
11. One plastic reading card for identification of positive probes.
12. Two data reporting sheets for storage of developed strips.

3. Methods (*see* Note 10)

3.1. Nucleic Acid Isolation

1. It is recommended to use the High Pure PCR Template Preparation Kit from Roche (cat. no. 1 796 828).
2. Take 200 µL of sample material (*see* **Note 11**).
3. Add 200 µL binding buffer (green cap) and 40 µL proteinase K (reconstituted); mix immediately and incubate for 10 min at 72°C.
4. Add 100 µL isopropanol and mix well.
5. Pipet the sample into the upper reservoir of a combined High Pure filter tube-collection tube assembly.
6. Centrifuge in a standard tabletop centrifuge for 1 min at 6800*g*.
7. Discard the flow-through and collection tube.
8. Combine the filter tube with a new collection tube.
9. Add 500-µL inhibitor removal buffer (black cap) to the upper reservoir.
10. Centrifuge for 1 min at 6800*g*.
11. Discard the flow-through and collection tube.
12. Combine the filter tube with a new collection tube.
13. Add 500-µL wash buffer (blue cap) to the upper reservoir.
14. Centrifuge for 1 min at 6800*g*.
15. Discard the flow-through and collection tube.
16. Combine the filter tube with a new collection tube.
17. Add 500-µL wash buffer (blue cap) to the upper reservoir.
18. Centrifuge for 1 min at 6800*g*.
19. Discard the flow-through.
20. Combine the filter tube with the same collection tube.
21. Centrifuge to remove residual wash buffer for 10 s at maximum speed.
22. Discard the collection tube.
23. Insert the filter tube in a clean microcentrifuge tube.
24. Add 200 µL prewarmed (70°C) elution buffer.
25. Centrifuge for 1 min at 6800*g*.
26. The microcentrifuge tube now contains the eluted DNA.
27. Use the eluted DNA directly or store the DNA at –20°C.

3.2. INNO-LiPA HBV Genotyping Amplification Procedure

Amplification of the HBV DNA can be achieved by different processes, including, but not limited to, transcription-mediated amplification (TMA), nucleic acid sequence–based amplification (NASBA), and polymerase chain reaction (PCR). In this chapter, we present PCR as an example.

3.2.1. Outer Amplification

1. Prepare master mix containing:
   N = number of samples + 1 negative control + 1 positive control + 1 ($N \times 32.4$ µL) autoclaved distilled water

   + ($N \times 5$ µL) 10X Taq2000 amplification buffer (Stratagene, cat. no. 600 196)
   + ($N \times 0.4$ µL) deoxynucleoside triphorphate (dNTP) mix (25 m*M*)

+ ($N \times 2.0$ μL) INNO-LiPA HBV Genotyping outer primer mix
+ ($N \times 0.2$ μL) Taq2000 DNA Polymerase 5 U/μL (Stratagene, cat. no. 600 196).

2. Aliquot 40 μL of this master mix into autoclaved amplification tubes.
3. Add 10 μL purified DNA.
4. Insert the samples in the calibrated thermal block.
5. Start the INNO-LiPA HBV Genotyping amplification profile (cycler type PE2400, PE9600): (1) Denature 94°C 4 min, (2) denature 94°C 30 s, (3) anneal primers 45°C 30 s, (4) extend primers 72°C 30 s, (5) repeat cycle steps 2 to 4, 40 times, (6) elongate 72°C 10 min, (7) cool to 4°C.

3.2.2. Nested Amplification

1. Prepare master mix containing:
   N = number of outer amplified samples + outer amplified negative control + 1 negative control + 1 positive control.
   ($N \times 40.4$ μL) autoclaved distilled water.
   + ($N \times 0.4$ μL) dNTP mix (25 m*M*)
   + ($N \times 5.0$ μL) 10X Taq2000 amplification buffer (Stratagene, cat. no. 600 196)
   + ($N \times 2.0$ μL) INNO-LiPA HBV Genotyping NP mix
   + ($N \times 0.2$ μL) Taq2000 DNA polymerase (5 U/μL) (Stratagene, cat. no. 600 196).
2. Aliquot 48 μL of this master mix into autoclaved amplification tubes.
3. Add 2 μL of the outer amplified product.
4. Insert the samples in the calibrated thermal block.
5. Start the INNO-LiPA HBV Genotyping nested amplification profile (cycler type PE2400, PE9600): (1) Denature 94°C 4 min, (2) denature 94°C 30 s, (3) anneal primers 45°C 30 s, (4) extend primers 72°C 30 s, (5) repeat cycle steps 2 to 4, 35 times, (6) elongate 72°C 10 min, (7) cool to 4°C.

Check outer and nested amplified products on a 2% agarose gel (use 5 μL). Based upon in-house observations, it is advised that if the outer amplified product gives a band of around 409 bp, an interpretable result should be given by the LiPA assay. If no band is visible for the outer amplified product, use the nested amplified product with the INNO-LiPA HBV Genotyping.

3.3. The INNO-LiPA HBV Genotyping Hybridization Procedure

3.3.1. Manual Procedure

3.3.1.1. Reagent Preparation

1. Allow all test materials to reach room temperature (20–25°C) before use.
2. The HS and the SW solution should be prewarmed to at least 40°C and must not exceed 50°C, the hybridization temperature.
3. Rinse solution should be prepared by diluting the concentrated rinse solution fivefold in distilled or deionized water (one part RS + four parts H_2O). Prepare 8-mL RS for each test trough + 10 mL in excess. The RS is stable for 2 wk at 2–8°C.
4. Conjugate solution should be prepared by diluting the concentrated conjugate (C) 100-fold in CD. Prepare 2-mL conjugate solution for each test trough + 2 mL in excess. (The conjugate solution can be prepared during the stringent wash.) The conjugate solution is stable for 24 h at room temperature (20–25°C).

5. Substrate solution should be prepared by diluting the concentrated BCIP/NBT substrate solution (S) 100-fold in SB. Prepare 2-mL substrate solution for each test trough + 2 mL in excess. (The substrate solution can be prepared during conjugate incubation.) The substrate solution is stable for 24 h at room temperature (20–25°C) if stored in the dark.

3.3.1.2. Denaturation and Hybridization (*see* **Note 12**)

1. Heat the shaking water bath to exactly 50°C. Check the temperature using a calibrated thermometer, and adjust the temperature if necessary. Do not exceed the indicated temperature. Prewarm the HS and the SW solution to at least 40°C but do not exceed 50°C. Mix before use. All crystals should be dissolved.
2. Using tweezers, remove the required number of INNO-LiPA HBV Genotyping strips from the tube (one strip per test sample and one strip for the blank amplified control sample). Pencil an identification number above the red marker line on the strip.
3. Take the required number of test troughs (one trough per test sample) and place them in the tray.
4. As shown in **Fig. 2** (step 1), pipet 10-μL DS into the upper corner of each trough (*see* **Note 13**).
5. Add 10-μL sample and carefully mix by pipetting up and down (**Fig. 2**, step 2). Always use sterile pipet tips. Allow denaturation to proceed for 5 min at 20–25°C.
6. Shake the prewarmed HS and gently add 2 mL to the denatured amplified product into each trough. Mix by gentle shaking (**Fig. 2**, step 3). Take care not to contaminate neighboring troughs during pipetting.
7. Immediately place the strip with the marked side of the membrane upward into the trough, as shown in **Fig. 2** (step 4). The strips should be completely submerged in the solution.
8. **Note**: Wear disposable gloves and use tweezers.
9. Place the tray into the 50°C shaking water bath (approx 80 rpm; see directions for incubation), close the lid, and incubate for 60 min. **Note**: Avoid splashing water from the water bath into the trough.

3.3.1.3. Stringent Wash (*see* **Note 12**)

1. After hybridization, remove the tray from the water bath.
2. Hold the tray at a low angle and aspirate the liquid from the trough with a pipet, preferably attached to a vacuum aspirator. Add 2 mL prewarmed SW solution into each trough and rinse by rocking the tray briefly (10–20 s) at 20–25°C. Aspirate the solution from each trough.
3. Repeat this washing step once.
4. Finally, aspirate the solution and incubate each strip in 2 mL prewarmed SW solution in the shaking water bath at 50°C for 30 min. Close the lid of the water bath. Before incubation, check the temperature of the water bath using a calibrated thermometer, and adjust the temperature if necessary. Always close the lid.

3.3.1.4. Color Development

1. All subsequent incubations are performed at room temperature (20–25°C) on a shaker. During the incubations, the liquid and test strips should move back and forth in the trough for homogeneous staining.
2. Wash each strip twice for 1 min using 2 mL of the diluted RS (*see* **Subheading 3.3.1.1.**).
3. Add 2 mL of the diluted conjugate (*see* **Subheading 3.3.1.1.**) to each trough and incubate for 30 min while agitating the tray on the shaker. **Note**: Dilute the BCIP/NBT substrate solution (S) about 10 min prior to the end of the conjugate incubation (*see* **Subheading 3.3.1.1.**).

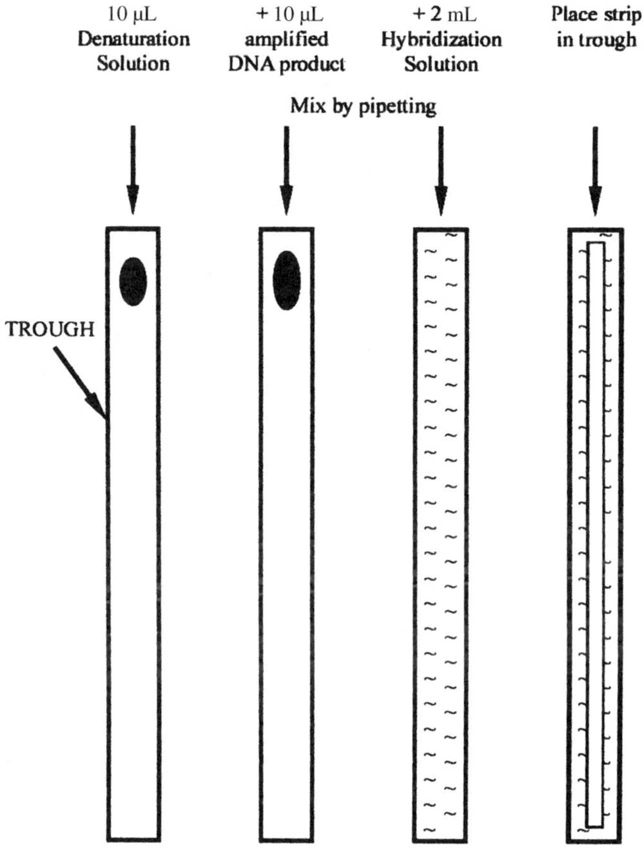

Fig. 2. Instructions for pipetting.

4. Wash each strip twice for 1 min using 2 mL of the diluted RS and wash once more using 2 mL SB.
5. Add 2 mL of the diluted substrate solution (*see* **Subheading 3.3.1.1.**) to each trough and incubate for 30 min while agitating the tray on the shaker.
6. Stop the color development by washing the strips twice in 2 mL distilled water while agitating the tray on the shaker for at least 3 min.
7. Using tweezers, remove the strips from the troughs and place them on absorbent paper. Let the strips dry completely before reading the results. Store the developed and dried strips in the dark.
8. Fix the strips on the data reporting sheet; do not put adhesive tape over the total length of the strip. The reading card will facilitate the identification of the lines.
9. Developed strips will retain their color if stored in the dark.

3.3.2. Auto-*LiPA Procedure*

The *Auto*-LiPA procedure allows automated processing of 30 strips in one run. After denaturation of the sample, the system proceeds automatically with the full procedure until final coloration of the strips. Manipulation errors are therefore excluded. One total run takes approx 3 h. The procedure allows highly standardized and reliable testing.

3.3.3. Interpretation and Storage of the Strips

Let the strips dry completely before reading the results **(Fig. 3)**. Store the developed and dried strips in the dark. The uppermost red line is the marker line. The first positive line should be lined up with the "conjugate control" line on the plastic reading card. This line controls for the addition of reactive conjugate and substrate solution during the detection procedure. It should always be positive and should have approximately the same intensity on each strip in the same test run. The second positive line ("amplification control" on the reading chart) controls for the addition of amplified material for hybridization.

If HBV DNA is present in the sample, and correct sample processing and amplification have been performed, the target amplicon hybridizes to this "amplification control" line. The negative control strip should be blank except for the conjugate control line. This demonstrates the absence of contamination in the negative control or kit reagents by HBV amplicons. With the plastic reading card, the HBV genotype can be determined based on the observed line reactivity. At least one line positive for a given genotype means the presence of this HBV genotype in the sample, except for genotype G (*see* **Subheading 1.1.**).

4. Notes

1. For purposes of verification, HBsAg region sequences (nt 328–619) of 364 HBV isolates derived from the public databases and in-house sequencing efforts, including sequences derived from 169 complete HBV genomes and covering HBV genotypes A through G, were analyzed for the presence of the chosen genotype-specific motifs. No genotype could be assigned in only 16 of 364 cases (4%) (IND: indeterminate result) due to additional sequence polymorphisms, resulting in an accuracy of 96%. Correct genotype assignment was verified by phylogenetic analysis in all cases.
2. For purposes of validation, 222 HBV-positive samples collected from Europe, North and South America, Asia, and the Middle East were analyzed using the INNO-LiPA HBV Genotyping, resulting in the correct assignment of 220 HBV genotypes (accuracy of 99%) and only two IND results.
3. The probes have been designed to be specific at the "one-nucleotide" level, meaning that the difference of one nucleotide between the target sequence and the probe sequence will interfere with the hybridization, and hence with the staining.
4. Infections with more than one HBV genotype could be detected in certain samples. The presence of these multiple genotypes was verified and proven correct by clonal sequencing. In all cases, multiple genotypes detected with the current version of the INNO-LiPA HBV Genotyping could be confirmed by analyzing the different clonal sequences. The INNO-LiPA HBV Genotyping is thus capable of correctly identifying mixed-genotype HBV infections.
5. The kit should be stored isolated from any source of contaminating DNA, especially amplified DNA products.
6. LiPA HS, SW solution, RS, CD, C, and SB contain N-methylisothiazolone HCl/2-chloroacetamide (MIT/CAA) as a preservative.
7. The strips are designed to be used only once! Do not touch the strips with bare hands; use clean tweezers. Do not allow the strips to dry between the washing steps.

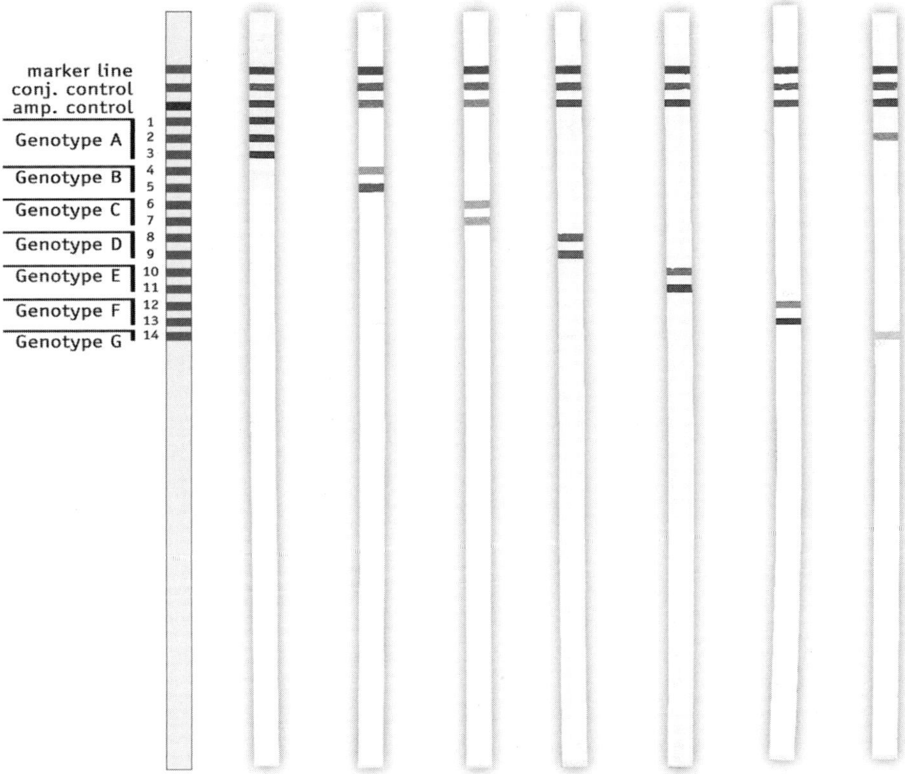

Fig. 3. Example of INNO-LIPA HBV Genotyping strips.

8. DS contains sodium hydroxide and is irritating to the eyes and the skin. Wear gloves and protective goggles.
9. BCIP/NBT substrate solution (S) contains dimethylformamide and BCIP. This solution may harm the fetus and may cause cancer. Furthermore, this solution is harmful by inhalation and by contact with skin and is also irritating to the eyes. Wear gloves and protective goggles.
10. To control contamination during extraction/amplification/hybridization, include at least one positive and one negative control sample each time these steps are performed.
11. Specimens should always be handled as potentially infectious.
12. The hybridization and stringent wash incubations at exactly 50°C (± 0.5°C) are the most critical steps to avoid false-positive (temperature too low) or false-negative/very weak signals (temperature too high). A shaking water bath with inclined lid allows a good control of temperature variations. Strict temperature control with a calibrated thermometer is necessary. Always close the lid of the water bath during incubations to avoid false-positive signals. Do not use hot-air shakers for the hybridization or stringent wash, because heat exchange is too slow, and optimal hybridization cannot be reached within the indicated time span. The amplitude of the motion generated by both the shaking water bath (hybridization procedure) and the shaker (color development procedure) is critical for achieving maximum sensitivity

and homogeneous staining. The strip surface should be completely submerged. The amplitude should be as high as possible. However, spilling of liquid over the edges of the troughs should be avoided! This spillage can lead to cross-contamination and invalid results.

13. The vial containing the DS should be closed immediately after use; prolonged exposure of this solution to air leads to a rapid deterioration of the denaturing strength.

References

1. Maddrey, W. C. (2000) Hepatitis B: an important public health issue. *J. Med. Virol.* **61**, 362–366.
2. Swenson, P. D., Riess, J. T., and Krueger, L. E. (1991) Determination of HBsAg subtypes in different high risk populations using monoclonal antibodies. *J. Virol. Methods* **33**, 27–28.
3. Okamoto, H., Tsuda, F., Sakugawa, H., et al. (1988) Typing hepatitis B virus by homology in nucleotide sequence: comparison of surface antigen subtypes. *J. Gen. Virol.* **69**, 2575–2583.
4. Magnius, L. O., and Norder, H. (1995) Subtypes, genotypes and molecular epidemiology of the hepatitis B virus as reflected by sequence variability of the S-gene. *Intervirology* **38**, 24–34.
5. Stuyver, L., De Gendt, S., Van Geyt, C., et al. (2000) A new genotype of hepatitis B virus: complete genome and phylogenetic relatedness. *J. Gen. Virol.* **81**, 67–74.
6. Swenson, P. D., Van Geyt, C., Alexander, E. R., et al. (2001) Hepatitis B virus genotypes and HBsAg subtypes in refugees and injection drug users in the United States determined by LiPA and monoclonal EIA. *J. Med. Virol.* **64**, 305–311.
7. Odemuyiwa, S. O., Mulders, M. N., Oyedele, O. I., et al. (2001) Phylogenetic analysis of new hepatitis B virus isolates from Nigeria supports endemicity of genotype E in West Africa. *J. Med. Virol.* ***65***, 463–469.
8. Tsubota, A., Arase, Y., Ren, F., Tanaka, H., Ikeda, K., and Kumada, H. (2001) Genotype may correlate with liver carcinogenesis and tumor characteristics in cirrhotic patients infected with hepatitis B virus subtype adw. *J. Med. Virol.* ***65***, 257–265.
9. Orito, E., Ichida, T., Sakugawa, H., et al. (2001) Geographic distribution of hepatitis B virus (HBV) genotype in patients with chronic HBV infection in Japan. *Hepatology* **34**, 590–594.
10. Kao, J. H., Chen, P. J., Lai, M. Y., and Chen, D. S. (2000) Hepatitis B genotypes correlate with clinical outcomes in patients with chronic hepatitis B. *Gastroenterology* **118**, 554–559.
11. Kao, J. H., Wu, N. H., Chen, P. J., Lai, M. Y., and Chen, D. S. (2000) Hepatitis B genotypes and the response to interferon therapy. *J. Hepatol.* ***33***, 998–1002.
12. Van Geyt, C., De Gendt, S., Rombout, A., et al. (1998) A line probe assay for hepatitis B virus genotypes. In: Schinazi, R. F., Sommadossi, J.-P., and Thomas, C. (eds), *Therapies for Viral Hepatitis,* International Medical Press, London, 139–145.

III

Molecular Biological Characterization

19

Processing of Hepatitis B Virus Surface Proteins

Volker Bruss

1. Introduction

The hepatitis B virus (HBV) can cause acute as well as chronic infections of the human liver. More than 300 million individuals are chronically infected worldwide, and it has been estimated that about 1 million of them die annually as a consequence of the infection *(1)*.

The hepatitis B surface antigen (HBsAg) formed by proteins of the viral particle that are located in the outer envelope surrounding the central nucleocapsid plays a central role in the control of the infection; the appearance of antibodies (anti-HBs) directed against HBsAg during the course of an infection is strongly correlated with elimination of the virus. HBV surface proteins are released from the infected liver into the blood not only as components of the viral envelope which has a diameter of 42 nm, but also as part of noninfectious subviral lipoprotein particles having a diameter of 22 nm which are produced in large excess relative to virions. Detection of these HBsAg particles in serum by commonly available tests allows a sensitive assessment of the carrier stage and is important for diagnostic and public health purposes. Prophylaxis against hepatitis B by active vaccination uses subviral HBsAg particles expressed by recombinant DNA technologies, e.g., in yeast as the active component.

The HBV envelope and subviral particles contain three different proteins, referred to as large (L), middle (M), and small (S) HBV surface proteins **(Fig. 1A)** *(2)*. They are expressed from one open reading frame (ORF), comprising 389 or 400 codons of the HBV genome depending on the virus subtype. The L protein corresponds to the entire ORF, whereas the expression of M starts at an internal initiation site at codon 108 or 119 of the ORF. Therefore, the M protein is coterminal with L. The N-terminal domain unique to L is named preS1. Expression of S starts at a second internal initiation site, 55 codons downstream of the M protein's start site. This 55-amino-acid domain N-terminal in M and internal in L is named preS2. The viral promoter for L expression is liver-cell specific *(3)* and is usually replaced by heterologous promoters like the simian virus 40 (SV40) early promoter for efficient expression in other cell types. The HBV

From: *Methods in Molecular Medicine, vol. 95: Hepatitis B and D Protocols, volume 1*
Edited by: R. K. Hamatake and J. Y. N. Lau © Humana Press Inc., Totowa, NJ

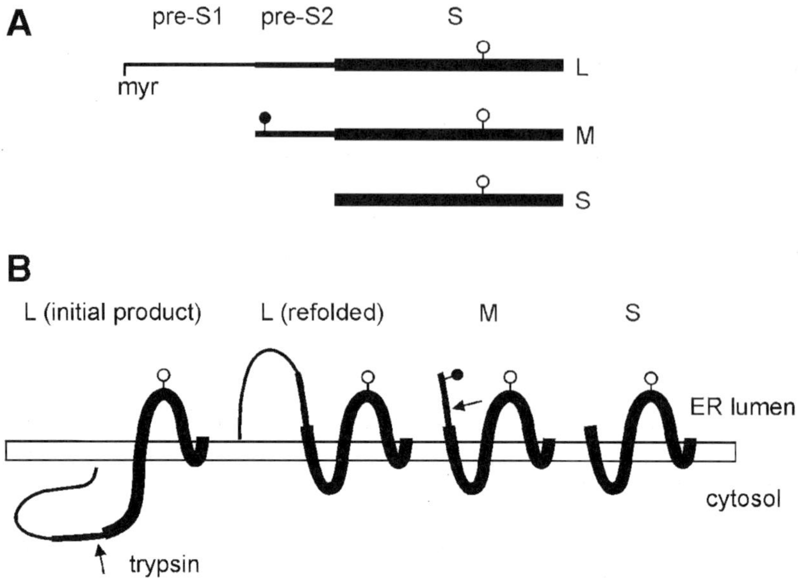

Fig. 1. Hepatitis B virus surface proteins. **(A)** Primary structure. The three coterminal surface proteins S (small), M (middle), and L (large) are related to each other and organized in a domain structure comprising the regions preS1, preS2, and S. The facultative N-glycosylation site in the S domain is indicated by an open circle; the N-glycosylation site in preS2 of M is indicated by a closed circle. The N terminus of L is myristylated. **(B)** Transmembrane topology. Co-translationally, the HBV surface proteins gain a complex transmembrane topology. The topology of approximately half of the L proteins changes during maturation. The arrows point to a trypsin-sensitive site in preS2.

DNA encoding the preS1 sequence contains a second promoter driving the expression of both the M and S proteins. This promoter functions in a variety of cell types. Therefore, the heterologous expression of the L protein is usually accompanied by M and S expression. The mRNAs for L, M, and S protein are not spliced. They contain a *cis*-acting element downstream of the ORF *(4)*, which is required for export of the mRNA from the nucleus and efficient translation.

During translation, the HBV surface proteins are inserted into the endoplasmic reticulum (ER) membrane, and generate a complex transmembrane folding **(Fig. 1B)**. The situation is even more complicated because the topology of the L protein changes during maturation of the protein: The preS domain is initially located at the cytosolic side of the ER membrane, corresponding to the internal side of the viral envelope *(5,7)*, but in approximately half of the L chains, the preS domain traverses the membrane post-translationally and appears on the outer surface of viral particles, which corresponds topologically to the luminal side of the ER membrane.

The HBV envelope proteins are modified by covalent linkages. A glycan residue is bound to asparagine residue 146 in approximately half of the S domains. Another glycan residue is bound to asparagine residue 4 of the preS2 domain in case of the M but not in case of the L protein (**Figs. 1A** and **2**) *(2)*. Early after synthesis, the HBV envelope proteins form disulfide linked hetero- and homodimers by cystine bridges *(8)*. Some cysteine residues are probably involved in intramolecular disulfide bridges.

How the HBV envelope proteins are transported from the intracellular membrane during subviral lipoprotein particle formation without engaging the viral nucleocapsid is an unresolved question. Also, the role of lipids in this process has not yet been investigated.

As a result of the importance of HBsAg, the expression, structure, and function of HBV surface proteins have been studied with great effort and are still objects of investigation. This chapter will concentrate on the description of a technique for efficient transient expression of HBV surface proteins in a eukaryotic cell line and on the following three basic experimental techniques for the analysis of some aspects of HBsAg biogenesis: protease protection experiments for characterizing the transmembrane topology of the proteins, treatment with endoglycosidase H to investigate N-glycosylation, and detection of the antigen in the culture medium after pulse/chase labeling for studying HBsAg secretion.

2. Materials

1. COS7 cells are grown on 8-cm dishes in culture medium at 37°C in an atmosphere containing 5 % CO_2. One or 2 d after they reach confluency, cells are subcultured by removing the medium, rinsing the cells first with 10 mL of warm (37°C) phosphate-buffered saline (PBS) and then with 3 mL of trypsin/ethylenediaminetetraacetic acid (EDTA) solution, incubating the dish for 2 min in the CO_2 incubator, suspending the cells in 8 mL warm medium, transferring 2 mL of this suspension into a fresh 10-cm dish containing 10 mL fresh warm medium, and placing the fresh dish into a CO_2 incubator. For smaller cultures, the volumes are reduced proportionally to the area of the dishes (e.g., for a 3.5-cm dish of a six-well plate, one-fifth of the volumes are used) (*see* **Note 1**).
2. Plasmid purity has been reported to be important for efficient transfection. We routinely use the polyethylene precipitation method for plasmid preparation *(9)* with yields around 1 mg pBluescript-based plasmid per 30 mL of culture.
3. Divide antisera (goat anti-HBs and rabbit anti-HBc, DAKO Diagnostika GmbH, Hamburg, Germany, cat. nos. B0560 and B0586, respectively) into 0.1-mL portions and stored at –70°C. Thaw one aliquot and store at 4°C until used up.
4. Protein A Sepharose CL-4B powder (Sigma Chemical Co., St. Louis, MO, cat. no. P-3391). Store at 4°C.
5. Culture medium: Dulbecco's modified Eagle's medium (DMEM; Life Technologies Ltd, Paisley, UK, cat. no. 41966-029) supplemented with antibiotic/antimycotic solution (Life Technologies Ltd, cat. no. 415240-096) and 10 % (v/v) fetal calf serum (Life Technologies Ltd, cat. no. 10091-148). Store at 4°C.
6. PBS: Prepare a 20X stock solution by dissolving 5.8 g of KH_2PO_4, 30.6 g of $Na_2HPO_4 \cdot 2\ H_2O$, and 151.8 of NaCl in distilled water; adjust the volume to 1 L; store at room temperature. To prepare a working solution, add 20 mL of the stock solution to 380 mL distilled water and sterilize by heat.
7. 10 X Trypsin/EDTA solution: 5 g/L trypsin, 2 g/L EDTA, 8.5 g/L NaCl (Life Technologies Ltd, cat. no. 35400-027). Store at –20°C. Prepare a working solution by diluting, e.g., 10 mL with 90 mL of distilled water, and filter sterilize. Store at 4°C.

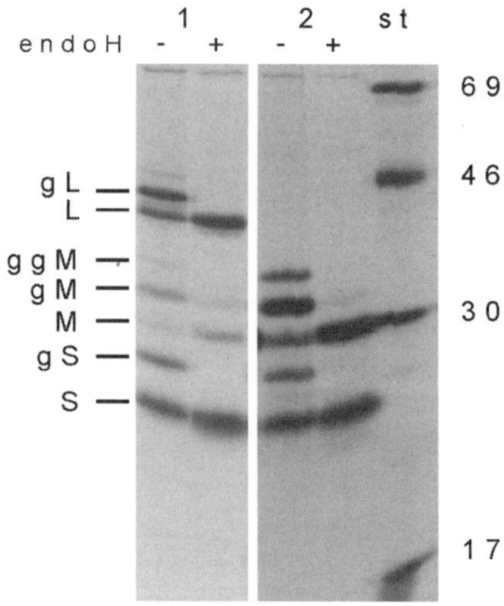

Fig. 2. N-Glycosylation of HBV surface proteins. The L, M, and S (lane 1) or M and S (lane 2) proteins were transiently expressed in COS7 cells, metabolically labeled, immunoprecipitated with anti-HBs, and treated with endoglycosidase H (+) or mock treated (–). The treatment converts the single N-glycosylated proteins gS (27 kDa), gM (33 kDa), and gL (42 kDa) as well as the double N-glycosylated protein ggM (36 kDa) into the nonglycosylated peptides S (24 kDa), M (30 kDa), and L (39 kDa), respectively. st: [^{14}C]-labeled molecular weight standard, numbers indicate molecular weight in kDa. Exposure on autoradiography film for 3 d.

8. Transfection solution: Dissolve 1 g of diethylaminoethyl-dextran (DEAE; ICN Pharmaceuticals; Costa Mesa, cat. no. 195133; store at room temperature) and 129 mg of chloroquine (ICN Pharmaceuticals, cat. no. 193919; store at room temperature) in 100 mL of PBS; filter sterilize. Store at 4°C.
9. DMSO solution: Mix 10 mL of dimethylsulfoxide with 90 mL of PBS, filter sterilize, and store at room temperature.
10. Methionine/cysteine-deficient medium for labeling: Minimal essential Eagle's medium without glutamine, methionine, and cysteine (ICN Pharmaceuticals, cat. no. 1641449), supplement with 1/100 volume of 200 m*M* L-glutamine (ICN Pharmaceuticals, cat. no. 1680146); do not add fetal calf serum, and store at 4°C.
11. ^{35}S-labeled methionine/cysteine: Contain approx 10 μCi [^{35}S]/μL, 70% of the label is bound to methionine, 15% to cysteine; specific activity: 1000 Ci/mmol (ICN Pharmaceuticals, cat. no. 51009); store at 4°C.
12. Lysis buffer: Mix 89.5 mL distilled water with 3 mL of 5 *M* NaCl stock solution, 5 mL of 1 *M* Tris-HCl, pH 7.5 stock solution, 0.5 mL of 1 *M* $MgCl_2$ stock solution, and 2 mL of 10% (v/v) IGEPAL stock solution (total volume 100 mL); store at room temperature.

13. TBS (Tris-buffered saline): Prepare a 10X concentrated stock solution by mixing 4 mL of distilled water with 10 mL of 1 *M* Tris-HCl, pH 7.5 stock solution, and 6 mL of 5 *M* NaCl stock solution; store at 4°C for up to 2 wk.
14. 10% (w/v) sucrose/TBS: Prepare freshly by dissolving 10 g sucrose in distilled water, adjust the volume to 90 mL with distilled water, and add 10 mL 10X TBS.
15. 10% (v/v) IGEPAL: Mix 10 mL IGEPAL CA-630 (ICN Pharmaceuticals, cat. no. 198596), a mild non-ionic detergent, with 90 mL distilled water. Store at room temperature.
16. Trypsin: Dissolve 5 mg trypsin (ICN Pharmaceuticals, cat. no. 101192) in 1 mL of 1X TBS; prepare freshly.
17. PMSF: Prepare freshly by dissolving 4.4 mg phenylmethylsulfonyl fluoride (Roche Diagnostics GmbH, cat. no. 236608) in 1 mL methanol (25 m*M*).
18. Aprotinin: 24 trypsin inhibitor unit (TIU)/mL (Sigma-Aldrich Corp., Cat. no. A6279). Store at 4°C.
19. 0.5 % IGEPAL/PBS: Mix 90 mL distilled water with 5 mL of 20X PBS stock solution and 5 mL of 10 % (v/v) IGEPAL (total volume: 100 mL); store at room temperature.
20. Endo H buffer: Mix 470 µL distilled water with 20 µL of a 2.5 *M* K acetate, pH 5.2 stock solution, 5 µL of a 2% (w/v) sodium dodecyl sulfate (SDS) stock solution, and 5 µL of a 1 *M* dithiothreitol (DTT) stock solution (kept at –20°C). Prepare freshly each time.
21. Endoglycosidase H: 1 U/220 µL (Roche Diagnostics GmbH, cat. no. 1088726).
22. Wash buffer: Mix 379 mL distilled water with 15 mL of 5 *M* NaCl stock solution, 25 mL of 1 *M* Tris-HCl, pH 7.5 stock solution, 20 mL of 0.5 *M* EDTA, pH 8.0 stock solution, 10 mL of 10% (v/v) IGEPAL, 1.25 mL of 20% (w/v) SDS stock solution, and 50 mL of 10% (w/v) sodium deoxycholate (SDC) stock solution (total volume 500 mL). Store at room temperature.

Because many pieces of equipment are required for the techniques described in this chapter, only a general list is given. The following items are needed:

23. General equipment for cell culture.
24. Laboratory for handling radioactivity, including a CO_2 incubator for cell culture.
25. Glass homogenizer, (e.g., neoLab, Heidelberg, Germany, # E-6960).
26. Beckman ultrazentrifuge and Beckman SW60 rotor.
27. Equipment for polyacrylamide gel electrophoresis, gel drying, and autoradiography or phosphoimaging.

3. Methods

*3.1. Transient Transfection (see **Note 2**)*

1. For studying the secretion of HBV surface proteins, it is usually sufficient to use a 35-mm dish in a six-well plate as starting material, as described in **Subheadings 3.1.** and **3.2.** For protease protection experiments, 80-mm dishes usually are sufficient. In such cases, all volumes mentioned in **Subheadings 3.1.** and **3.2.** should be scaled up by a factor of 5.
2. Split COS7 cells and seed them into 35-mm dishes (six-well plates) in such a way that they will be subconfluent by the following day. Incubate the culture overnight in a CO_2 incubator at 37°C.
3. Mix 1 mL of fresh warm culture medium with 40 µL of transfection solution in a test tube and add 2 µL of plasmid DNA with a sterile pipet tip. Remove the culture medium from the culture dish and add the mixture of medium, transfection solution, and plasmid to the cells. Place the dish into the CO_2 incubator for 3.5 to 4 h.

4. When cells start to look "sick," remove the plasmid solution and add cautiously 1 mL of warm DMSO solution. Incubate for 2 min at room temperature. Remove the DMSO solution and wash cells carefully with 2 mL of warm PBS. Avoid detaching cells during this procedure. Carefully add 2 mL of warm culture medium and place the dish into the CO_2 incubator for 2 d (*see* **Note 3**).

3.2. Metabolic Pulse/Chase Labeling

For sensitive and specific detection of the HBV surface proteins in transfected cells, we use radioactive metabolic labeling of the proteins with [^{35}S]methionine/cysteine followed by immunoprecipitation with polyclonal anti-HBs, polyacrylamide gel electrophoresis, and autoradiography. The S protein, comprising 226-amino-acid residues, contains 5 methionine and 14 cysteine residues. Detection of this protein by Western blotting is not very successful because all dominant epitopes are conformational. However, fusion of epitope tags, e.g., from the influenza virus hemagglutinin to the C terminus, allows detection by Western blotting and may be a way to circumvent radioactive labeling ***(10)***.

1. Remove the medium and wash cells once with 2 mL of warm PBS. Add 0.6 mL of warm methionine/cysteine-deficient medium for labeling, and place cells for 40 min into the CO_2 incubator.
2. Add 8 μL (80 μCi) of ^{35}S-labeled methionine/cysteine. Leave the pipet tip in a radioactive plastic waste container and collect all disposable plastic items contaminated during the experiment. Place the dish into the CO_2 incubator during the labeling period (between 10 min and 1 h) (*see* **Note 4**)
3. Remove the medium and dispose of it in a liquid radioactive waste container. Collect all radioactive liquid waste during the experiment. If a chase period follows, add 1 mL of warm culture medium and place the dish into the CO_2 incubator for the appropriate time period (between minutes and 24 h).

3.3. Further Procedures

3.3.1. Harvest for Direct Immunoprecipitation

Use this procedure to investigate the secretion of HBV surface proteins as subviral particles after a 24-h chase period.

1. Transfer the culture medium after the chase period into a test tube.
2. Prepare a cell lysate by rinsing the cells with 2 mL of cold PBS, incubating the cells with 1 mL of lysis buffer for 15 min at room temperature, detaching the cells by pipetting, and transferring the cell lysate into a test tube.
3. Cell lysate and medium are now ready for immunoprecipitation (**Subheading 3.4.**).

3.3.2. Preparation of Microsomes and Protease-Protection Experiment

For protease-protection experiments, right-side-out microsomes need to be prepared from transfected cells. Protein domains exposed to the cytosolic side of the membrane are located at the outer side of the microsomes and therefore are vulnerable to exogenously added proteases. On the other hand, luminal protein domains are located at the inside of microsomes and therefore are protected from protease attack. By mapping protease-accessible sites of proteins, their transmembrane folding can therefore be deduced. PreS domains **(Fig. 1B)** and the antigen loop of the S protein contain trypsin cleavage sites. The luminal loop of S between transmembrane region I and II is resistant to protease digestion **(Fig. 1B)**. For an example of a protease protection experiment, see **Fig 3**.

1. For a protease-protection experiment, use 85-mm culture dishes for transfection and labeling. Scale up all volumes used in **Subheadings 3.1.** and **3.2.**, by a factor of 5.
2. After removing the labeling medium, place the dish on ice. Wash the cells with 5 mL of cold 1X TBS.
3. Add 1 mL of cold 0.1X TBS to the cells and incubate the dish for further 10 min on ice. Detach the cells by scraping them off using the upper blunt end of a 1-mL pipet tip. Transfer the cell suspension into a cold 2-mL glass homogenizer placed on ice. Rinse the culture dish with 0.2 mL of 0.1X TBS and add this volume to the homogenizer. Lyse the cells by pushing the pestle 20 times up and down. Add 130 μL of cold 10X TBS, transfer the homogenate into a test tube, spin for 15 min at 500*g* in a microfuge at 4°C, and transfer the postnuclear supernatant into a fresh tube.
4. Add 2.7 mL of cold 10 % (w/v) sucrose/1X TBS into a Beckman SW60 ultracentrifuge tube. Add the postnuclear supernatant (approx 1.2 mL) onto the sucrose solution and sediment the microsomes by spinning for 30 min at 4°C and 37,000 rpm in a Beckman ultracentrifuge.
5. Remove the supernatant, wash the pellet with 1 mL of cold 1X TBS, and resuspend the pellet in 1 mL of cold 1X TBS using a syringe and a 23-gauge needle (push 10 times up and down).
6. Divide the microsome preparation into three aliquots (A, B, and C). Add nothing to A, add the protease to B (e.g., 7 μL of 5 mg trypsin/mL in 1X TBS), and add the protease plus 18 μL 10 % (v/v) IGEPAL to C. Incubate for 30 min at 37°C and for another 30 min on ice.
7. In case of trypsin, add 40 μL of PMSF solution and 40 μL of aprotinin to inhibit the protease and incubate 10 min on ice.
8. Add 18 μL of 10 % (v/v) IGEGAL to A and B, add 300 μL of 0.5 % IGEPAL/PBS to all three samples, and incubate for 20 min on ice. Use this material for immunoprecipitation with 2-μL antiserum and 20-μL swollen protein A Sepharose beads.

3.4. Immunoprecipitation

Antibodies for immunoprecipitation are prebound to protein A Sepharose CL-4B bead before use (*see* **Note 5**). For immunoprecipitation using a cell lysate or medium from a 3.5-cm dish, we routinely use 1 μL of antiserum and 2.5 mg of protein A Sepharose CL-4B beads for each sample. This amount of beads will provide 10 μL of swollen gel. For material from an 8-cm culture dish 3 μL of antiserum and 7.5 mg of beads are used.

1. Put the dry Sepharose CL-4B beads into a 1.5-mL test tube.
2. Add 1 mL of PBS, vortex for 30 s; sediment the beads by spinning at 15,000g for 5 s; remove the supernatant but leave 0.1 mL in the tube.
3. Repeat step 2.
4. Add a suitable volume (e.g., 0.6 mL) of PBS and the antiserum. Incubate on a rolling incubator for 2 h at room temperature or overnight at 4°C. If the volume of the protein A gel suspension is too high for the following steps, the beads might be sedimented by short centifugation after the incubation and PBS might be removed from this suspension.

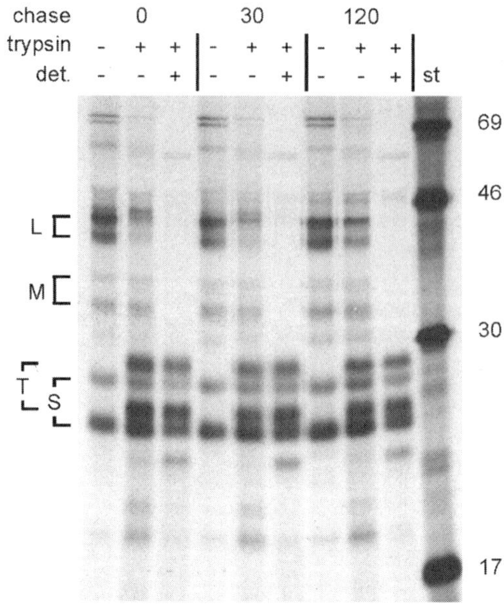

Fig. 3. Protease protection experiment after pulse/chase labeling of HBV S, M, and L protein. COS7 cells transiently transfected with an SV40 early-promoter expression plasmid for HBV S, M, and L protein *(5)* were metabolically labeled with [^{35}S]-methionine/cysteine for 10 min. Microsomes were prepared after 0, 30, and 120 min of chase. One-third of the samples were not treated, one-third were treated with trypsin in the absence, and one-third were treated in the presence of detergent. The preS2 domain of M is not cleaved unless detergent is added, indicating that this domain is in the luminal compartment. After 0 or 30 min of chase, the L protein is cleaved, even in the absence of detergent, indicating the cytosolic location of this domain. The two cleavage products are labeled with "T" and represent the nonglycosylated peptide and glycosylated derivative. After 120 min, a substantial fraction of L is protected, probably because the preS domain of L is transported post-translationally into the ER lumen. st: [^{14}C]-labeled molecular weight standard, numbers indicate molecular weight in kDa. Exposure on autoradiography film for 7 d.

5. Spin the solution containing the antigen for immunoprecipitation for 10 min at full speed and 4°C in a microfuge. Transfer the liquid phase into a fresh test tube and discard the pellet into the radioactive waste.
6. Add the preincubated protein A Sepharose/antibody/PBS mixture corresponding to 1-μL antiserum and 10-μL swollen protein A gel to the antigen (*see* **Note 6**). Incubate with agitation for 2 h at room temperature or overnight at 4°C.
7. Sediment the beads by centrifugation for 5 s and transfer the liquid phase to the radioactive waste. Leave approx 20 μL of liquid in the test tube from aspirating the Sepharose beads. Add 1-mL washing buffer and vortex for 10 s.
8. Repeat **step 7** once or twice, depending on the unspecific background resulting from this experimental procedure in your hands (*see* **Note 7**).
9. Skip **Subheading 3.5.** if endoglycosidase H treatment is not desired.

3.5. Endoglycosidase H Treatment

1. Remove all liquid from the Sepharose beads with a capillary. Add 30 μL endo H buffer and incubate for 5 min at 95°C.
2. Add 2 μL of 1.5 % (v/v) IGEPAL, mix, and divide the sample into two equal parts by transferring 16 μL of the supernatant into a fresh tube. Ignore the Sepharose beads. Add 0.5 μL of endo H to one sample and incubate both samples at 37°C overnight.
3. Spin the tubes briefly and add 4 μL water to each sample to adjust the volume to 20 μL.

3.6. Polyacrylamide Gel Electrophoresis and Autoradiography (see Note 8)

1. Add 20 μL of 2X gel-loading buffer containing SDS and 10% (w/v) DTT.
2. Boil the sample for 5 min and load it onto a 13% polyacrylamide gel. It does not matter whether Sepharose beads are transferred or not.
3. Place the gel on a piece of Whatman paper after electrophoresis and dry the gel at 80°C in a vacuum gel drier.
4. Expose the dried gel to an autoradiography film or a phosphoimager screen.

4. Notes

1. The HBV surface proteins can be expressed in a variety of cell lines. In our laboratory, we routinely use plasmids carrying the SV40 origin of replication/early promoter for the expression of foreign proteins. This promoter is efficient in COS7 cells, which constitutively express the SV40 large T-antigen mediating episome amplification and strong transcription.
2. Transfection efficiencies vary strongly between different cell types. For other cell lines, different transfection procedure might be more efficient. In our hands, using COS7 cells, the transfection efficiency of the described procedure is similar to some commercially available transfection kits.
3. A convenient way to test the transfection efficiency using HBV surface protein–expression vectors is to measure the amount of HBsAg secreted into the culture medium by commercially available HBsAg enzyme-linked immunosorbent assays. Using wild-type S protein and the protocol described here, the amount of HBsAg in the medium should reach approx 3 μg/mL 2 d after transient transfection. A 1:200 dilution of the medium should give a signal in the upper linear range of the test.
4. To avoid radioactive contamination of the CO_2 incubator during the labeling and chase period, we place the culture dish into a plastic box in the incubator together with an open dish containing active charcoal. The charcoal will bind low amounts of radioactive gasses that might evaporate from the culture dish.
5. Antibodies bind to protein A with different affinities, depending on the isotype and species. The light and heavy chains of immunoglobulin G isolated from 1 μL of antiserum by protein-A binding should result in two clearly visible bands around 30 kDa and 60 kDa in a polyacrylamide gel after Coomassie staining.
6. Aliquotting of a suspension of Sepharose CL-4B beads requires continuous resuspension of the beads because they sediment rather quickly simply by gravitation. Sepharose CL-4B beads have a large diameter. Therefore, for pipetting the pipet tips should be shortened by approx 5 mm with a scissors to increase their aperture.
7. If the background on the autoradiogram is low, PBS might be used for washing the immune complexes bound to protein A instead of washing buffer. This step might enhance the specific signal but might also enhance the background signal.

8. Use a mock transfection with a plasmid carrying no relevant insertion or preimmune serum as a negative control.

References

1. Blumberg, B. S. (1997) Hepatitis B virus, the vaccine, and the control of primary cancer of the liver. *Proc. Natl. Acad. Sci. USA* **94**, 7121–7125.
2. Heermann, K. H., Goldmann U., Schwartz, W., Seyffarth, T., Baumgarten H., and Gerlich, W. H. (1984) Large surface proteins of hepatitis B virus containing the pre-S sequence. *J. Virol.* **52**, 396–402.
3. Cattaneo, R., Will, H., Hernandez, N., and Schaller, H. (1983) Signals regulating hepatitis B surface antigen transcription. *Nature* **305**, 336–338.
4. Zang, W. O., and Yen, T. S. (1999) Distinct export pathway utilized by the hepatitis B virus posttranscriptional regulatory element. *Virology* **259**, 299–304.
5. Bruss, V., Lu, X., Thomssen, R., and Gerlich, W. H. (1994) Post-translational alterations in transmembrane topology of the hepatitis B virus large envelope protein. *EMBO J.* **13**, 2273–2279.
6. Ostapchuck, P., Hearing, P., and Ganem, D. (1994) A dramatic shift in the transmembrane topology of a viral envelope glycoprotein accompanies hepatitis B viral morphogenesis. *EMBO J.* **13**, 1048–1057.
7. Prange, R., and Streeck, R. E. (1995) Novel transmembrane topology of the hepatitis B virus envelope proteins. *EMBO J.* **14**, 247–356.
8. Wunderlich, G., and Bruss, V. (1996) Characterization of early hepatitis B virus surface protein oligomers. *Arch. Virol.* **141**, 1191–1205.
9. Sambrook, J., Fritsch, E. F., and Maniatis, T. (1989) *Molecular Cloning: A Laboratory Manual.* Cold Spring Harbor Laboratory, Cold Spring Harbor, NY.
10. Loeffler-Mary, H., Dumortier, J., Klentsch-Zimmer, C., and Prange, R. (2000) Hepatitis B virus assembly is sensitive to changes in the cytosolic S loop of the envelope proteins. *Virology* **270**, 359–367.

20

Binding of Duck Carboxypeptidase D to Duck Hepatitis B Virus

Stephan Urban

1. Introduction

The initial step in viral infection is binding of the particle to a receptor on the host-cell surface. The specificity of this process is the outcome of an evolutionary adaptation of the pathogen to its host. Receptor recognition frequently determines host specificity and tissue tropism. For enveloped viruses, binding is followed by fusion of the virus membrane with either the plasma or an endosomal membrane. The general mechanism of membrane fusion involves conformational changes of virus-encoded fusion proteins, leading to physical approximation and finally merging of viral and cellular membranes. A detailed understanding of receptor binding and membrane fusion is not only of general interest for molecular virologists, it also provides the basis for therapeutics that interfere with infection.

Hepatitis B viruses are a group of small, enveloped DNA viruses that cause acute and chronic liver infection in mammals and birds. Biochemical approaches combined with functional studies led to the discovery of one receptor component in the duck hepatitis B virus (DHBV) model system: carboxypeptidase D (CPD; formerly gp180; ***1–4***). Duck CPD (duCPD) turned out to be the prototype of a family of membrane-bound regulatory carboxypeptidases with a unique domain architecture (**Fig. 1**). The highly glycosylated extracytosolic/luminal part of duCPD comprises about 170 kDa of its molecular weight and consists of three homologous carboxypeptidase E-like domains. Two of them, domains 1 and 2 (also called A and B), have enzymatic activity, whereas domain 3 (or C) is inactive as a carboxypeptidase *(5)* but binds duck, heron, and probably all other avian hepatitis B viruses *(6)*.

Virus binding does not depend on glycosylation and is mediated by only one of the two viral envelope proteins: the L protein *(1)*. The L (or large) protein contains a hydrophobic C-terminal transmembrane region, the so-called S part that serves as an anchor in the virus membrane, and a hydrophilic N-terminal extension of 161 amino

From: *Methods in Molecular Medicine, vol. 95: Hepatitis B and D Protocols, volume 1*
Edited by: R. K. Hamatake and J. Y. N. Lau © Humana Press Inc., Totowa, NJ

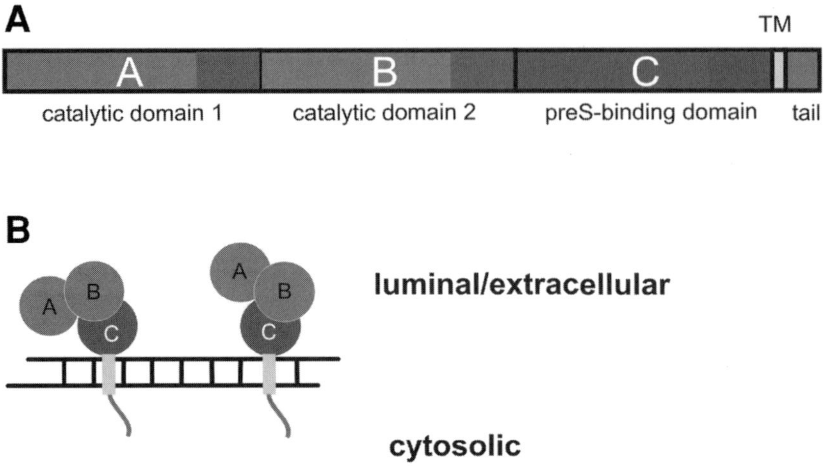

Fig. 1. **(A)** Domain structure of duCPD. The carboxypeptidase E-like catalytic domains are marked with A and B, the enzymatically inactive DHBV-binding domain with C. The transmembrane domain is designated TM, and the highly conserved 60 amino-acid cytoplasmic tail is designated tail. **(B)** Topology of duCPD. Note that the DHBV-binding domain is closest to the cellular membrane.

acids, termed preS. Within preS, an internal subdomain encompassing amino acids 30–115 is sufficient for CPD binding *(7)*. This receptor-binding domain consists of a partly α-helical essential region and a stabilizing element **(Fig. 2)**. C terminal to the three luminal carboxypeptidase domains is a transmembrane-anchor sequence and a highly conserved cytoplasmic tail of 60 amino acids **(Fig. 1)**. The tail sequence and its modification determine vesicular trafficking of CPDs, including endocytosis from the cell surface to their place of residence, the *trans*-Golgi network *(8,9)*.

Before describing the methods and techniques that have successfully been applied to purify DHBV preS (DpreS) and duCPD and to investigate the interaction of both proteins, it is worthwhile to stress some noticeable features when compared with receptor interactions of other viruses. Virus-binding domains of proteinaceous attachment receptors are usually located opposite to the domain that is linked to the transmembrane region. Conversely, DHBV binds the membrane adjacent to domain 3 of duCPD *(6,10)*.

The monomeric DpreS ligand is able to complex with duCPD with an exceptionally high affinity. At 37°C, the dissociation constant K_d was determined to be 1.5 n*M*, which is about 30 times lower than that for poliovirus at 4°C *(10)*. Thus, the bimolecular interaction of DpreS and duCPD provides an affinity that is usually obtained for an entire viral particle when contacting several receptor molecules.

The preS subdomain involved in high affinity duCPD binding comprises about 85 amino acids (amino acids 30–115). This receptor-binding site is predominantly unstructured in solution (80% random coil, 20% α-helix) *(10)*. Thus, DHBV/receptor interaction represents one of the few examples involving a protein ligand with a random conformation.

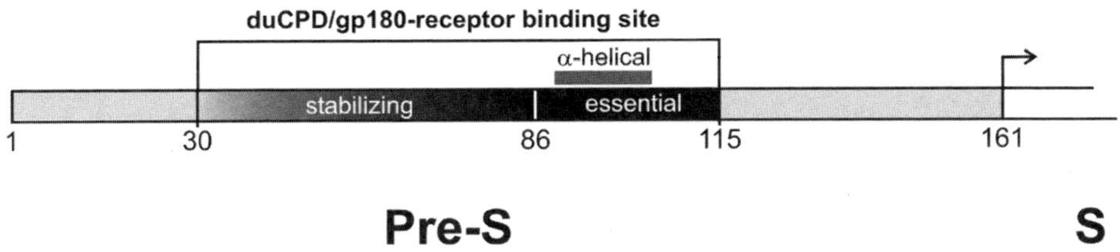

Fig. 2. Schematic representation of the preS domain of the DHBV L protein. PreS consists of 161 hydrophilic amino acids. Amino acids 30–115 represent the duCPD–receptor-binding domain. This domain contains a partially α-helical essential element (amino acids 86–115) and an N terminally located part that contributes to complex stabilization (amino acids 30–85). The hydrophobic S part (shown only as an outline) anchors preS in the viral membrane.

Binding of DpreS to duCPD induces conformational alterations of the receptor structure itself. This fact points to a function of duCPD that exceeds its function as only an attachment receptor and raises the possibility that it actively takes part in the formation of a prefusion complex.

1.1. Purification of CPD from Tissues

CPD was initially isolated from whole duck-liver lysates by DpreS-affinity chromatography. The specific binding of duCPD to DpreS was the first indication that CPD may function as a DHBV receptor *(1)*. **Figure 3** shows the result of a related experiment, described in detail in **Subheading 3.3.** With this method, duCPD can be partially purified from duck-liver extracts. However, for preparative purposes, the standard purification of CPDs, described by Song and Fricker *(5)* using PABA (para-amino-benzoyl-arginine) Sepharose, is recommended. PABA-affinity chromatography allows the enrichment of the regulatory carboxypeptidases from probably all species that both express these enzymes and contain an enzymatically active CPE-like carboxypeptidase domain.

1.2. Purification of Recombinant Soluble Forms of duCPD

To quantitatively investigate the interaction of duCPD with DHBV-preS, it is much more suitable to use soluble CPD variants that can be obtained in reasonable amounts (1–5 mg per 500-mL cell culture) and excellent purity from recombinant sources. One expression system used to acquire the complete extracellular portion of duCPD or the duCPD C domain is the baculovirus expression system *(7,* and *see* **Subheading 3.**). In addition, the yeast *Pichia pastoris* has successfully been used as a source for domain 2 for crystallization purposes *(11)*.

In addition to baculoviruses, recombinant adenoviruses encoding complete duCPD as well as fragments and mutants thereof are suitable for transduced expression in hepatocytes in vitro *(12)* and also in vivo. This approach allows studies of receptor function by means of transdominant expression of mutants. However, our attempts to obtain duCPD from *Escherichia coli* in a functional form, even when directed to the

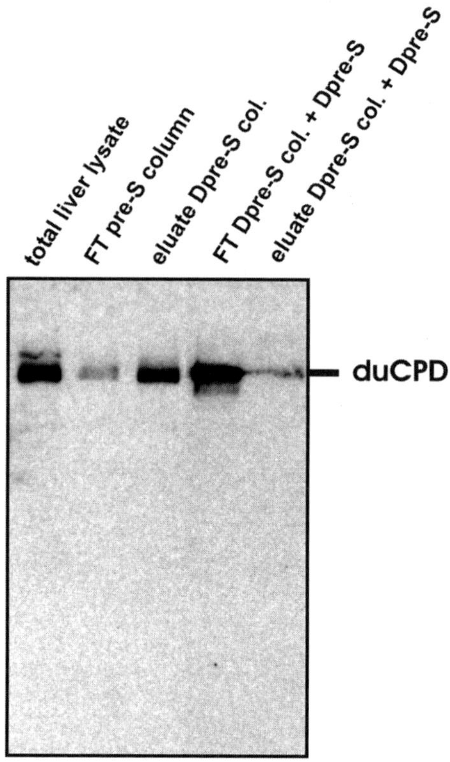

Fig. 3. Binding of duck liver–derived CPD to a DpreS affinity column. A solubilized duck-liver lysate was applied to a DpreS Sepharose column in the absence and presence of DpreS as described in **Subheading 3.3.1.** Flow-through (FT) fractions and eluates were separated on a 7.5% SDS gel and blotted, and duCPD was detected with a specific antibody.

periplasm, failed. This failure is not the result of low protein levels but rather to improper folding of the highly disulfide-bridged domains. Nevertheless, this approach can be used to generate large amounts of denatured protein for immunization purposes.

As for full-length CPD, purification of variants that lack the transmembrane region but contain an active carboxypeptidase domain 1 or 2 is best performed on PABA Sepharose. We routinely use the buffers described for purification of the complete protein without detergent (*see* **Subheading 3.4.**). Subfragments of CPD (e.g., the C domain) that do not contain at least one active carboxypeptidase domain either have to be purified by conventional chromatography or as described in **Subheading 3.5.** by DpreS-affinity chromatography ***(10)***. Disruption of the DpreS–duCPD complex can be achieved by a pH shift to 4.5–4.0. This critical step allows a complete recovery of active C domain provided that the eluted protein is immediately rebuffered to a neutral pH. This process is best performed by adding 1/10 volume of 1 *M* Tris-HCl pH 8.0 to the eluate.

1.3. Binding of DHBV PreS to Duck CPD

Binding of DpreS polypeptides or DHBV particles to duCPD has been performed by several different methods. The easiest and most convenient methods take advantage of *E. coli*–derived preS polypeptides that have been purified by some kind of affinity tag, e.g., glutathione-*S*-transferase (GST) ***(1)*** or histidine ***(3)***. In the case of a hexahistidine fusion, most DpreS fragments are targeted to inclusion bodies and need to be solubilized and purified under denaturing conditions ***(3)***. However, because the preS domain is not folded in an extensive three-dimensional structure ***(10)***, complete renaturation can be achieved by simple dialysis against the appropriate buffer (highest solubility was obtained in 25 m*M* NaP_i, pH 6.3). For binding assays, these tags can be used to coprecipitate duCPD ***(1,2)***. Alternatively, the fusion proteins can be covalently immobilized on plastic wells or activated CH Sepharose (*see* **Subheading 3.2.**). For elaborate studies on the binding kinetics of DHBV preS and duCPD, it is recommended that surface plasmon resonance spectroscopy (BIAcore) be used as described ***(7,10)***. Because this technique is not applicable in most laboratories, we developed a semiquantitative assay based on covalent immobilization of DHBV preS on 96-well plates (covalink plates) containing free amino groups (*see* **Subheading 3.6.**).

An approach that more closely resembles the natural situation is the recombinant expression of duCPD in primary duck hepatocytes or heterologous cell lines (such as HepG2 and HuH7) followed by the measurement of DHBV-particle or DpreS binding and uptake. Labeling of the respective ligand with ^{125}I, rhodamine, or other fluorescent dyes allows the quantification of ligand binding/uptake and facilitates studies on receptor trafficking ***(12)***.

An example of this kind of assay is shown in **Fig. 4** and is described in **Subheading 3.7.** This approach has also been used to map sequence elements within CPD that are important for DHBV interaction ***(13)***. Binding of duCPD-specific antibodies to cell-surface–exposed duCPD results in uptake of the antibody and retrieval to the *trans*-Golgi network ***(8)***. Interestingly, duCPD-mediated uptake of DHBV particles leads to a redirection of the receptor/particle complex to the lysosomal pathway, indicating that virus binding induces signaling pathways that interfere with the default retrieval pathway of duCPD ***(12)***.

2. Materials (*see* Note 1)

Unless otherwise stated, all reagents used are of analytical grade.

2.1. DpreS Purification

1. TB medium: Dissolve 24 g Bacto-Trypton (Gibco), 48 g Bacto Yeast-Extract (Gibco), and 8 mL 100% glycerol in 1.8-L distilled water and sterilize at 120°C for 30 min. Add 200 mL sterile 10X phosphate buffer (170 m*M* KH_2PO_4, 720 m*M* K_2HPO_4) prior to use.
2. 1,000-Fold IPTG-stock solution: Dissolve 2.38 g IPTG (BTS Biotech, cat. no. CH8102) in 10 mL water. Prepare aliquots of 1 mL and store at –70°C.

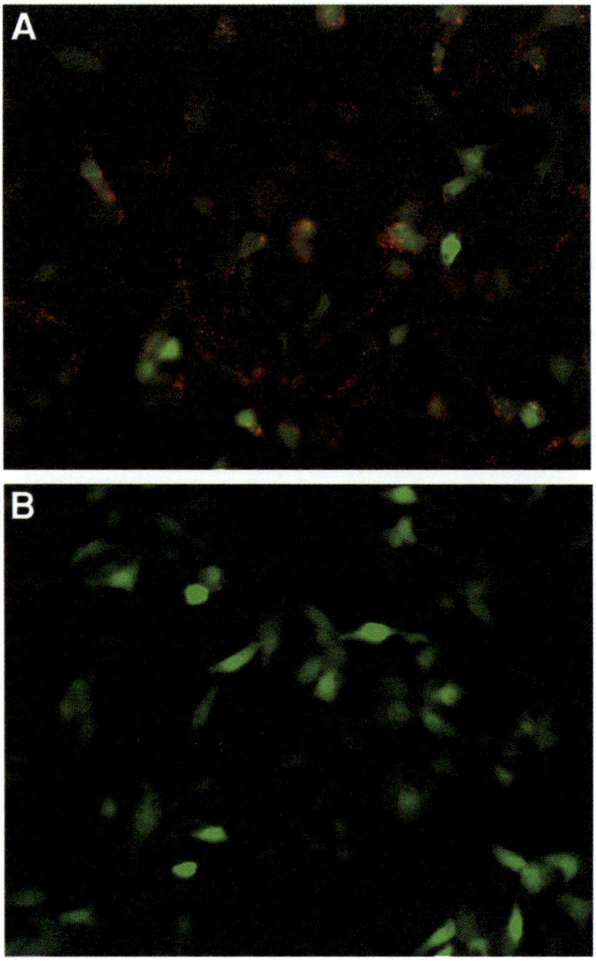

Fig. 4. Binding of rhodamine–labeled DpreS to HepG2 cells that express a cell surface–located mutant of duCPD. HepG2 cells were infected with recombinant adenoviruses encoding a CPD mutant that lacks the cytosolic tail and is therefore localized at the cell surface and GFP as a marker. **(A)** Binding of rhodamine labeled DpreS (red) to CPD-expressing HepG2 cells (green). **(B)** Binding can be inhibited with the monoclonal antibody mAb 4F8 that recognizes an epitope within the essential part of the DHBV–receptor-binding site.

3. PreS solubilization buffer A: 6 *M* guanidine hydrochloride, 100 m*M* NaP_i, 10 m*M* Tris-HCl, pH 8.0. Sterile filter this solution through a 0.45-μm nitrocellulose filter to remove fine particles and store at 4°C. The solution is stable for several months.
4. Buffer B: 7 *M* urea, 100 m*M* NaP_i, 10 m*M* Tris-HCl, pH 8.0. Sterile filter this solution prior to use. Do not store this solution longer than 1 wk.

5. Buffer C: 7 *M* urea, 100 m*M* NaP_i, 10 m*M* Tris-HCl, pH 6.30. Sterile filter this solution prior to use. Carefully control the pH before use and do not store this solution longer than 1 wk.
6. Elution buffer D: 7 *M* urea, 250 m*M* imidazole (Sigma I 0250), 100 m*M* NaP_i, 10 m*M* Tris-HCl, pH 6.30. Sterile filter this solution prior to use and do not store longer than 1 wk. Use pure imidazole, otherwise there will be absorption by contaminants at 280 nm.
7. S 200 running buffer: Add 100 mL 10X phosphate-buffered saline (PBS), pH 7.4, to 240 g urea, and fill up with distilled water to 1 L. Remove fines by sterile filtration. Use immediately.
8. preS dialysis buffer: 25 m*M* NaP_i, pH 6.3.
9. Ni^{2+}NTA-agarose superflow, Qiagen, cat. no. 1004493.
10. Dialysis tube SpectraPor, Serva, cat. no. 44185.
11. Column, XK16/20, Amersham Bioscience, cat. no. 18-8773-01.

2.2. Covalent Immobilization of DpreS and PABA to Fixed Matrices

1. Sulfo-NHS solution: Dissolve 3.48 mg *N*-hydroxysulfosuccinimide (Pierce, cat. no. 24510) in 1 mL pure water. Make fresh as required.
2. EDC solution: Dissolve 3.07 mg 1-ethyl-3-[3-dimethylaminopropyl] carbodiimide hydrochloride (Pierce, cat. no. 22980) in 1 mL double-distilled water. Make fresh as required.
3. Covalink immunoplates NH modules (Nunc, cat. no. 478042).
4. Activated CH Sepharose 4B (Amersham Bioscience, cat. no. 17-0490-01).
5. PABA coupling buffer: 0.1 *M* $NaHCO_3$, 0.5 *M* NaCl.
6. NHS-rhodamine solution: Dissolve 1 mg NHS-rhodamine (Pierce, cat. no. 46102) in 100 μL dimenthy-l-formamide DMSO. Do not store this solution.
7. PD10 size exclusion column (Amersham Bioscience, cat. no. 17-0851-01).

2.3. Purification of duCPD from Duck Liver

1. CPD solubilization buffer: 1% octylglucoside, 50 m*M* NaP_i, 150 m*M* NaCl, 0.5 m*M* DTT, 1 tablet Roche protease inhibitors (Roche, cat. no. 1697498), pH 7.4.
2. preS elution buffer: 1% octylglucoside, 100 m*M* NaAc, 0, 5 m*M* DTT, pH 4.0.
3. PABA buffer: 1% octylglycoside, 20 m*M* NaAc, 1 *M* NaCl, 1 m*M* PMSF, pH 5.5.
4. CP elution buffer 1: 50 m*M* Tris-HCl, pH 8.0, 100 m*M* NaCl, and 0.1% octylglycoside.
5. CP elution buffer 2: 20 m*M* Tris-HCl pH 8.0, 25 m*M* arginine, and 0.1 % octylglycoside.
6. CPD dialysis buffer: 50 m*M* Tris-HCl, pH 8.0, 100 m*M* NaCl, and 0.1% octylglycoside.

2.4. Recombinant Expression and Purification of Soluble duCPD Variants

1. High Five insect cells, Invitrogen, cat. no. B855-02.
2. TNM-FH, insect medium, Sigma, cat. no. T 3285, add 10 mL/500 mL 200 m*M* glutamine and 5 mL/500 mL Pen/Strep prior to use (for flask cultures).
3. ExCell 405 medium, JRH Bioscience, cat. no. 14405-79P, add 10 mL/500 mL 200 m*M* glutamine and 5 mL/500 mL Pen/Strep prior to use (for spinner cultures).
4. PABA equilibration buffer B: 20 m*M* NaAc, 1 *M* NaCl, pH 5.5.
5. PABA wash buffer: 10 m*M* NaAc, pH 5.5.
6. PABA elution buffer B: 50 m*M* L-arginine in 20 m*M* Tris-HCl, pH 8.0.
7. HiLoad 16/60 Superdex 200 prep grade column (Amersham Bioscience, cat. no. 17-1069-01).
8. S 200 running buffer: 25 m*M* NaP_i, 150 m*M* NaCl, pH 6.8.

2.5. Recombinant Expression and Purification of a Soluble CPD C Domain

1. CPD-C washing buffer: 50 m*M* Tris-HCl, 150 m*M* NaCl, pH 7.4.
2. CPD-C elution buffer: 100 m*M* NaAc, pH 4.0.
3. CPD-C dialysis buffer: 25 m*M* NaP_i, pH 7.0.

3. Methods

3.1. Recombinant Expression and Purification of DHBV PreS Polypeptides (*see* Note 2)

3.1.1. Expression of PreS in *E. coli*

1. Transform *E. coli* M15pREP4 cells (Qiagen) with pQE expression plasmids encoding the respective hexahistidine preS sequences.
2. Grow this culture in 2 L TB medium in a 5 L Erlenmeyer flask in the presence of 100 μg/mL ampicillin and 25 μg/mL kanamycin to an OD_{600} of 1.0 and induce with 2 mL IPTG-stock solution (final concentration: 1 m*M*) for 4 h at 37°C. Ensure sufficient air supply by rapidly shaking the culture.
3. Harvest the cells by centrifugation at 4,500*g* for 20 min in a Sorvall preparative centrifuge and wash the bacterial pellet in 200 mL PBS.
4. Centrifuge the bacterial pellet and either freeze bacteria at –20°C or proceed with **Subheading 3.1.2.**

3.1.2. Purification of Hexahistidine PreS Fusion Proteins

1. Lyse the bacterial pellet in 75 mL preS solubilization buffer A through gentle agitation for 15 min in a bacterial shaker. Make sure that all bacteria have been released from the tube and centrifuge at 50,000*g* for 30 min (SW 28 rotor).
2. Apply the supernatant to a 10 mL Ni^{2+}NTA-agarose superflow column (flow rate 0.5 mL/min) connected to a peristaltic pump (or, if available, to an FPLC chromatography system).
3. Wash with 100-mL buffer B (flow rate 2 mL/min) and subsequently with 30-mL buffer C to get rid of most nonspecifically bound *E. coli* proteins. (This step will also lead to a partial loss of DpreS, which should be taken into account.)
4. Elute the denatured hexahistidine-tagged preS polypeptide with elution buffer D.
5. Collect the eluate in 2–3 mL fractions, determine the OD_{280}, and pool fractions with the highest protein content (OD_{280} will exceed 2.0 for the main fractions, OD = 1 corresponds to about 0.9 mg/mL).
6. For further purification and removal of imidazole, apply 2 mL of the pooled protein fractions to a Superdex S 200 gel-filtration column (1.6 × 60 cm), connected to a chromatography device (FPLC) equilibrated with S 200 running buffer.
7. Discard minor peak fractions and pool the major peak, eluting at an apparent molecular weight of about 35 kDa (V_e/V_0 of about 2). Note that the high proline content of the preS sequence leads to an increase of apparent molecular weight in gel filtration and SDS PAGE.
8. For long-term storage, freeze the pooled fractions at –20°C.
9. To remove urea and induce folding of the few secondary structural elements within DpreS, dialyze three times against 5 L preS dialysis buffer. It is important to use dialysis tubes with an exclusion size below 3.5 kDa (e.g., SpectraPor 3500).
10. Store the purified protein at 4°C in the presence of 0.05% sodium azide. This protocol is suitable for all DHBV and HBV preS constructs.

3.2. Covalent Coupling and Labeling of DHBV PreS and PABA to Fixed Matrices

3.2.1. Coupling of DpreS to Covalink Immunoplates

1. Analytical binding studies of DpreS to duCPD are best performed using covalink 96-well immunoplate NH modules. To prepare these plates, place 15–30 μg DpreS or variants thereof in 100 μL 25 m*M* NaP_i, pH 6.3 per well, add 50 μL sulfo-NHS solution followed by 50 μL EDC solution and incubate for 60 min at room temperature with gentle agitation.
2. Wash the plates three times with 300 μL distilled water and three times with 300 μL PBS.
3. Block with 200 μL 2% bovine serum albumin (BSA) in PBS for 30 min.
4. It is suggested to immobilize a DpreS deletion mutant that is completely deficient in duCPD binding (e.g., DpreSΔ85-96) as a control.
5. PreS-coated wells can be stored at 4°C in 20% EtOH or PBS containing 0.05% sodium azide for several days. It is worthwhile to note that preS-coated wells can be regenerated by washing three times with 1 m*M* HCl and re-equilibration with binding buffer without loss of binding activity.

3.2.2. Coupling of DHBV PreS Polypeptides to Activated CH Sepharose 4B

1. Soak 3.5 g activated CH Sepharose in 25 mL of 1 m*M* HCl for 10 min.
2. Place the swollen gel (about 10 mL) onto a fine-glass-sintered filter and continuously wash with 1 L of 1 m*M* HCl to remove the stabilizers of the reactive groups.
3. Resuspend the wet gel matrix in 30 mL dialyzed DpreS (about 0.25–0.5 mg/mL in 50 m*M* NaP_i, pH 7.0–7.5) and gently shake the suspension for 4 h at room temperature. It is important to extensively dialyze DpreS prior to coupling to remove all traces of urea, otherwise the free NH_2 groups of urea compete with DpreS for the reactive CH groups of the gel.
4. Fill the gel suspension into a suitable column (e.g., XK 16/20), equilibrate with 0.5 *M* Tris-HCl, pH 7.5 (neutralization of uncoupled reactive groups), and incubate overnight. Alternatively, wash the column with 1 m*M* HCl and 0.1 *M* Tris-HCl, pH 8.5, and equilibrate with binding buffer.
5. Monitor the coupling efficiency by SDS-PAGE and Coomassie staining of the matrix supernatant. No free DpreS should be detectable in the supernatant after the reaction.
6. If not in use, store the column in 20% EtOH at 4°C.

3.2.3. Synthesis and Preparative Coupling of PABA to Activated CH Sepharose

1. PABA was synthesized by a combination of the methods described by Hitchcock et al. ***(14)*** as well as Plummer and Horwitz ***(15)***. The product was recrystallized and its structure was verified by ^{3}H-nuclear magnetic resonance (NMR), ^{13}C NMR, and mass spectrometry.
2. Soak 3.5 g activated CH Sepharose 4B in 50 mL of 1 m*M* HCl for 10 min.
3. Place the gel onto a sintered glass filter and wash for additional 15 min with 1 L of 1 m*M* HCl.
4. Dissolve 225–450 mg PABA. $H_2SO_4 \cdot H_2O$ (500 μmol to 1 mmol) in 15 mL PABA-coupling buffer.
5. Adjust the pH to 8.0 by adding 1 *M* $NaHCO_3$ (about 2.5 mL required).
6. Incubate the mixture for 3 h at room temperature (gentle agitation) and pour the gel into a suitable column (e.g., XK 16/20, Amersham Bioscience).
7. Wash with 100 mL coupling buffer and block remaining active sites with 1 *M* Tris-HCl, pH 8.0 (or as an alternative 250 m*M* ethanolamine, pH 8.0).
8. After washing with 100 m*M* NaAc, 500 m*M* NaCl pH 4.0, and 100 m*M* Tris-HCl/500 m*M* NaCl pH 8.0, store the column in 20% ethanol.

3.2.4. Labeling of DpreS Polypeptides and DHBV Particles with Rhodamine

1. Add 10 μL freshly prepared NHS-rhodamine stock solution to 1 mL DpreS (0.5 mg/mL), buffered in 100 m*M* Na-borate, pH 8.5.
2. Incubate for 1 h at room temperature.
3. Separate the labeled preS from the unreacted dye by a PD-10 size exclusion column (Amersham Bioscience). To do this, equilibrate the column with 25 m*M* NaP_i, pH 6.3 (25 mL), apply 1 mL of the reaction mixture, and collect in 1-mL fractions. Rhodamine-labeled DpreS elutes in fractions 3 and 4. The same approach is suitable for labeling of purified subviral particles.

3.3. Partial Purification of duCPD from Duck Liver (*see* Note 3)

3.3.1. Enrichment of duCPD from Duck Liver by DpreS Affinity Chromatography

1. Cut 10 g of a DHBV-negative duck liver (*see* **Note 4**) into small pieces, add 50 mL of ice cold CPD-solubilization buffer, and homogenize with about 50 strokes using a Dounce homogenizer.
2. Allow membrane proteins to dissolve for about 30 min under gentle agitation on ice and remove debris by centrifugation at 200,000*g* for 30 min.
3. Fill a suitable column (e.g., XK16/20) with 5 mL DpreS Sepharose and extensively recirculate the protein extract for 10–14 h at 4°C with a peristaltic pump.
4. Wash with 20 bed volumes CPD-solubilization buffer and elute with preS elution buffer.
5. As a control for binding specificity, perform a parallel experiment in the presence of a surplus of free DpreS (50 μg/mL) added to the membrane extract as a competitor prior to the application to the column **(Fig. 3).**

3.3.2. Purification of duCPD by PABA Affinity Chromatography

1. Alternatively apply the liver extract (or extracts from other organs) onto a PABA column, prepared according to the protocol described in **Subheading 3.2.3.**
2. After 10-fold recircularization of the solubilized cell extract, wash with 10 column volumes PABA buffer and elute carboxypeptidase E with CP elution buffer 1.
3. Subsequently elute CPD with CP elution buffer 2.
4. To remove arginine and to rebuffer, dialyze protein-containing fractions against CPD dialysis buffer and monitor the purity of the protein on a 7.5 % SDS gel.
5. Store purified duCPD at –70°C in 50% glycerol.

3.4. Recombinant Expression and Purification of Soluble CPD Variants that Contain an Active Carboxypeptidase Domain from a Baculovirus Expression System (*see* Note 5)

3.4.1. Expression and Partial Purification of Soluble CPD

1. Infect 1.8×10^7 High Five insect cells (Invitrogen), per one T175 flask with 2×10^8 recombinant baculoviruses encoding the respective duCPD fragment under control of the polyhedrin promoter (MOI = 10). Alternatively, grow suspension culture–adapted High Five insect cells (250–500 mL) using Fernbach flasks. To avoid contamination with serum albumin, it is recommended that serum-free medium be used as described in **Subheading 2.4.**
2. Incubate infected cells at 27°C for 72 h to allow protein expression.

3. Centrifuge the culture at 3000*g* for 15 min to remove cells and pass the supernatant through a 0.45-μm nitrocellulose filter.
4. Adjust the pH of the cell culture supernatant to 5.5 with acetic acid and apply it to a PABA–Sepharose column (15 mL bed volume, flow rate of 0.5 mL/min). For preparation of the column, see **Subheading 3.2.3.** Perform all purification steps at 4°C.
5. To remove nonspecifically bound proteins, wash the column extensively (at least 15 bed volumes) with PABA equilibration buffer B.
6. Subsequently wash with five bed volumes of PABA wash buffer and elute the soluble duCPD fragment in 1-mL fractions through PABA elution buffer B.
7. Measure the OD_{280} of each fraction, perform standard SDS-PAGE and pool accordingly. Protein-containing fractions will be highly enriched in soluble CPD. However, we have noted that they contain baculovirus-encoded chitinase, which binds PABA for unknown reasons. Moreover, the soluble CPD consists of monomeric and oligomeric forms that differ in their preS binding affinities for hitherto unknown reasons. For qualitative analyses, the purity of this preparation is sufficient.

3.4.2. Separation of Oligomeric and Monomeric Forms of CPD

For quantitative analytical purposes, it is necessary to separate the oligomeric and monomeric forms of duCPD and to remove the contaminating chitinase. This process can easily be performed on a Superdex 200 HR gel filtration column connected to a chromatographic device.

1. Apply 2 mL of the pooled CPD-containing fractions from **Subheading 3.4.1.** onto the column equilibrated with S 200 running buffer and elute at a flow rate of 2.2 mL/min.
2. Oligomeric duCPD elutes shortly after the void volume at about 50 mL, monomeric duCPD at an apparent molecular weight of 250 kDA, and chitinase at about 50 kDA.
3. The monomeric duCPD is of high purity and can be used for DHBV preS-binding studies *(7)*.
4. To determine the protein concentration, measure the OD_{280}. Calculate the protein concentration on the basis of a molar extinction coefficient ϵ = 159,400 as described in ref. ***16***.

3.5. Recombinant Expression and Purification of a Soluble CPD C Domain Without an Active Carboxypeptidase Domain.

1. Use the respective baculoviruses encoding a secretable duCPD C domain to infect High Five insect cells and prepare cell-culture supernatants according to the protocol described in **Subheading 3.4.1.**
2. Adjust the pH of the cell-culture supernatant to 7.4 with 0.1 *N* NaOH and apply it to the DHBV preS-affinity column prepared as described in **Subheading 3.2.2.** (bed volume 10 mL, flow rate 0.5 mL/min, 4°C).
3. Wash with 20 bed volumes CPD-C washing buffer (flow rate: 1mL/min, 4°C).
4. Warm up the column to 37°C (use a fan) and elute with CPD-C elution buffer (*see* **Note 6**).
5. Immediately dialyze the duCPD-C–containing fractions against CPD-C dialysis buffer. The protein is of high purity, consists exclusively of its monomeric form, and can be stored at 70°C after addition of 50% sucrose.
6. Determine the protein concentrations by measuring the extinction at 280nm. The theoretical molar extinction coefficient ϵ for duCPD-C is 43,960. Eventually, concentrate the protein in Amicon ultracentrifugation tubes.

3.6. Binding of duCPD to DHBV PreS

3.6.1. In Vitro Binding Assays Using Recombinant DpreS Proteins

Binding and binding-competition assays are performed using DpreS-coated covalink plates prepared as described in **Subheading 3.2.1.**

1. Add 100 μL of duCPD-containing fractions (e.g., crude-cell extracts and duCPD-containing media supernatants) and incubate overnight at 4°C. To avoid evaporation, seal the wells with parafilm.
2. Collect the supernatant and wash five times with PBS or binding buffer.
3. Elute bound proteins with 100 μL SDS sample buffer at about 80°C. This is best accomplished by placing the wells on a heated metal plate and gentle shaking.
4. Perform SDS-PAGE and CPD-specific Western blots with the supernatant and the eluted fractions (*see* **Note 7**).

3.6.2. Binding and Uptake of DpreS and DHBV Particles in CPD-expressing Cells

To perform binding and uptake studies in a cellular context, duCPD can be expressed in a variety of cell lines followed by incubation with fluorescently labeled DpreS polypeptides or labeled particles. This process is exemplarily described for transduced HepG2 cells below and depicted in **Fig. 4.**

1. Grow HepG2 cells to 40% confluence and infect them with a recombinant adenovirus that encodes duCPD and green fluorescent protein (GFP) as a marker (MOI 1–5).
2. Incubate cells until the GFP fluorescence is clearly detectable (24–36 h) and add 5–10 μL rhodamine-labeled DpreS.
3. Incubate for another 1–4 h at 37°C, wash twice with PBS, and visualize DpreS-rhodamine binding in a fluorescence microscope through excitation at 544 nm.
4. As an alternative to adenovirus-mediated transduction of duCPD, transfect cells by either standard calcium phosphate procedures or lipofection. Ensure the specificity of this assay by addition of antibodies that interfere with binding (e.g., mAb 4F8) or the utilization of binding-deficient–DpreS mutants (e.g., rhodamine-labeled DpreSΔ85–96). Variations of these kinds of experiments not only facilitate studies of receptor binding in living cells but also provide the basis for detailed analyses of DHBV/receptor trafficking. Since we are far away from a comparable state of knowledge for the human hepatitis B virus, we might still learn fascinating lessons from this unique mode of hepadnavirus-receptor usage.

4. Notes

1. Plasmids for recombinant expression of preS polypeptides, antibodies for detection of duCPD and DHBV-surface proteins, as well as baculoviruses encoding soluble CPD and fragment thereof can be obtained from the author upon request.
2. Denaturation of DpreS polypeptides for purification and regeneration purposes is not critical for subsequent binding analyses. Denatured DpreS can be completely renatured to its CPD-binding active form by simple dialysis or fast rebuffering. In a quantitative BIAcore experiment ***(10)***, we have treated covalently immobilized DpreS 50 times with 1 m*M* HCl without a measurable loss of binding activity after rebuffering.

3. Duck livers should be prepared from Pekin ducks only and should be tested for DHBV infection before CPD preparation. This can be performed by Western blotting of total liver lysates on DHBV L protein. Be aware that hepatocytes from DHBV-infected ducks contain only very small amounts of duCPD, because of receptor downregulation ***(17)***.
4. Liver samples should be either processed immediately at 4°C or stored in sliced pieces at –80°C. Do not refreeze after thawing. Homogenize rapidly.
5. Expression of soluble CPD and CPD fragments is best performed in High Five insect cells (Invitrogen). Compared with Sf9 or Sf21 insect cells, High Five cells express significantly higher levels of CPD (5-fold to 10-fold). In addition, they can be grown in serum-free media and can be adapted to spinner cultures. However, these cells cannot be used to propagate virus stocks. To this aim, Sf9 cells are required.
6. duCPD cannot be reasonably renatured after contact with highly acidic buffers. Once treated with 1 m*M* HCl, duCPD lost its ability to interact with DpreS. However, the short incubation with 100 m*M* NaAc pH 4.0 to release duCPD C from immobilized DpreS does not result in irreversible denaturation.
7. This simple binding assay can be modified according to the specific question that should be addressed. For example, it allows the easy measurement of pH and salt dependence of binding by adding appropriate 10X buffers that determine the pH and salt conditions. Immobilization of the respective DpreS mutants allow the identification of sequence elements within DpreS that are required for CPD binding. Addition of reagents (e.g., anti-duCPD antibodies, DHBV particles, or free DpreS mutants) to the reaction mixture facilitates quantification of the interference with binding. The latter method is especially useful when stoichiometric mixtures of recombinant soluble duCPD and DpreS variants are used, because variation of the stoichiometry also allows detection of weak interactions.

Acknowledgments

The author is grateful to Heinz Schaller, Christa Kuhn, and Klaus Breiner for the monoclonal antibody 4F8 and recombinant adenoviruses encoding duCPD. He also thanks Nicole Schmut and Matthias Engelke for the preparation of **Figs. 3 and 4.** This work was supported by a grant from the Deutsche Forschungsgemeinschaft, DFG (UR 72/1-1).

References

1. Kuroki, K., Cheung, R., Marion, P. L., and Ganem, D. (1994) A cell surface protein that binds avian hepatitis B virus particles. *J. Virol.* **68**, 2091–2096.
2. Tong, S., Li, J., and Wands, J. R. (1995) Interaction between duck hepatitis B virus and a 170-kilodalton cellular protein is mediated through a neutralizing epitope of the pre-S region and occurs during viral infection. *J. Virol.* **69**, 7106–7112.
3. Urban, S., Breiner, K. M., Fehler, F., Klingmüller, U., and Schaller, H. (1998) Avian hepatitis B virus infection is initiated by the interaction of a distinct pre-S subdomain with the cellular receptor gp180. *J. Virol.* **72**, 8089–8097.
4. Breiner, K. M., Urban, S., and Schaller, H. (1998) Carboxypeptidase D (gp180), a Golgi-resident protein, functions in the attachment and entry of avian hepatitis B viruses. *J. Virol.* **72**, 8098–8104.
5. Song, L. and Fricker, L. D. (1995) Purification and characterization of carboxypeptidase D, a novel carboxypeptidase E-like enzyme, from bovine pituitary. *J. Biol. Chem.* **270**, 25,007–25,013.

6. Eng, F. J., Novikova, E. G., Kuroki, K., Ganem, D., and Fricker, L. D. (1998) gp180, a protein that binds duck hepatitis B virus particles, has metallocarboxypeptidase D-like enzymatic activity. *J. Biol. Chem.* **273**, 8382–8388.
7. Urban, S., Kruse, C., and Multhaup, G. (1999) A soluble form of the avian hepatitis B virus receptor: biochemical characterization and functional analysis of the receptor ligand complex. *J. Biol. Chem.* **274**, 5707–5715.
8. Eng, F. J., Varlamov, O., and Fricker, L. D. (1999) Sequences within the cytoplasmic domain of gp180/carboxypeptidase D mediate localization to the trans-Golgi network. *Mol Biol. Cell,* **10**, 35–46.
9. Kalinina, E., Varlamov, O., and Fricker, L. D. (2002) Analysis of the carboxypeptidase D cytoplasmic domain: implications in intracellular trafficking. *J. Cell. Biochem.* **85**, 101–111.
10. Urban, S., Schwarz, C., Marx, U. C., Zentgraf, H., Schaller, H., and Multhaup, G. (2000) Receptor recognition by a hepatitis B virus reveals a novel mode of high affinity virus-receptor interaction. *EMBO J.* **19**, 1217–1227.
11. Gomis-Ruth, F.X., Companys, V., Qian, Y., et al. (1999) Crystal structure of avian carboxypeptidase D domain II: a prototype for the regulatory metallocarboxypeptidase subfamily. *EMBO J.* **18**, 5817–5826.
12. Breiner, K. M. and Schaller, H. (2000) Cellular receptor traffic is essential for productive duck hepatitis B virus infection. *J. Virol.* **74**, 2203–2209.
13. Spangenberg, H. C., Lee, H. B., Li, J., et al. (2001) A short sequence within domain C of duck carboxypeptidase D is critical for duck hepatitis B virus binding and determines host specificity. *J Virol.* **75**, 10,630–10,642.
14. Hitchcock, M. and Smith, J. N. (1964) Comparative detoxication: 13. detoxication of aromatic acids in arachnids: arginine, glutamic acid and glutamine conjugations. *Biochem. J.* **93**, 392–400.
15. Plummer, T. H. and Hurwitz, M. Y. (1978) Human plasma carboxypeptidase N: isolation and characterization. *J. Biol. Chem.* **253**, 3907–3912.
16. Gill, S. C., and von Hippel, P. H. (1989) Calculation of protein extinction coefficients from amino acid sequence data. *Anal. Biochem.* **182**, 319–326.
17. Breiner, K. M., Urban, S., Glass, B., and Schaller, H. (2001) Envelope protein-mediated down-regulation of hepatitis B virus receptor in infected hepatocytes. *J. Virol.* **75**, 143–150.

21

Nucleoprotein Transport of HBV Capsid Particles

Michael Kann

1. Introduction

Eukaryotic cells are compartmentalized and therefore possess mechanisms to transport molecules between the different organelles. Viruses take advantage of cellular transcription and translation machinery for their multiplication. Consequently, they utilize cellular routes for transporting their proteins and genome into the correct compartments.

Hepatitis B viruses (HBVs) contain a DNA genome that is multiplied by reverse transcription of a pregenomic mRNA (PG) precursor (for review of the viral life cycle see ref. *1*). The PG is synthesized by using the cellular RNA polymerases within the nucleus of an infected hepatocyte. After being exported into the cytoplasm, the PG acts as the precursor for DNA synthesis and also serves as the template for translation of the viral capsid (core) proteins and the viral polymerase (Pol). After translation, Pol binds to the PG, which mediates the specific encapsidation into the viral capsid that is formed by the core proteins. Capsid formation occurs spontaneously, even when expressing the capsid protein in heterologous systems such as *Escherichia coli*. In the absence of Pol, however, only host RNA is nonspecifically encapsidated.

In addition to Pol and PG, a cellular protein kinase becomes trapped when the viral capsids are expressed in eukaryotic cells. These immature capsids undergo a maturation process during which the PG is converted into partially double-stranded DNA. A mature capsid has two possible fates: it can be enveloped by the viral surface proteins, forming a progeny virus that is secreted, or it can deliver its encapsidated genome into the nucleus of the infected cell. The latter step contributes to amplification of the episomal nuclear viral DNA and leads to persistent infection of the cell.

These elements of the viral life cycle require the following transport processes: During initial infection the viral genome must be transported from the plasma membrane into the cytosol, which occurs by endocytosis; it must be transported through the cytoplasm toward the nuclear pore complexes (NPCs) and the genome must pass the nuclear pore to reach the karyoplasm.

From: *Methods in Molecular Medicine, vol. 95: Hepatitis B and D Protocols, volume 1*
Edited by: R. K. Hamatake and J. Y. N. Lau © Humana Press Inc., Totowa, NJ

None of the HBV-related intracellular transport events are well understood. This lack of knowledge is the result of the lack of a suitable experimental system. Whereas infectable cell lines exist for all well-studied viruses, allowing the determination of the entry steps in detail, only primary human hepatocytes are susceptible to HBV and then only for a short period of approx 3 d *(2)*. In addition, only a few viruses become incorporated into primary hepatocytes during infection. Thus, visualization techniques are of limited use for studying the import events during natural infection. Tracing the viral proteins and genome therefore requires other techniques derived from nuclear import studies in cell biology. These techniques comprise transfection, microinjection, and the use of permeabilized cells.

Transfection studies can readily be performed to determine whether a protein is karyophilic or not. As a result of the long delay between transfection of the DNA and observation of encoded proteins, however, this system suffers from serious disadvantages. Small proteins with a molecular weight below 80 (such as the hepatitis B capsid protein) may enter the nucleus by diffusion. When these proteins interact with components of the karyoplasm, the diffusion may result in a nuclear accumulation that mimics active nuclear transport. In addition, successful transfection requires cell division. Thus, proteins may become passively trapped in the nuclei during reconstitution of the nuclear envelopes.

Localization of a protein after microinjection allows transport studies minutes after injection. Thus, diffusion can be differentiated from active transport. The disadvantage, however, is that microinjection requires a high protein concentration because of the limited injection volume (50–100 fL per somatic cell culture cell; 50–100 nL per *Xenopus laevis* oocyte). In addition, microinjection allows only limited modifications of cellular-transport pathways so that detailed information on nuclear import is difficult to obtain.

An alternative is the use of digitonin-permeabilized cells *(3)*. Since this is an in vitro system, it allows deciphering import pathways on the molecular level. However, as with all in vitro systems, the assay is artificial and thus requires correlation with phenomena observed in vivo.

1.1. Overview of Nuclear Import

This section is a brief overview of nuclear import. For detailed information on the mechanisms of nuclear import and export, I strongly recommend the study of specialized reviews, e.g., ref. ***4***. Because of the intensive interest in this topic and the rapid growth of knowledge, these reviews are frequently updated.

The nuclear membrane segregates the cytoplasm from the nucleus. As a result of its impermeability, the only means by which molecules can be exchanged between these compartments in nondividing cells is through the NPCs. Transport between the cytoplasm and the nucleus is highly regulated and is facilitated by soluble transport receptors. The key elements of these transport receptors are proteins of the importin β superfamily, comprising importin β (karyopherin β) and its homolog, transportin. Both proteins bind directly or indirectly via adaptor protein(s) to the karyophilic protein (cargo). After formation of such a cargo-import receptor complex, the importin β or transportin mediates binding to the cytosolic face of the NPC and subsequent transport through the nuclear pore into the nuclear basket. The basket is part of the NPC and is a cage-like structure formed by eight fibers derived from the karyoplasmatic face of the NPC. The imported complex becomes arrested at these fibers until the import reaction is terminated by interaction of importin β or transportin with Ran in its GTP-bound form (RanGTP). The formation of the import receptor–RanGTP heterodimer dissociates the import complex so that the cargo enters the free karyoplasm. In contrast, the importin β– or transportin–RanGTP complex is exported through the pore.

Reaching RanGAP, which is associated with the cytosolic fibers of the NPC, the Ran-bound GTP becomes hydrolyzed to GDP, which lowers the affinity to the import receptor. Whereas transportin dissociates from RanGDP, importin β needs an additional transient interaction with RanBP. The released RanGDP interacts with NTF2, which facilitates its nuclear import. Inside the karyoplasm GDP is replaced by GTP at the major GTP-exchange factor RanGEF (RCC1), which is bound to chromatin. In summary, the import receptors as well as Ran are recycled and can participate in another round of nuclear import and export.

Although transportin and importin β show sequence and in particular functional homologies, they differ with regard to the cargos they bind. Transportin interacts with so-called M9 domains, which comprise a stretch of leucine-rich amino acids, as is present on the prototype protein A1 of hnRNPs. In contrast, importin β binds to basic amino acid-rich importin β-binding (IBB) domains.

It is currently thought that karyophilic proteins do not frequently expose an IBB but are bound via an IBB-exposing adaptor protein, called importin α, to importin β. Thus far, seven isoforms of importin α have been identified, all recognizing a nuclear localization sequence (NLS) on the surface of the karyophilic cargo. An NLS consists of basic amino acids with the consensus sequence K K/R X K/R; this sequence, however, is not always conserved. Apparently, all importin α isoforms accept most NLS, but some exceptions are known (STAT1, influenza NP).

Viruses, which replicate within the nucleus of nondividing cells, use the cellular transport machinery for the import of their genomes into the nucleus. Nucleic acids are not karyophilic. Their nuclear import is thus mediated by karyophilic proteins, to which they are attached. In a consistent manner, viral genomes are imported as a complex with karyophilic viral proteins using the same recognition motifs and regulation mechanisms as cellular proteins (for review on nuclear transport of viruses, see ref. ***5***). In addition to the generally smaller cellular proteins, they might only bind to the NPC without being imported if their size exceeds the maximal functional diameter of the nuclear pore of 39 nm ***(6)***.

1.2. Overview of HBV–Related Transport Processes

HBV is a relatively simple virus. The number of proteins that might be involved in the nuclear import of the viral genome is limited to Pol, which is covalently attached to the viral DNA, and the capsid proteins surrounding the viral DNA. In fact, both proteins have been shown to be karyophilic. Subjection of the Pol–DNA complex, isolated from the woodchuck hepatitis virus (a close relative of human HBV), to cells permeabilized by digitonin results in a nuclear localization of the viral genome *(7)*. It must be considered, however, that the isolation of the Pol–DNA complex requires harsh treatment so the folding of Pol does not necessarily reflect the authentic in vivo conformation. Thus, there may be protein domains exposed to the transport receptors that are hidden in the native form. This hypothesis may explain why after transfection only truncated mutants of Pol are transported into the nucleus (R. Schilling and H. Will, personal communication).

Empty capsids accumulate in nuclei of HBV-infected human livers. Corresponding to these observations, positively charged NLSs could be identified within the carboxy terminus of the capsid protein. Transfection, however, cannot provide an answer to the question of whether the capsids found in the nucleus of infected livers have been transported as intact particles or as isolated proteins, which might assemble into particles within the nucleus.

To resolve this uncertainty and to circumvent the lack of a suitable infection system, the system of digitonin-permeabilized cells as described below was used. Addition of *E. coli*-expressed capsids and their in vitro phosphorylated equivalents revealed that capsids become bound to the NPC only after phosphorylation of at least some capsid subunits at one or more phosphorylation sites. The binding was found to be dependent on the transport receptors importin α and importin β. Consistent with and supporting the in vivo relevance of this finding, importin β was found to co-immunoprecipitate with capsids derived from authentic HBV *(8)*.

The most frequently used model for HBV infection is the duck hepatitis B virus (DHBV), which replicates in a manner that is similar to that of the human pathogen. In contrast to HBV, the phosphorylation of DHBV capsid proteins results in a different migration pattern during sodium dodecyl sulfate (SDS) gel electrophoresis, thus being easy to determine. The DHBV system showed that, in contrast to HBV, the exposure of the capsid NLS does not depend on phosphorylation *(9)*. In fact, mature capsids are poorly phosphorylated, although they contain a protein kinase, as do HBV capsids. It is, however, difficult to apply these observations to HBV. First, in DHBV capsid proteins, the NLS and the phosphorylation sites do not overlap. Second, the limited extent of phosphorylation in mature capsids might be the result of an external dephosphorylation by cellular phosphatases.

Although no data exist for HBV capsids, unpublished observations with HBV NLS linked to fluorescent-labeled proteins showed that the NLS itself should not be phosphorylated, so dephosphorylation of the HBV capsid may occur, as in the DHBV system. Examples in which phosphorylation adjacent to an NLS supports its function, whereas phosphorylation within the NLS inhibits its functions, have been well studied, such as for the prototype NLS present on the simian virus 40 (SV40) TAg.

As described above, the function of the individual phosphorylation sites is poorly understood. However, in addition to the mechanism of nuclear import of the viral genome, there are more HBV-related nuclear transport processes that may play a crucial role in HBV replication. In addition to the core protein itself, little is known about the localization of the viral X protein, which may have significant impact on its still unknown function(s).

2. Materials

2.1. Solutions and Reagents

1. Material and reagents required for cell culture.
2. Material and reagents for immune fluorescence.
3. 10X transport buffer: 20 m*M* Mg-acetate, 200 m*M* HEPES pH 7.3, 1100 m*M* K-acetate, 10 m*M* EGTA, 50 m*M* Na-acetate. Store at 4°C.
4. Washing buffer: 1X transport buffer, 2 m*M* dithiothreitol (DTT), 0.5% bovine serum albumin (BSA), 5% goat serum. Store on ice until use.
5. 500X proteinase inhibitor mix: 5 mg/mL aprotinin, 5 mg/mL leupeptin, 5 mg/mL pepstatin (Sigma-Aldrich, Taufenkirchen, Germany). Store in aliquots at –20°C.
6. Collagen (Sigma-Aldrich, Taufenkirchen, Germany) or tissue adhesive (e.g., Cell-Tak, Becton Dickinson, NJ, USA).
7. Goat serum (Dianova, Hamburg, Germany).
8. Digitonin (Fluka/RdH; Sigma-Aldrich, Taufenkirchen, Germany). Dissolve in dimethyl sulfoxide (DMSO) at 10 mg/mL. Store at room temperature.
9. Creatine phosphate (Calbiochem, Bad Soden, Germany). Store in aliquots at –20°C.
10. Creatine phosphokinase (Calbiochem, Bad Soden, Germany). Store in aliquots at –20°C.
11. Cytosol (rabbit reticulocyte lysate [retic lysate], Promega, Madison, USA). Store in aliquots at –70°C.
12. Anti-NPC antibody (e.g., mAb414, BAbCO, Richmond, CA, USA).
13. Anti-HBV capsid antibodies (e.g. anti-HBc, Dako, Hamburg, Germany).
14. 3% paraformaldehyde (Merck, Darmstadt, Germany)/phosphate buffered saline (PBS). Store in aliquots at –20°C.
15. DTT, ATP, GTP, BSA.

2.1.1. Optional Reagents

1. RanGDP (not commercially available).
2. Ran mutants (not commercially available).
3. Importin α (not commercially available).
4. Importin β (not commercially available).
5. Transportin (not commercially available).
6. Hexokinase (Sigma-Aldrich, Taufenkirchen, Germany).
7. Peptides for inhibition experiments or generation of conjugates, according to Görlich et al. ***(10)***.
8. Fluorophore-labeled BSA (Sigma-Aldrich, Taufenkirchen, Germany).
9. Fluorophore-labeled lysine-fixable dextrane, MW 150000 (Sigma-Aldrich, Taufenkirchen, Germany).
10. GTPγS (Sigma-Aldrich, Taufenkirchen, Germany).
11. Wheat-germ agglutinin (WGA) (Boehringer-Mannheim, Mannheim, Germany).

2.2. Equipment

1. Equipment for cell culture and for immune fluorescence microscopy (preferably including a confocal laser scan microscope).
2. Water bath.
3. Incubators for 37°C and 30°C.
4. Glass cover slips (12 mm).
5. 20-G Needle.

6. Jeweler's forceps.
7. Humidified box.
8. Filter paper.
9. Parafilm.

2.3. Cells

1. In principle, all adherent mammalian cell lines are suitable. However, if the cells are not growing as a monolayer, only the cells on the surface may become permeabilized. Thus, in the cells sticking to the cover slip on the bottom, the cargo may not be able to enter the cytoplasm. In microscopy following the transport assay, these cells look negative, which could cause inconsistent results, even within one sample.
2. Although nuclear transport seems to be conserved in all eukaryotic cells ***(11)***, it must be considered that post-translational events like phosphorylation of the cargo may interfere with the exposure of a functional NLS. Thus, the choice of the cytosolic source may affect the outcome of a transport assay.

3. Methods (*see* Note 1)

3.1. Growing of the Cells

1. Permeabilized cells do not stick to the surface as well as unpermeabilized cells do. A pretreatment of the glass surface of the cover slips with collagen (1% collagen for 20 min at room temperature, followed by rinsing the cover slips with PBS) or with a tissue adhesive may be extremely helpful (*see* **Note 2**).
2. Seeding of the cells: Wash the dish on which the cells have been grown once with serum-free medium. Replace the medium by trypsin/PBS, which has been preincubated at 37°C. Incubate the dish with the cells at room temperature or 37°C. Meanwhile, add 1 mL of serum-containing medium to each well of the 24-well dish containing collagen-treated cover slips. When the cells round off, remove the trypsin and wash the cells off the dish by pipetting using serum-containing medium. If the cells of a 16-cm dish have been harvested in 10 mL, one drop of the suspension is sufficient per cover slip when using rapidly dividing cells, such as HeLa cells.
3. Allow the cells to grow overnight at 37°C in a humidified incubator with 5% CO_2 (*see* **Note 3**).

3.2. Permeabilization of the Cells

The following steps are described for one 12-mm cover slip in a 24-well dish.

1. Prepare the following solutions and material immediately before permeabilization:
   i. Washing buffer (dependent upon the protocol from **Subheading 3.3., steps 8** or **9**, 1.2 mL or 2.5 mL of washing buffer are required per sample).
   ii. Serum-free medium: 2.5 mL are required per sample. Store at 37°C until use.
   iii. Serum-free medium containing 40 µg/mL digitonin: 0.5 mL are required per sample. Store at 37°C until use.
   iv. Eppendorf cups for the individual transport reactions (*see* **Note 4**).
   v. Reagents for the transport reactions (**Subheading 3.3.**) (*see* **Note 5**).
   vi. Humidified box with parafilm: Put filter paper on the bottom of a flat container, and rinse with an excess of water. Wait some moments and remove the air bubbles. Take parafilm and label the individual positions where the cover slips will be placed. Place the labeled

side on the filter paper. The parafilm must be flat without any bubbles or nicks because the fluid film below the cover slips in the transport reaction is only 0.18 mm thick.

vii. Equipment for removal of the cover slips from the wells: 20-G needle with a barb, jeweler's forceps for microscopy.

viii. Incubators at 37°C and/or 30°C required for thawing the transport reagents and for control reaction containing an energy-depletion system.

2. Wash the cells twice with 1 mL of serum-free medium to remove the fetal calf serum (FCS) present in the growth medium. The volume of each wash should be at least the same as the growth medium.
3. Add 0.5 mL of digitonin-containing medium and incubate the cells for approx 5 min at 37°C (*see* **Note 6**).
4. Put the cells on ice and replace the digitonin-containing medium immediately by 0.3–0.5 mL of ice-cold washing buffer. Leave the dish on ice and incubate the cover slips for 10 min with gentle shaking. Be aware that permeabilized cells dry out very quickly. Therefore, do not remove the medium from a large number of wells and add the washing buffer afterward.
5. Repeat the washing twice. Do not add too much washing buffer during the last washing step or it will be difficult to see the edge of the cover slip when picking it up for transfer to the humidified box.

3.3. Transport Reactions

All solutions and material as well as pipetting steps should be stored or mixed on ice!

The transport mixture consists of the transported cargo, salts reflecting the intracellular environment, DTT to mimic the reducing intracytosolic atmosphere, an ATP/GTP-generating system, recombinant isolated transport receptors, or cytosol containing these transport factors and proteinase inhibitors. The most frequently used source of cytosol is rabbit reticulocyte lysate (*see* **Note 7**), which has the advantage of a high protein concentration of approx 70 mg/mL. Because the kinetics of nuclear import depend on the concentration of the transport receptors, by using reticulocyte lysate, only a small percentage of the reaction volume is needed for the cytosolic proteins, allowing higher volumes of the cargo (e.g., if its concentration is low).

A "typical" reaction mixture contains: 1X transport buffer, 2 m*M* DTT, 15–25 μg/μL reticulocyte lysate, 10 μg/mL aprotinin, 10 μg/mL leupeptin, 10 μg/mL pepstatin, 1 m*M* ATP, 5 m*M* creatine phosphate, 20 U/mL creatine phosphokinase, and the cargo. For fluorophore-linked cargoes like NLS-linked FITC–BSA, a concentration of 20 ng/μL is usually sufficient. When using HBV capsids and subsequent indirect immunofluorescence detection, 2.5 ng/μL is the lowest limit, assuming that a highly reactive antibody like the rabbit-anti-HBc from Dako is used.

1. Make up a master mix that will result in the following volumes being added for each transport reaction: 2 μL 10X transport buffer, 0.04 μL 1 *M* DTT, 0.04 μL 50X proteinase inhibitor mix, 0.2 μL 100 m*M* ATP, 0.25 μL 400 m*M* creatine phosphate, 0.4 μL 1 U/μL creatine phosphokinase, 4.3–7.1 μL 70 mg/mL reticulocyte lysate (*see* **Note 8**).
2. Add aliquots of the master mix to 10–12.8 μL of cargo (*see* **Note 9**) to obtain a final volume of 20 μL, and load the reaction mixtures onto parafilm in a humidified box that is placed on ice (*see* **Note 10**).

3. Remove the cover slips from the wells (*see* **Note 11**). Remove excess washing fluid quickly by touching the edge of the cover slip with filter paper.
4. Transfer the cover slips onto the drop with the reaction mixture. As a result of the residual amounts of washing fluid, especially at the downward oriented edge of the cover slip, it is best to place the cover slip on the drop at an oblique angle, with the washing fluid covered edge first. This approach guarantees a homogeneous dilution of the washing solution and homogeneous transport conditions throughout all cells. Keep in mind: The cell-covered surface must face the reaction mixture (cell-covered surface down)!
5. Transfer the humidified box to the appropriate reaction temperature (30°C or 37°C) incubator (*see* **Note 12**).
6. After 20 min, put it back on ice (*see* **Note 13**).
7. During this incubation period, thaw an aliquot of 3% paraformaldehyde/PBS at 37°C. After the solution becomes clear, store it on ice until use.

There are two possible ways to proceed:

8. If you have a strong import and would like to see the increased concentration within the nucleus, in comparison to the concentration within the cytosolic space, add 100 μL of cold 3% paraformaldehyde/PBS to the reaction mixture under the cover slips. This step can be accomplished by placing the tip of the pipet close to the edge of the cover slip (approx 0.5 mm, without touching it) and carefully letting the paraformaldehyde/PBS flow under the cover slip. After finishing, remove the humidified box from the ice and place it for 20–30 min at room temperature. During incubation, the cells become fixed and ready for further staining.
9. If the goal is to analyze the import reaction by conventional fluorescence microscopy, a low nuclear fluorescence is expected, or you want to see your cargo bound to the NPC, remove the excess cargo prior to visualization. Therefore, allow 100 μL of washing buffer to flow under the cover slips, as described for the paraformaldehyde/PBS solution in **step 8**. Afterward, remove the cover slips from the drops with forceps (*see* **Note 14**); remove the excess fluid and place the cover slips (cell-covered side upward!) in washing buffer-filled wells of a 24-well dish. Wash the cells three times on ice, as described in **Subheading 3.2**. Fix the cells by replacing the washing buffer with 0.4 mL of 3% paraformaldehyde/PBS and subsequent incubation for 20 to 30 min at room temperature.

3.4. Immune Stain and Microscopy

The possibilities of visualizing the cargoes and cellular structures are too vast to be described in this chapter. However, there are some aspects regarding nuclear transport that should be mentioned.

To verify nuclear localization, either the nucleus or the nuclear envelope may be stained. Propidium iodide stain may show the chromatin and thus the nucleus but cannot show the integrity of the nuclear membrane and morphological changes caused by mechanical maltreatment of the cells. The same is true for the frequently used DAPI stain. DAPI, in addition, needs short-wavelength excitation, and most confocal laser scan microscopes do not have an ultraviolet source.

Optical serial sections of the nucleus using confocal laser scan microscopy after staining of the nuclear envelope are more reliable. Whether the staining is achieved by anti-

NPC antibodies or by anti-lamin antibodies depends on the species of the cell line (e.g., the mAb 414 does not recognize mouse NPCs), the availability of the antibody, and personal experience with the antibody.

3.5. Control Reactions Confirming Active Transport

A number of control reactions exist with which it is possible to confirm that an observed nuclear transport has been an active one. The hypothesis that an active nuclear import has occurred should never be based on just one type of control experiment.

1. Transport at 4°C. The same reaction mixture is used as for the positive reaction. Instead of incubating at 30°C or 37°C, perform the assay at 4°C.
2. Energy depletion. In this control, use the protocol for the positive reaction mixture but do not add ATP and replace the ATP-generating system by an ATP/GTP-depleting system. The depleting system consists of 7 m*M* glucose and 1 U/mL hexokinase. To remove ATP and GTP, the reaction mixture has to be incubated for 10 min at 30°C prior to use. The system of glucose and hexokinase is frequently called an ATP-depleting system. However, most frequently hexokinase from baker's yeast is used, which accepts both ATP and GTP.
3. Blocking the NPC by WGA. By adding WGA at a final concentration of 50 μg/mL, the nuclear import reaction is blocked by the binding of WGA to N-glycosylated proteins of the NPCs (e.g., p62); (*see* **Note 15**).
4. Blocking the NPC by antibodies. More specific is the inhibition of the nuclear transport by monoclonal antibodies directed against the NPC. At the same time, this experiment can confirm that an observed binding to the nuclear envelope is caused by an interaction with the NPC. The experimental protocol requires that the NPC become blocked prior to addition of the cargo, i.e., during the initial washing steps. Because of the limited time and the low temperature, high concentrations of antibodies, like 200 μg/mL mAb 414 (BaBCo, CA, USA), are required.
5. Dependence on cytosolic transport receptors. For this experiment, the cells are prepared as described, but during the transport reaction, the cytosol is replaced by the same concentration of BSA.
6. Dependence on recycling of the soluble transport receptors. To prevent the recycling of the soluble transport receptors, the addition of a nonhydrolyzable GTP analog can be added to a positive reaction mixture. One example is the use of GTPγS at 1 m*M* (*see* **Note 16**).
7. Inhibition of specific import pathways. These assays are based on the competition between the cargo and an excess of other karyophilic proteins. Thus, they are suitable to decipher the soluble import receptors required for the transport of the cargo. In these experiments, peptides (less than 1 m*M*) are added to a positive reaction mixture (**Subheading 3.3., step 1**). When in excess, the peptides will interact predominantly with the corresponding transport receptors, which depletes the number of available transport receptors for the cargo if the cargo uses the same transport pathway. Examples for such peptides are the M9 domain of the protein A1 of hnRNP (YNNQSSNFGPMK) interfering with the transportin-mediated nuclear import, or the NLS of the SV40 TAg (PKKKRKVED) inhibiting the importin β–mediated nuclear uptake (*see* **Note 17**).
8. Inhibition by selective addition of transport factors. When isolated transport receptors are used to confirm the route of one distinct pathway, one of the transport receptors can be left out. In particular, this approach helps to confirm that the cargo interacts directly with the transport receptors.

3.6. Internal Controls

Differences observed between positive and negative samples are promising, but sometimes the results observed on one single cover slip may be inconsistent (*see* **Subheading 3.7.**). In addition, the microscope shows just a few selected cells and not a large overview. It is thus a great help and more convincing to use internal controls, which allow interpretation of the results for every single cell.

1. Exclusion of diffusion. To exclude the possibility that the observed cells contain a nuclear membrane that is defective, include large molecules directly linked to fluorophore to the reaction mixture containing the cargo. One example is lysine-fixable dextran with a molecular weight of 150 kDa.
2. Control of active import. Include a cargo that is actively imported. Examples are conjugates between FITC–labeled BSA and peptides, which mediate established active nuclear import (*see* **Note 18**).

3.7. Troubleshooting

3.7.1. No Cells

1. Monolayer. Cells have grown as a monolayer and were detached from the glass surface during the washing steps.
2. Excessive permeabilization. The permeabilization lysed the bottom membrane required to attach the cell on the cover slip. In this case, usually some remaining remnants of the plasma membrane sticking on the cover slip can be observed.
3. Insufficient fixation. There are several reasons for an insufficient fixation; such as too long storage of paraformaldehyde/PBS aliquots, too short or too cold incubation during fixation.
4. Traces of detergents. Some cargo preparations like HBV capsids require a detergent treatment. The remaining traces of detergent lyse all membranes. However, detergent contaminations are usually obvious because of the flat form of the drops after pipetting the reaction mixture onto the parafilm.

3.7.2. Loss of Most Cells

1. Harsh washing by direct pipetting onto the cells. In this case, usually a loss of cells in a defined large central area is observed.
2. If there are only single cells left on the cover slip, consider an excessive permeabilization of cells that were not growing as a monolayer. In this scenario, the digitonin-accessible cells were washed off, and only those cells that were protected by surrounding cells from digitonin are left on the cover slip. In these cells, however, no import reaction should have occurred.

3.7.3. No Staining

1. Insensitive detection method or not enough cargo in the transport reaction. Include a positive internal control to test whether the assay has worked. If the cargo is directly labeled, compare the fluorescence of the cargo and the control onto a fluoroimager.
2. However, consider that the cargo may not be karyophilic.
3. Alternatively, it may be possible that a post-translational modification of the cargo makes the NLS nonfunctional. One possibility is phosphorylation within the NLS. For investigation, it is possible to add [γ^{32}P]ATP to the assay and analyze the phosphorylation of the cargo after the assay (*see* **Subheading 3.3., step 9**). If there is evidence or phosphorylation, protein

kinase inhibitors can be added to the assay but consequences for the in vivo situation should be considered.

4. No nuclear staining after immune detection. Especially when a fluorescent positive control is nuclear localized, the detergent treatment after fixation may be forgotten, so the antibodies have not had access to the nuclear cargo.

3.7.4. Inhomogeneous Staining Throughout the Cover Slip

1. Sharply defined areas with and without import. Bubbles in the transport mixture or during immune staining.
2. Nuclear accumulation changes smoothly from one to the other side of the cover slip. The cover slip may not have been placed flatly on the drop during transport assay or immune staining. Alternatively, residual amounts of washing fluid may have accumulated on one side of the cover slip as a result of the method of putting the cover slip onto the drop.
3. Isolated cells or small areas without nuclear staining. An inhomogeneous permeabilization may have occurred. One reason may be that some cells have not grown as a monolayer.
4. Flat nuclei. The cells dried during the transfer from the wells onto the drops. However, this phenomenon can also be frequently observed when using a wrong fixation method, e.g., MetOH–acetone fixation.
5. No nuclear binding in the absence of Ran. In the presence of the cytosolic transport receptors but in the absence of Ran, the cargo should bind to the NPC without becoming imported into the karyoplasm. However, there may be only single molecules binding to the NPC, in contrast to the nuclear accumulation in the presence of Ran. Thus, the sensitivity of cargo detection is a plausible reason. However, check whether the soluble import receptors are functional; they are fairly sensitive to degradation.
6. Cargo sticks to extranuclear matrix. Some proteins stick to the extranuclear matrix. This process usually becomes prominent when the cytosolic extract is replaced by isolated transport factors. Alternative blocking other than BSA should be considered or the concentration of the blocking reagent increased. If the problem occurs with directly fluorophore-linked substrates, try the unlabeled cargo and immune detection; fluorophores increase the unspecific association with membranes. In addition, check whether the cargo is aggregated.
7. Import in the negative controls. Test whether the nuclear membrane remained intact during the assay. Problems may occur as a result of excessive permeabilization. The easiest way is to add a nonkaryophilic substrate, such as fluorophore-labeled, lysine-fixable dextran. However, when using small proteins, the active import overlaps with diffusion. Thus, consider decreasing the incubation time.

4. Notes

1. During the setup of the transport reaction, it is necessary to permeabilize and wash the cover slips in parallel to prepare the individual transport reactions. Some of the components used in the assay are unstable, and thus the reaction mixtures cannot be prepared in advance. When the assay is being performed for the first time, it is highly recommended to use only a limited number of reactions (four to six) to become familiar with the sequence of the different steps. Even with practice, it is important to note where every single component is stored as there will be no time to search for reagents.
2. I prefer the use of 12-mm cover slips in 24-well dishes, which need a volume per well of not more than 20 μL of transport solution in the assay and 20 μL of antibody mixture for indirect immune fluorescence staining. Although the usage of smaller cover slips or trays for

immune staining with up to 36 wells requires even smaller volumes in the transport reaction, their use cannot be recommended because the relatively large amount of washing buffer remaining on the cover slips after permeabilization dilutes the reaction mixture in an unpredictable manner.

3. Avoid allowing the cells to become confluent because mechanical detachment of a part of a monolayer during the assay usually results in the loss of the entire layer.
4. It is a good idea to label the cups in advance, especially if 50 cups have to be labeled and several transport mixtures have to be prepared at the same time.
5. Be aware that some reagents are unstable. Thus, do not thaw them in advance.
6. The batches of digitonin differ in their content of saponin. Thus, it is recommended to test each batch prior to its first use. A more time-consuming alternative is crystallization of the digitonin. After successful permeabilization, the nuclei of the cells have a speckled appearance in the light microscope (see **Fig. 1**), but there should not be any cells detached from the surface.
7. When the import pathway is known, the reticulocyte lysate can be replaced by individual transport factors. In this case, importin α, importin β, and RanGDP should be added at a concentration of at least 15 ng/μL, 30 ng/μL, and 50 ng/μL, respectively. RanGDP must be added, because washed cells are basically free of Ran, which is removed from the karyoplasm by diffusion. In this reaction, ATP should be replaced by the same amount of GTP. To prevent unspecific binding to cellular structures and the extracellular matrix, BSA should be added at a final concentration of 20 μg/μL.
8. The reagent most sensitive to degradation is the reticulocyte lysate. Thus immediately before use it should be thawed at 37°C and stored on ice. Avoid any additional freezing and thawing cycles; the transport capacity is completely gone after two or three cycles!
9. Reflect about the salts present in the solution containing the cargo! The protocol above can only be used if the cargo is diluted in H_2O! Since this solution is not a physiological buffer, I recommend storing the cargo in 1X transport buffer and reducing the amount of 10X transport buffer by one-tenth of the cargo volume.
10. Do not put the box onto ice too early or the parafilm will be covered with condensation. After addition of the reaction mixture, the humidified surface will cause dispersion of the drops. Under all circumstances, avoid all—even small—air bubbles!
11. To remove the cover slips from the wells, I prefer the use of a 20-G needle with a small barb (prepared by pressing the tip of the needle on a hard surface). I use this needle to lift one edge of the cover slip so the cover slip can be grasped with a forceps.
12. Active transport does not occur at 4°C or on ice. To subject the cells at the same time to a transport reaction, no import should have occurred prior to warming up the cells with the reaction mixture. Thus, the drops on the parafilm in the humidified box must be cooled down prior to addition of the cover slips. When using small transport cargos, the active import, however, overlaps with passive diffusion. Thus, work as quickly as possible.
13. Import reactions take place within minutes. To obtain reproducible results, it is required that the reaction temperature be reached quickly and that the reaction be terminated in all cells at the same time. Thus, I prefer the use of a water bath for incubation and termination of the reaction on ice. As mentioned above, the active import overlaps with passive diffusion. Thus, a prolonged incubation period usually does not result in an increased active import but in an increased diffusion, which impairs the signal–noise ratio.
14. The remaining drops of buffer-diluted reaction mixtures can be used for further biochemical analysis.

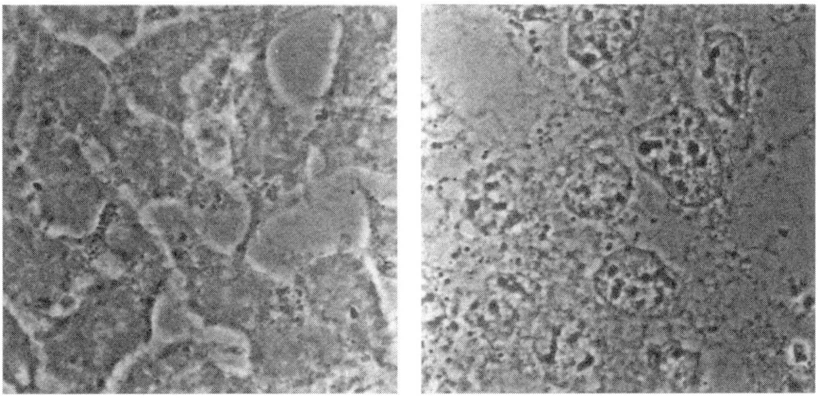

unpermeabilized **permeabilized**

Fig. 1. Light microscopy of unpermeablized and digitonin-permeabilized Huh7 cells.

15. If the detection system is sensitive, even small amounts of nuclear-localized protein, which have been transported before the WGA has blocked the pores, may be seen. In this case, the addition of WGA during the initial washing steps may be helpful.
16. In this experiment, the import receptors can mediate the first round of nuclear import. Thus, the stoichiometry of transport receptors, cargo, and the detection limit is essential. When low amounts of substrate are used and the detection limit is low, no inhibition may be observable. In contrast, with an insensitive detection and large amounts of cargo, which require several rounds of import before an import can be observed, there is a dramatic reduction.
17. Be aware that although SV40 TAg interacts with importin a, it depletes the amount of available importin β indirectly. Thus, an observed inhibition just means that importin β is involved, not necessarily importin α. The addition of peptides sometimes results in unspecific effects. Thus, the use of conjugates between nonkaryophilic proteins and the peptides has to be favored. The conjugates can be synthesized by chemical conjugation of BSA with a peptide comprising the signal sequence, which is separated from the reactive amino acid, e.g., cysteine, by a GGG spacer ***(10)***. These conjugations may transfer 19 peptides to 1 BSA molecule. In general, the inhibitory concentration of the conjugates is much lower than that for the peptides (50 μg/mL).
18. This type of internal control is useful in competition experiments. For example, when a transport assay includes the cargo, which is labeled or indirectly stained with Texas Red, you may add FITC-labeled BSA–SV40 TAg conjugate plus a Cy5 labeled BSA–M9 conjugate plus an unlabeled M9 competitor. In this assay, the reduction of nuclear Cy5 label would indicate that the inhibition has worked and that the Cy5 substrate did not enter the nucleus passively, the nuclear FITC label provides evidence that the transport reaction has taken place, and an import of cargo would mean that transportin is not required for its import.

References

1. Seeger, C. and Mason, W. S. (2000) Hepatitis B virus biology. *Microbiol. Mol. Biol. Rev.* **64**, 51–68.
2. Tuttleman, J. S., Pugh, J. C., and Summers, J. W. (1986) In vitro experimental infection of primary duck hepatocyte cultures with duck hepatitis B virus. *J. Virol.* **58**, 17–25.
3. Adam, S. A., Marr, R. S., and Gerace, L. (1990) Nuclear protein import in permeabilized mammalian cells requires soluble cytoplasmic factors. *J. Cell. Biol.* **111**, 807–816.
4. Görlich, D. and Kutay, U. (1999) Transport between the cell nucleus and the cytoplasm. *Annu. Rev. Cell. Dev. Biol.* **15**, 607–660.
5. Whittaker, G. R., Kann, M., and Helenius, A. (2000) Viral entry into the nucleus. *Annu. Rev. Cell. Dev. Biol.* **16**, 627–657.
6. Pante, N. and Kann, M. (2002) Nuclear pore complex is able to transport macromolecules with diameters of ~39 nm. *Mol. Biol. Cell.* **13**, 425–434.
7. Kann, M., Bischof, A., and Gerlich, W. H. (1997) In vitro model for the nuclear transport of the hepadnavirus genome. *J. Virol.* **71**.
8. Kann, M., Sodeik, B., Vlachou, A., Gerlich, W. H., and Helenius, A. (1999) Phosphorylation-dependent binding of hepatitis B virus core particles to the nuclear pore complex. *J. Cell. Biol.* **145**, 45–55.
9. Mabit, H., Breiner, K. M., Knaust, A., Zachmann-Brand, B., and Schaller, H. (2001) Signals for bidirectional nucleocytoplasmic transport in the duck hepatitis B virus capsid protein. *J. Virol.* **75**, 1968–1977.
10. Görlich, D., Prehn, S., Laskey, R. A., and Hartmann, E. (1994) Isolation of a protein that is essential for the first step of nuclear protein import. *Cell* **79**, 767–778.
11. Siomi, M. C., Fromont, M., Rain, J. C., et al. (1998) Functional conservation of the transportin nuclear import pathway in divergent organisms. *Mol. Cell. Biol.* **18**, 4141–4148.

22

Phosphorylation Analysis of Hepatitis B Virus Core Protein in Mammalian Cells

Jie Li, Yanyan Zheng, Jinah Choi, and Jing-hsiung Ou

1. Introduction

The hepatitis B virus (HBV) C gene encodes the core protein and the precore protein. The core protein, also known as the core antigen, is an important serologic marker for HBV infection. Although this protein is rarely detected in free forms in patients with HBV, the antibody directed against this protein is almost always found in people who have been exposed to HBV.

The core protein is a structural protein. It packages its own messenger RNA, which is larger than the length of the genome and is also known as the pregenomic RNA (pgRNA), to form the core particle. The pgRNA is subsequently converted to the viral DNA genome by the viral DNA polymerase that is also packaged in the core particle. The core particle will then interact with the viral envelope protein, also known as the surface antigen, on the membrane of the endoplasmic reticulum (ER). This interaction results in the budding of the core particle into the ER lumen. During this budding process, the virus acquires its envelope and is released into the ER lumen and subsequently secreted from infected hepatocytes.

The core protein is a phosphoprotein. Recent studies indicate that the phosphorylation of the core protein may be important for the packaging of the pgRNA, and its dephosphorylation may be important for viral DNA replication *(1,2)*. Furthermore, the phosphorylation of the core protein by protein kinase C in the early phase of infection has also been suggested to be important for the transport of the core protein and its DNA cargo into the nucleus *(3)*.

The precore protein contains the entire sequence of the core protein plus an amino-terminal extension of 29 amino acids. The first 19 amino acids of this amino-terminal extension ("the precore region") constitute a signal sequence, which targets the precore protein to the ER for secretion *(4–6)*. This signal sequence is removed from the precore protein sequence by the signal peptidase located in the ER lumen. The precore protein

From: *Methods in Molecular Medicine, vol. 95: Hepatitis B and D Protocols, volume 1*
Edited by: R. K. Hamatake and J. Y. N. Lau © Humana Press Inc., Totowa, NJ

derivative is further cleaved at the arginine-rich sequence at its carboxy terminus and secreted ***(7,8)***. The secreted precore protein derivatives are known as the e antigen ***(9)***. The function of the e antigen is not totally understood. It likely plays an important role in the establishment of chronic infection following neonatal infection ***(9)***. Although the great majority of the precore protein is translocated across the ER membrane and secreted, a small, but not insignificant, fraction of the precore protein is released back into the cytosol following the signal peptidase cleavage ***(10,11)***. This cytosolic precore protein can also be phosphorylated and is thought to serve as a dominant negative factor for the packaging of the viral pgRNA ***(12)***.

The phosphoamino-acid analysis indicates that the core protein is phosphorylated primarily on serine residues ***(13)***. Further analysis identified three major phosphorylation sites—serines 157, 164, and 172—in the carboxy-terminal arginine-rich region ***(14)***. Although the phosphorylation sites in the precore protein have not been identified, they are likely also located in the carboxy terminus, as the truncation of the carboxy terminus of the precore protein abolished the phosphorylation of the precore protein ***(15)***. In this chapter, we will describe the procedures for the analysis of the phosphorylation of the core protein. However, the same procedures can also be used to analyze the phosphorylation of the precore protein.

2. Materials

2.1. Reagents and Solutions

1. ^{32}P orthophosphate: ICN (cat. no. 64014). Store at room temperature.
2. Trans-^{35}S-Label: ICN (cat. no. 51006). Store at –80°C.
3. 100 m*M* phenylmethylsulfonyl fluoride (PMSF) solution: Dissolve 17.4 g of PMSF (Roche Diagnostics, cat. no. 837091) in 100 mL of isopropanol. Store at room temperature.
4. 1 *M* HEPES, pH 7.0: Invitrogen/Gibco (cat. no. 15630-080).
5. 1 *M* phosphate buffer, pH 7.0: Dissolve 23 g $NaH_2PO_4{\cdot}H_2O$ (Fisher Scientific, cat. no. BP330-500) and 47.3 g Na_2HPO_4 (Fisher Scientific, cat. no. S374-500) in 450 mL H_2O, titrate to pH 7.0 with 4 *N* NaOH, then add H_2O to a final volume of 500 mL. Autoclave to sterilize.
6. 1 *M* Tris-HCl, pH 7.0: Dissolve 60.5 g Tris-base in 450 mL H_2O; titrate with concentrated HCl to pH 7.0; add H_2O to a final volume of 500 mL. Autoclave to sterilize.
7. 5 *M* NaCl: Dissolve 146.1 g NaCl in 500 mL H_2O. Autoclave to sterilize.
8. 0.5 *M* ethylenediaminetetraacetic acid (EDTA), pH 8.0: Dissolve 93.1 g disodium EDTA (Fisher Scientific, cat. no. S311-500) in 400 mL H_2O; adjust pH to 8.0 with 10 *N* NaOH; add H_2O to a final volume of 500 mL. Autoclave to sterilize. Store at room temperature.
9. TE: 10 m*M* Tris-HCl, pH.7.0, 1 m*M* EDTA.
10. Tris-buffered saline (TBS): 10 m*M* Tris-HCl, pH 7.0, 150 m*M* NaCl. Add 5 mL 1 *M* Tris-HCl, pH 7.0, and 15 mL 5 *M* NaCl to sterile H_2O to a final volume of 500 mL. Store at room temperature or 4°C.
11. Radioimmunoprecipitation assay (RIPA) buffer: 10 m*M* Tris-HCl, pH 7.0, 150 m*M* sodium chloride, 1% Triton X-100 (Sigma, cat. no. X100), 1% sodium deoxycholate (SDC), 0.1% sodium dodecyl sulfate (SDS). Store at 4°C.
12. Phosphate-buffered saline (PBS): Invitrogen/Gibco (cat. no. 14280036). Store at 4°C.
13. Dulbecco's modified Eagle's medium (DMEM): Invitrogen/Gibco (cat. no. 11965-092).
14. Phosphate-free medium: Invitrogen/Gibco (cat. no. 11971-025).

15. Methionine-free medium: Invitrogen/Gibco (cat. no. 21013-024).
16. Fetal bovine serum (FBS): Invitrogen/Gibco (cat. no. 16000-044).
17. Dialyzed fetal bovine serum (dFBS): Invitrogen/Gibco (cat. no. 10440014).
18. Trypsin-EDTA: Invitrogen/Gibco (cat. no. 25300054).
19. Pansorbin: Calbiochem (cat. no. 507858). Store at 4°C.
20. Prewashed and preblocked Pansorbin: add 1 mL of FBS to 100 μL of Pansorbin; incubate at 4°C overnight; microfuge 2 min at full speed (15,000*g*) to pellet Pansorbin; resuspend Pansorbin in 1 mL of RIPA; vortex well; microfuge again to pellet Pansorbin; repeat the wash with RIPA two more times; finally resuspend Pansorbin in 100 μL of RIPA.
21. 2X HBS: 50 m*M* HEPES, pH 7.0, 280 m*M* NaCl, 10 m*M* KCl, 1.5 m*M* sodium phosphate buffer, pH 7.0, 12 m*M* dextrose. For 100 mL, add 5 mL 1 *M* HEPES, pH 7.0, 5.6 mL 5 *M* NaCl, 1 mL 1 *M* KCl, 150 μL 1 *M* sodium phosphate buffer, pH 7.0, 0.2 g dextrose; add H_2O to 100 mL. Filter sterilize.
22. 2X Laemmli buffer: 0.135 *M* Tris-HCl, pH 6.8, 6% SDS, 10% β-mercaptoethanol, 20% glycerol.
23. The rabbit anticore antibody: This antibody was made against a recombinant HBV core protein in our laboratory ***(11)***. However, the anticore antibodies are also commercially available (e.g., the mouse monoclonal anticore antibodies from Virogen, cat. no. 016-A or 017-A).

2.2. Cells and Plasmids

1. The Huh7 cell is a well-differentiated hepatoma cell line. This cell line is maintained in DMEM containing 10% FBS.
2. The plasmid pHBV2 contains a head-to-tail dimer of the HBV genome (adw2 subtype) joined at the unique *Eco*RI site ***(16)***. This HBV genomic dimer was inserted into pUC19 at the *Eco*RI site. pCMV-Core contains the HBV core protein coding sequence inserted into the pRc/CMV vector (Invitrogen) ***(17)***. The expression of the core protein sequence in this plasmid is under the control of the immediate early promoter of the cytomegalovirus. For the control transfections, we routinely use the parental vector pUC19 or pRc/CMV.

3. Methods

3.1. DNA Transfection of Huh7 Cells by Calcium Phosphate Precipitation (see Notes 1 and 2)

1. Split a confluent plate of Huh7 cells the day before transfection. Plate the cells in a 10-cm dish at a density that will allow the cells to become 80% confluent at the time of transfection (*see* **Note 3**).
2. Calcium phosphate precipitation of the DNA: Mix 20 μg of pHBV2 or pCMV-core (*see* **Note 4**) with H_2O in an Eppendorf tube to a final volume of 219 μL; add 31 μL of 2 *M* $CaCl_2$ to the bottom of the tube below the DNA solution, allow two phases to form and do not mix with the DNA sample at this step; add 250 μL of 2X HBS to the bottom of the tube and gently mix the samples by bubbling with the pipet. Sit at room temperature for 30 min for DNA to precipitate (*see* **Note 5**).
3. Remove the medium from the cells; add 9.5 mL of the fresh medium; pipet the DNA precipitates onto the cells. Swirl the plates gently to spread the DNA precipitates to the entire plate. Incubate cells at 37°C in a humidified CO_2 incubator for 8–16 h.
4. Remove the medium that contains the DNA precipitates. Rinse the cells twice with 5 mL PBS each and once with 4 mL trypsin-EDTA. Add 2 mL trypsin-EDTA to the cells (*see* **Note 6**). Incubate the cells in the 37°C CO_2 incubator for 5 min. Add 4 mL DMEM containing 10%

FBS. Pipet up and down gently to resuspend and disperse the cells. Split the cells into two 60-mm plates and incubate the cells in the 37°C CO_2 incubator until 48 h after the beginning of the transfection procedures. One plate of the cells will be used for ^{32}P labeling and the other plate will be used for Western blotting or ^{35}S labeling.

3.2. Metabolic Labeling of Cells with ^{32}P Orthophosphate (see Note 7)

1. Rinse one plate of cells once with 4 mL of the phosphate-free medium. Starve cells for 2 h for phosphate in 4 mL of the phosphate-free medium containing 10% dFBS (*see* **Note 8**).
2. Label the cells at 37°C for 1–3 h with 2 mL of phosphate-free medium containing 10% dFBS and 0.5 mCi of ^{32}P orthophosphate (*see* **Note 9**).
3. Remove the ^{32}P medium. Rinse the cells twice with PBS. Remove the residual PBS. Add 1 mL of RIPA containing 1 m*M* PMSF to the Petri dish to lyse the cells. Because of the short half-life of PMSF in aqueous solutions, PMSF should be freshly diluted in RIPA before use.
4. Scrape the cells off to one corner of the Petri dish with a disposable cell scraper (Falcon, cat. no. 08-773-1).
5. Pipet up and down first with a 1-mL Pipetman and next with a 200-µL Pipetman to shear the chromosomal DNA. Pipetting should be continued until the cell lysates are clear and no longer viscous (*see* **Note 10**).
6. Transfer the cell lysates to an Eppendorf tube.
7. Spin the samples in a microfuge at full speed (15,000*g*) for 5 min to pellet the cell debris.
8. Transfer the supernatant to a new Eppendorf tube. Centrifuge in a microfuge one more time (*see* **Note 11**).
9. Transfer the supernatant to a new Eppendorf tube. Add 1 µL of the anticore antibody to the cell lysates. Incubate at 4°C overnight.
10. Add 15 µL of the preblocked, prewashed Pansorbin (*see* **Note 12**) to the sample. Incubate at 4°C for 1 h to allow binding of the immune complex to Pansorbin (*see* **Note 13**).
11. Microfuge for 2 min to pellet Pansorbin.
12. Discard the supernatant in a radioactive waste container. Resuspend the pellet in 100 µL of RIPA by extensive vortexing. Add 900 µL of RIPA and vortex briefly again.
13. Microfuge to pellet Pansorbin and the immune complexes that bind to it.
14. Repeat the wash of the Pansorbin pellet. Repeat these wash and pelleting procedures for a total of four times. Transfer the resuspended Pansorbin after the third wash to a new Eppendorf tube. Microfuge for 2 min.
15. Discard the supernatant and resuspend the pellet in 15 µL 2X Laemmli buffer. Boil the sample at 100°C for 5 min and then chill on ice. Microfuge to pellet Pansorbin. The supernatant, which contains the ^{32}P-labeled core protein, is ready for gel electrophoresis (*see* **Note 14**). A typical phosphorylation result is shown in **Fig. 1**.

3.3. Western Blot Analysis and ^{35}S Labeling of the Core Protein

1. Use the second plate of cells for Western blot analysis or ^{35}S-methionine labeling.
2. For Western blotting, rinse the cells twice with PBS. Scrape the cells off from the plate in 1 mL of PBS with a cell scraper.
3. Transfer the cells to an Eppendorf tube. Microfuge the cells at 1500*g* at 4°C for 3 min. Discard the supernatant.
4. Resuspend the cell pellet in 200 µL of 2X Laemmli buffer. Sonicate to shear the chromosomal DNA. Boil at 100°C for 5 min and immediately chill on ice afterward. The samples can be stored at –80°C until used for the Western blotting.

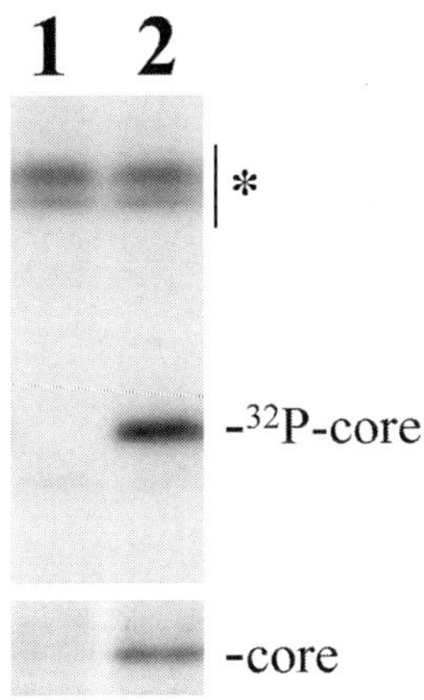

Fig. 1. Phosphorylation analysis of the HBV core protein in Huh7 cells. Lane 1, Huh7 cells transfected with pRc/CMV; lane 2, Huh7 cells transfected with pCMV-Core. Upper Panel: Cells were labeled with ^{32}P orthophosphate followed by radioimmunoprecipitation with the anticore antibody. Lower Panel: Cells were lysed and used directly for Western blotting. The locations of the core protein labeled by ^{32}P and the core protein detected by Western blotting are marked. The asterisk marks the locations of nonspecific bands.

5. For ^{35}S-methionine labeling, rinse the cells with 4 mL of the methionine-free medium and starve the cells for methionine with 4 mL of the methionine-free medium containing 10% dFBS for 2 h. (*see* **Note 8**).
6. Label the cells at 37°C for 1 h with 2 mL of methionine-free medium containing 10% dFBS and 0.2 mCi of ^{35}S-methionine (Trans-^{35}S-Label); (*see* **Note 9**). Follow the same procedures as used for ^{32}P-labeling for the preparation of the cell lysates for immunoprecipitation (*see* **Notes 15** and **16**).

4. Notes

1. Huh7 cells can be replaced with other cells, such as HepG2 cells or NIH3T3 cells. We prefer Huh7 cells for our experiments because they have a higher transfection efficiency.
2. Although the above procedures are described for the transient transfection experiments, they can also be used to study stable cell lines that express the core protein or the complete HBV genome.
3. For transfection, splitting a confluent plate of Huh7 cells 1:4 in the afternoon will typically give rise to the cells that are 80% confluent the next morning. This is an ideal density for DNA transfection.
4. We usually store our DNA sample in TE at a concentration of 1 μg/μL. It is important not to keep the DNA concentration too low, as the EDTA in TE will interfere with the $CaPO_4$ precipitation and reduce the transfection efficiency.
5. 2X HBS and 2 *M* $CaCl_2$ should be warmed to room temperature before use.
6. The trypsinization step to split the cells after transfection can be omitted if there is no need to perform Western blot analysis or ^{35}S-methionine labeling.
7. The ^{32}P work should be conducted behind a beta-shield for proper radiation protection. The liquid and solid wastes should be properly disposed in radioactive-waste containers.

8. The phosphate or methionine starvation time may vary from 1 to 3 h without significant difference of the results.
9. The ^{32}P- or ^{35}S-labeling time may also vary, depending on the nature of the experiments. Fifteen minutes of pulse-labeling time for ^{35}S-methionine is sufficient to generate a decent signal for the core protein.
10. Using pipetting to shear the chromosomal DNA is a laborious step. It may take 2–5 min to shear the DNA of each Petri dish. Because this pipetting procedure generates foams, care should be taken to avoid the radiation contamination of the Pipetman.
11. After lysing the cells and shearing the chromosomal DNA, the cell debris should be removed carefully by centrifugation twice. Any residual cell debris that is not removed will increase the background signals substantially.
12. As Pansorbin precipitates from the solution, it should be vortexed extensively before use. Pansorbin may also be replaced with Protein A Sepharose (Amersham Pharmacia, cat. no. 17-0780-01) or, if the mouse anticore antibody is used, GammaBind Plus Sepharose (Amersham Pharmacia Biotech, cat. no. 17-0886-01).
13. A total of 15 μL of Pansorbin is used for each sample in the radioimmunoprecipitation experiment, because the binding capacity of Pansorbin for IgG is usually near 2 mg/mL. Thus, 15 μL of Pansorbin will bind nearly 30 μg of IgG, which is more than the amount of IgG in 1 μL of antiserum.
14. For the analysis of the core protein, we routinely use a 12.5% polyacrylamide gel.
15. It is possible to perform subcellular fractionation to separate cytoplasm and nuclei. This process will require modification of the procedures. For example, the cells can be lysed in TBS containing 0.5% Nonidet P-40. The insoluble nuclear pellet can then be separated from the cytoplasmic supernatant by centrifugation in a microfuge. The nuclear lysates can be extracted with RIPA followed by radioimmunoprecipitation. The cytoplasmic lysates, however, will need to be mixed with an equal volume of RIPA prior to immunoprecipitation.
16. The same labeling procedures can also be used to study the phosphorylation of the precore protein, although in general, the labeling efficiency for the precore protein is much lower than that for the core protein, likely because most of the precore protein is secreted.

References

1. Lan, Y. T., Li, J., Liao, W., and Ou J. H. (1999) Roles of the three major phosphorylation sites of hepatitis B virus core protein in viral replication. *Virology* **259**, 342–348.
2. Gazina, E. V., Fielding, J. E., Lin, B., and Anderson, D. A. (2000) Core protein phosphorylation modulates pregenomic RNA encapsidation to different extents in human and duck hepatitis B viruses. *J. Virol.* **74**, 4721–4728.
3. Kann, M., Sodeik, B., Vlachou, A., Gerlich, W. H., and Helenius, A. (1999) Phosphorylation-dependent binding of hepatitis B virus core particles to the nuclear pore complex. *J. Cell Biol.* **145**, 45–55.
4. Ou, J. H., Laub, O., and Rutter, W. J. (1986) Hepatitis B virus gene function: the precore region targets the core antigen to cellular membranes and causes the secretion of the e antigen. *Proc. Natl. Acad. Sci. U. S. A.* **83**, 1578–1582.
5. Roossinck, M. J., Jameel, S., Loukin, S. H., and Siddiqui, A. (1986) Expression of hepatitis B viral core region in mammalian cells. *Mol. Cell. Biol.* **6**, 1393–1400.
6. Standring, D. N., Ou, J. H., Masiarz, F. R., and Rutter, W. J. (1988) A signal peptide encoded within the precore region of hepatitis B virus directs the secretion of a heterogeneous population of e antigens in Xenopus oocytes. *Proc. Natl. Acad. Sci. USA* **85**, 8405–8409.

7. Takahashi, K., Machida, A., Funatsu, G., et al. (1983) Immunochemical structure of hepatitis B e antigen in the serum. *J. Immunol.* **130**, 2903–2907.
8. Wang, J., Lee, A. S., and Ou, J. H. (1991) Proteolytic conversion of hepatitis B virus e antigen precursor to end product occurs in a postendoplasmic reticulum compartment. *J. Virol.* **65**, 5080–5083.
9. Ou, J. H. (1997) Molecular biology of hepatitis B virus e antigen. *J. Gastroenterol. Hepatol.* **12**, S178–S187.
10. Garcia, P. D., Ou, J. H., Rutter, W. J., and Walter, P. (1988) Targeting of the hepatitis B virus precore protein to the endoplasmic reticulum membrane: after signal peptide cleavage translocation can be aborted and the product released into the cytoplasm. *J. Cell Biol.* **106**, 1093–1104.
11. Ou, J. H., Yeh, C. T., and Yen, T. S. (1989) Transport of hepatitis B virus precore protein into the nucleus after cleavage of its signal peptide. *J. Virol.* **63**, 5238–5243.
12. Scaglioni, P. P., Melegari, M., and Wands, J. R. (1997) Posttranscriptional regulation of hepatitis B virus replication by the precore protein. *J. Virol.* **71**, 345–353.
13. Roossnck, M. J., and Siddiqui, A. (1987) In vivo phosphorylation and protein analysis of hepatitis B virus core protein. *J. Virol.* **61**, 955–961.
14. Liao, W., and Ou J. H. (1995) Phosphorylation and nuclear localization of the hepatitis B virus core protein: significance of serine in the three repeated SPRRR motifs. *J. Virol.* **69**, 1025–1029.
15. Yeh, C. T., and Ou, J. H. (1991) Phosphorylation of hepatitis B virus precore and core proteins. *J. Virol.* **65**, 2327–2331.
16. Valenzuela, P., Quiroga, M., Zaldivar, J., Gray, P., and Rutter, W. J. (1980) The nucleotide sequence of the hepatitis B virus viral genome and the identification of the major genes. In Field, B. N., Jaenisch, R., and Fox, C. F., (eds) *Animal Virus Genetics*, Academic Press, New York, 57–70.
17. Yeh, C. T., Wong, S. W., Fung, Y. K., and Ou, J. H. (1993) Cell cycle regulation of nuclear localization of hepatitis B virus core protein. *Proc. Natl. Acad. Sci. USA* **90**, 6459–6463.

23

Study of HBV Replication Capacity in Relation to Sequence Variation in the Precore and Core Promoter Regions

Fabien Zoulim, ShuPing Tong, and Christian Trépo

1. Introduction

Chronic hepatitis B virus (HBV) infection remains a major public health problem worldwide as well as a therapeutic challenge *(1)*. HBV belongs to the hepadnavirus family and replicates its DNA genome via a reverse transcription step *(2)*. The spontaneous error rate of the viral reverse transcriptase is responsible for the evolution of the viral genome during the course of infection under the antiviral pressure of the host immune response or specific therapy *(3)*. Eight major viral genotypes, A to H, have been identified *(4)* as well as many mutants, some of which have important clinical implications *(3)*. In clinical practice, the most frequently encountered variant form of chronic HBV infections is the hepatitis B e antigen (HBeAg)-minus chronic hepatitis B associated with the replication of precore stop codon mutants that terminate preC/C protein (HBeAg precursor) expression *(5–8)*.

Emergence of precore stop codon mutants is highly dependent on viral genotypes because of a structural restriction in the pregenome encapsidation signal *(9–11)*. Such variants are selected during seroconversion from HBeAg to anti-HBe and are responsible for the HBeAg-negative chronic hepatitis B, which represents up to 50–95% of the chronic hepatitis B cases followed in liver units in Europe and has an increasing prevalence from north to south *(12,13)*. In vivo evolution of the HBV genome from wild-type to HBe-minus mutant takes an intermediate step, i.e., the emergence of mutations in the core promoter region that downregulate the transcription of precore messenger RNA and reduce HBeAg expression *(14)*. The most common and best characterized core promoter mutations are A1762T and G1764A.

The core promoter mutants are independent of viral genotypes and are usually maintained following the development of precore mutation. Although it is clear that these variants are associated with viral persistence and chronic hepatitis in patients who test

From: *Methods in Molecular Medicine, vol. 95: Hepatitis B and D Protocols, volume 1*
Edited by: R. K. Hamatake and J. Y. N. Lau © Humana Press Inc., Totowa, NJ

positive for anti-HBe antibody, their relation to the severity of liver disease remains a matter of controversy ***(15–18)***. These mutants may also be associated with viral reactivation and ALT exacerbations in patients who are in a phase of remission.

Furthermore, therapy for patients with HBeAg-negative chronic HBV infection remains a clinical challenge. Interferon alpha is only moderately active, with approx 50% of patients responding during therapy and only 30% having a sustained response ***(19,20)***. There is also some molecular evidence suggesting that the precore stop codon mutants may be more resistant to interferon alpha ***(19,21)***.

There are only a few studies reporting the efficacy of a 12-mo course of lamivudine treatment in patients with HBeAg-negative chronic HBV infection. Approximately two-thirds of the patients showed a virological, biochemical, and histological response at mo 12, and selection of polymerase drug-resistant mutants was observed in one-quarter of the patients ***(22,23)***. The sensitivity of precore mutants and core promoter mutants to lamivudine by comparison with wild-type virus remains a matter of controversy ***(24–27)***.

The HBV genome circulates as a complex quasi-species of mutants that evolve constantly depending on the immune and/or antiviral pressure. Because the relative proportion of mutants versus wild-type virus may be of critical importance in the outcome of infection ***(13,28)***, there is a need to use optimal methods for the quantitative detection of HBV mutants. Molecular and functional studies of newly identified mutants in cell-culture system are warranted to gain insight into the mechanisms of viral clearance or persistence ***(3,29,30)***.

Moreover, the replication capacities of the precore and core promoter mutants may be an important determinant of their sensitivity to therapies. In this regard, viral titer in vivo may not accurately reflect viral replication capacity, because significant viral destruction by the immune system can take place. Thus, core promoter mutants and especially precore stop codon mutants are frequently detected in patients with low viremia titers, although these mutations do not reduce viral replication in cell culture ***(31)***. In fact, there are reports that precore and core promoter mutations enhance HBV replication ***(32–34)***, although this issue remains controversial. The study of the sensitivity of these mutants to lamivudine or interferon alpha in tissue culture and immunological studies during the course of antiviral therapy are required for better therapeutic design. In the future, it will be important to revisit the long-term consequences of polymerase mutants in the YMDD motif, conferring resistance to lamivudine according to viral genotype, and the precore/core promoter region sequence.

The study of viral dynamics in the context of viral quasi-species during the natural history of the disease or during antiviral therapy mainly depends on direct sequencing or sequencing polymerase chain reaction (PCR) clones or more rapid hybridization assays. The in vitro analysis of the replication capacity of these mutants in the presence or absence of nucleoside analogs relies on the transient transfection of eukaryotic cells with linear HBV genomes amplified by PCR directly from clinical isolates, plasmids containing an HBV–pregenome equivalent, or HBV–genome dimers. The methodology used depends mainly on the mutations under study. Some examples are illustrated below.

2. Materials

2.1. Molecular Biology Reagents

1. DNA from 200-μL serum sample are extracted using High Pure PCR Template Preparation Kit (Roche Diagnostics, Mannheim, Germany) according to the manufacturer's recommendations.
2. QIAEX II Gel Extraction Kit (Qiagen).
3. Plasmids: pGEMT Vector system II for direct cloning of PCR products (Promega, Madison, WI); pUC18 or pUC19 for whole HBV–genome cloning (New England Biolabs, Beverly, MA); pSEAP2 reporter vector (Clontech Inc, Palo Alto, CA).
4. Restriction enzymes: *Hind*III, *Sac*I (*Sst*I), *Sap*I (New England Biolabs, Beverly, MA).
5. Rapid DNA Ligation Kit (Roche Diagnostics Mannheim, Germany).
6. Quickchange Site Directed Mutagenesis Kit (Stratagene, La Jolla, CA).
7. FuGENE 6 transfection reagent (Roche Diagnostics, Mannheim, Germany) or Profection Mammalian Transfection System (Promega).
8. Agarose for gel electrophoresis of viral DNA.
9. Hybond-C membrane (Amersham Pharmacia Biotech, Little Chalfont, GB) or Hybond N+ for Southern blot analysis of viral DNA.
10. AUK 3 and EBK (DiaSorin srl, Saluggia, Italy) for measuring extracellular HBsAg and HBeAg, respectively.

2.2. PCR Amplification

2.2.1. Primers for Amplification of the Core- Promoter and Precore Region

1. p68: 5'-CAT AAG AGG ACT CTT GGA CT-3' (nt 1653–1672) for the first and second round.
2. pC7: 5'-AGG TAC AGT AGA AGA ATA AAG CC-3' (nt 2516–2492) for the first round.
3. pC6: 5'-CGT CTG CGA GGC GAG GGA GT-3' (2403–2384) for the second round when required.

2.2.2 Primers for Amplification of the Whole HBV Genome

1. P1:5'-CCGGAAAGCTTATGCTCTTCTTTTTCACCTCTGCCTAATCA-3' (*Hind*III and *Sap*I sites underlined).
2. P2:5'-CCGGAGAGCTCATGCTCTTC AAAAAGTTGCATGGTGCTGG-3' (*Sst*I and *Sap*I sites underlined).

2.2.3 Thermophilic DNA Polymerase

1. Taq DNA polymerase (Roche Diagnostics, Mannheim, Germany) for subgenomic amplification.
2. Expand™ High Fidelity PCR System (Roche Diagnostics, Mannheim Germany), which includes an enzyme mixture containing *Taq* DNA polymerase and 3'5' proofreading polymerase to ensure fidelity and yield for whole-genome amplification.

3. Methods

3.1. In Vivo Studies of the Replication of Mutants

3.1.1. Determination of the Core Promoter and Precore-Region Sequence by Direct Sequencing of PCR Products

The precore promoter, the precore region, and a part of the core gene of the HBV genome is amplified by PCR and sequenced (**Fig. 1**).

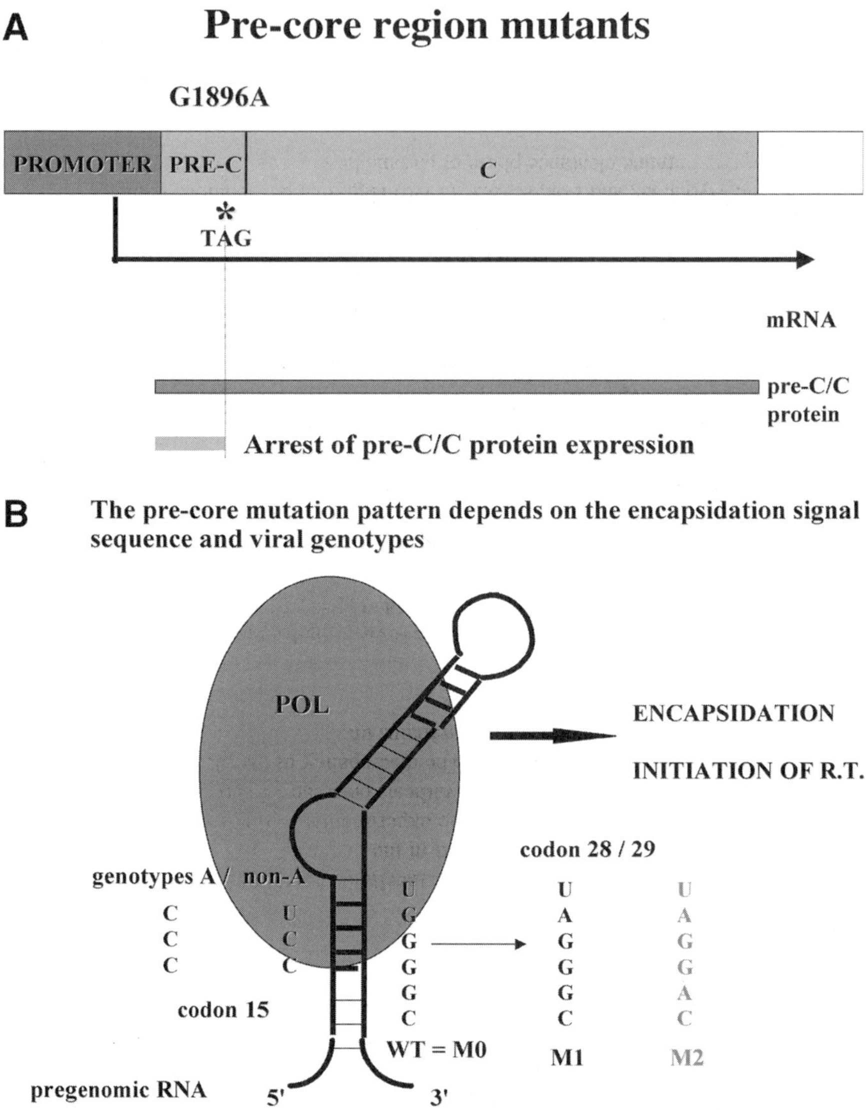

Fig. 1. Main mutation pattern in core promoter and precore regions.

Panels A and B: Mutations in the precore region result in the abrogation of HBeAg expression and depend on viral genotypes. **Panel C**: Mutations in the core promoter result in the decrease of precore messenger RNA transcription (*see* refs. ***9, 11, 14***).

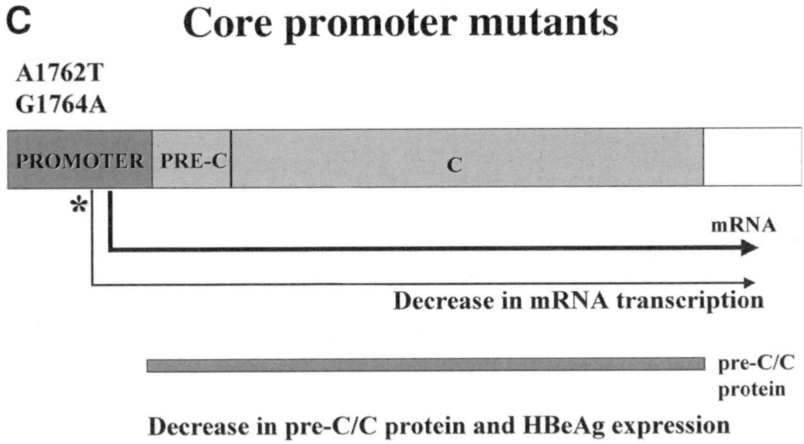

1. After nucleic-acid extraction of serum viral DNA, nested PCR amplification is performed using primers p68 and pC7 in the first round and primers p68 and pC6 in the second round.
2. This process is followed by direct DNA sequence analysis on PCR products, using an automated sequencer and primer p68, to analyze the promoter region as well as the precore and core regions.

3.1.2. Detection of Precore Mutants and Determination of Viral Genotypes by Reverse Hybridization Assay

To simplify the detection of the variability of the viral genome at codons 28 and 29 of the precore region, a research line-probe assay (LiPA) has been designed by Innogenetics (Ghent, Belgium). This assay uses specific probes covering the following motifs: 28W–29G (wild type); 28X–29G (mutant M2); 28W–29D (mutant M4); and 28X–29D (double mutant M2–M4). In addition, two specific probes for the precore promoter region covering the important variability at nucleotides 1762 and 1764 have also been designed.

1. Probes are applied on a nitrocellulose membrane as described ***(1)***.
2. The HBV precore region is amplified from a 10-µL aliquot of serum DNA extract, with biotinylated primers:
   HBPr8: 5'-GAAGGAAAGAAGTCAGAAGGC-3' (antisense) and
   HBPr69: 5'-ACATAAGAGGACTCTTGGAC-3' (sense) for first-round amplification
   HBPr70: 5'-TACTTCAAAGACTGTGTGTTTA-3' (sense), and
   HBPr7: 5'-CTCCACAGTAGCTCCAAATTC-3' (antisense) are used in a second round of amplification for nested PCR when required.
3. LiPA test performance is identical, as described for INNO-LiPA HCV II.
4. Viral genotypes are also determined by LiPA after amplification of the S gene and hybridization of the PCR products on 18 specific probes, allowing the determination of the six HBV genotypes (A to F) ***(16)***.

Perspectives: Initially, the in vivo studies of precore mutants relied on the cloning of the viral genome followed by sequence analysis. Once the main mutations were determined, rapid but nonsensitive and semiquantitative assays using specific oligoprobes were developed. The development of real-time PCR methodology should serve for the development of ultrasensitive and quantitative detection of the core promoter and precore mutants in vivo.

3.2. Analysis of the in Vitro Replication Capacity of the Precore and Core-Promoter Mutants

Overview: During the natural HBV life cycle, viral DNA replication is initiated from supercoiled, circular, double-stranded viral DNA (ccc DNA) present in the nucleus. This template for replication can be mimicked in vitro by tandem dimeric copies of HBV genome cloned into a plasmid (*see* **Subheading 3.2.3.**). The advantage of tandem dimers is that viral replication is under the endogenous enhancer/promoter elements, thus any mutation in the viral genome (including core promoter mutations) can be studied. However, use of tandem dimers is cumbersome in that each time a mutation is introduced through restriction sites, the dimer is reverted into a monomer and thus de novo construction of the dimer is required. The use of overlength HBV genome complementary to pregenomic RNA cloned downstream of a strong foreign promoter (such as cytomegalovirus [CMV]) allows abundant production of pregenomic RNA and hence extremely high replication efficiency (*see* **Subheading 3.2.2.**). However, this approach is unsuitable for the study of HBeAg expression (which requires the slightly longer precore mRNA) and for the effect of mutations in the core-promoter region (which is replaced by the foreign promoter in the over-length construct).

Finally, Dr. Will's group found that HBV replication, albeit inefficient, can be initiated from linearized full-length HBV genome *(35)*. Together with the full-length HBV PCR technique developed by this group, analysis of many naturally occurring HBV isolates becomes possible (*see* **Subheading 3.2.1.**). The major drawback of this approach is the requirement for *Sap*I (a low-concentration enzyme) digestion for each transfection, which together with the low-replication efficiency demands a highly efficient transfection system. Furthermore, it is possible to convert such a PCR-derived HBV monomer into dimers.

3.2.1. Whole HBV Genome PCR, Cloning, and Transfection of Eukaryotic Cells

1. Amplification of the whole HBV genome by PCR is conducted with Expand™ High Fidelity PCR System, as described by Günther et al. *(35)*. Briefly, HBV DNA isolated from 200 μL of serum is amplified by PCR in 50 μL of buffer containing 50 m*M* Tris-HCl, pH 8.3, 50 m*M* KCl, 1.5 m*M* $MgCl_2$, 200 μ*M* dNTP, 0.01% gelatin, 2.6 U of *Taq*–Pwo DNA polymerase mix, and 0.3 μ*M* primer P1 and primer P2. These primers differ from those described by Günther et al. *(35)* in that the *Sac*I site is removed from the P1 primer, whereas the *Hind*III site is deleted from the P2 primer; in this way, efficient directional cloning of the PCR products into the *Hind*III/*Sac*I sites of the vector becomes possible (*see* **Fig. 2**). The amplification is performed as previously described, with 30–40 cycles, including denaturation at 94°C for 40 s, annealing at 60°C for 1 min, and elongation at 72°C for 3 min, with an increment of 10 s at each cycle.
2. PCR products are analyzed by electrophoresis through 1.2% agarose gels and visualized by ethidium bromide staining. If necessary, Southern blot hybridization can be performed to confirm the specificity of the amplification products, as previously described *(35)*.

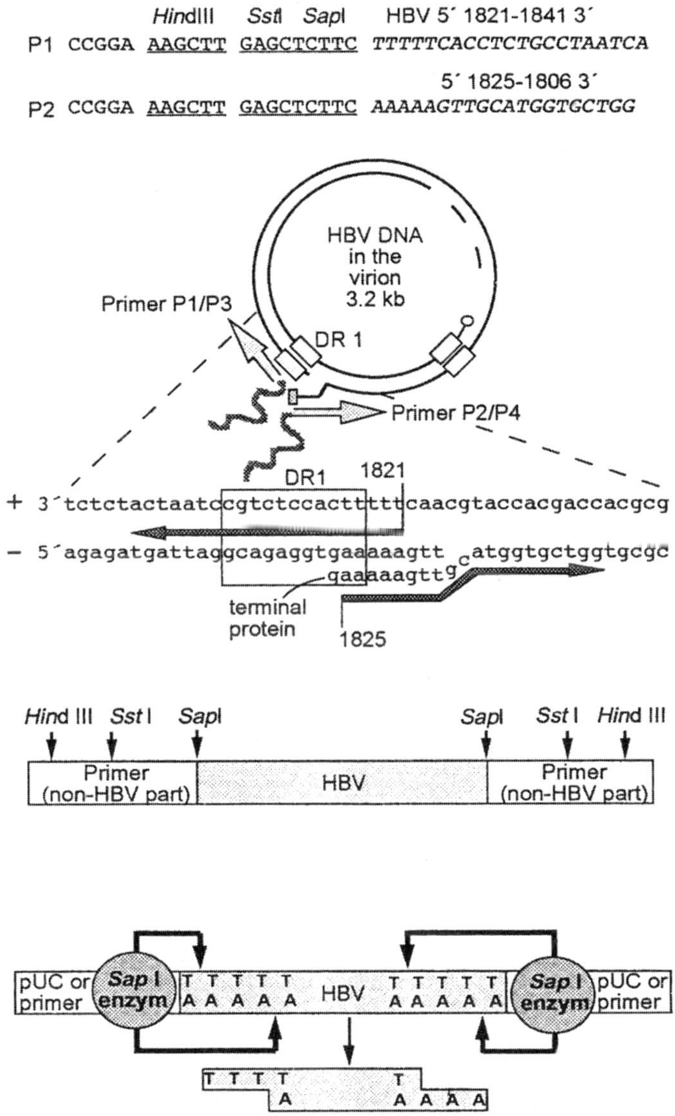

Fig. 2. Whole HBV genome amplification strategy by PCR *(35)*. Note that the original primers described by Günther et al. have been slightly modified to improve the cloning of the PCR products.

3. To clone the PCR product, the 3.2-kb HBV DNA is excised from the agarose gel and purified by the QIAEX II Gel Extraction Kit.
4. After double digestion with *Hind*III and *Sac*I, HBV DNA is purified by phenol/chloroform extraction and cloned into the *Hind*III and *Sac*I sites of the pUC18 or pUC19 vector.

5. Linear HBV genomes are released by cleavage with 0.5 U of *Sap*I per μg of DNA for at least 12 h.
6. Digested HBV DNA with *Sap*I sticky ends is purified by phenol/chloroform extraction and ethanol precipitation.
7. Transfection of 2 μg of linear HBV DNA is carried out using the Fugene procedure in Huh7 or HepG2 cells plated at a density of 1.3×10^6 cells per 60-mm diameter Petri dish. A marker gene such as one encoding alkaline phosphatase is co-transfected to control for transfection efficiency (*see* below).

3.2.2. Introduction of Precore Mutants into a Pregenome Expression Vector Followed by Transfection

1. A PBR vector containing an overlength HBV genome inserted behind the CMV immediate early promoter allows the transcription of the HBV pregenome and replication of viral DNA (kindly provided by Dr. Christoph Seeger, Fox Chase Cancer Center, Philadelphia, PA) ***(36)***.
2. Precore-region mutations are introduced into this plasmid by site-directed mutagenesis using the Stratagene kit. The presence of the mutations is confirmed by DNA sequence analysis.
3. Eight micrograms of the different plasmids are then transfected using the Fugene kit or the calcium-phosphate precipitation method, as previously described. Huh7 cells were plated at a density of 1.3×10^6 cells per 60-mm diameter Petri dish. The medium was changed 1 d after transfection, and cells were harvested at d 7 post-transfection. Transfection is performed at least three times for each construct.
4. Co-transfection with 2 μg of plasmid pSEAP (Clontech Laboratories, CA) encoding for alkaline phosphatase is performed as a control for the efficiency of transfection. Alkaline-phosphatase activity is assessed on 25 μL of cell-culture supernatant, following the manufacturer's recommendation.

3.2.3. Transfection Study of Core-Promoter Mutants Using HBV Dimers

1. Full-length HBV DNA was amplified from serum DNA and cloned into the *Sac*I/*Hind*III sites of pUC18 (*see* **Subheading 3.2.1.**).
2. HBV DNA was released from the pUC vector by overnight digestion with *Sap*I and *Bgl*I. The 3.2-kb HBV DNA was gel purified and ligated with T4 DNA ligase.
3. The HBV DNA is relinearized by digestion with *Eco*RI, gel purified again and ligated with *Eco*RI cut and dephosphorylated pUC18 vector at a 10:1 molar ratio. After transformation, colonies were screened by colony hybridization with an oligonucleotide probe covering the *Eco*RI junction of HBV genome (5'-GGCCATGCAGTGGAATTCCACWRCYTTCCA-3' where W=A+T; R=A+G; Y=C+T).
4. Positive clones were further verified by digestion with *Hind*III (yielding a 9-kb fragment for a dimer) and *Eco*RV (yielding a 3.2-kb fragment if the dimer is tandem).
5. Transfection is similar to the above methods.
6. To introduce core promoter mutations into the HBV genome, mutations are introduced by the overlap-extension PCR, with the outer sense primer upstream of the *Rsr*II site and the outer antisense primer downstream of the *Apa*I site. Next, the PCR product is digested with *Rsr*II/*Apa*I and cloned into the *Rsr*II/*Apa*I sites of HBV pUC18. The full-length HBV is released by *Eco*RI digestion and cloned back into pUC18 using a high insert-to-vector ratio to obtain the dimer (see the preceding steps).

3.3. Analysis of Viral Replication After Transfection of HBV DNA

3.3.1. Intracellular Core Particles

Intracellular core particles are isolated as described by Horwich et al. *(37)*.

1. Cells are washed once with ice-cold phosphate-buffered saline (PBS) and lysed with 500 µL of lysis buffer (50 m*M* Tris-HCl, pH 8, 1 m*M* ethylenediamine tetraacetic acid [EDTA], 1% NP40) per 60-mm Petri dish.
2. The lysed cells are transferred to Eppendorf tubes, vortexed, and subjected to centrifugation for 1 min at 14,000 rpm.
3. The supernatant is adjusted to 10 m*M* $MgCl_2$ and treated with 0.1 mg/mL of DNase (Boehringer) and 0.1 mg/mL of RNase (Boehringer) for 30 min at 37°C. The reaction is stopped by the addition of 25 m*M* of EDTA.
4. Core particles are then precipitated in 5% polyethyleneglycol for 1 h at 4°C. After centrifugation at 4°C for 5 min at 4000 rpm, the pellet is then subjected to proteinase-K digestion for 1 h at 45°C in 450 mL of a buffer containing 0.5% sodium dodecyl sulfate (SDS) and 0.5 mg/mL of proteinase K.
5. Nucleic acids are purified by phenol/chloroform extraction and ethanol precipitation after the addition of 10 mg of tRNA.
6. DNAs isolated from cytoplasmic core particles were separated on 1.5% agarose gels, blotted onto Hybond-C membranes (Amersham), hybridized with a α^{32}P-labeled full-length HBV fragment, followed by autoradiography of the blots. **Figure 3** shows examples of encapsidated replicative intermediates resulting from transfection of precore mutants.

3.3.2. Total Cellular RNA

1. Total cellular RNAs were extracted with Trizol (Gibco-BRL) and treated with RNase-free DNase.
2. Total RNAs were glyoxalated and separated on 1% agarose gels, using 10 m*M* sodium phosphate, pH 6.5, as a running buffer with constant buffer recirculation.
3. After capillary transfer to Hybond-C membranes, RNA was hybridized with a specific α^{32}P-labeled full-length HBV fragment, as described elsewhere.
4. Quantitation of viral nucleic acids after Northern or Southern blot analysis was performed by laser densitometry analysis after scanning the autoradiograms or phosphorimager analysis of the blots *(30,36,38)*.

3.3.3. HBV Protein Markers

HBsAg and HBeAg were assayed in the culture supernatant by using commercially available kits (AUK3 and EBK, DiaSorin, respectively).

Perspectives: HBV replication is most efficient with pregenome-expressing plasmid and least efficient with linearized HBV genome. Thus, in the latter case, a high-efficiency transfection system, such as Fugene 6 system, and a highly transfectable cell line, such as Huh7, are critical. Whether to transfect full-length, naturally occurring precore or core promoter mutants or to introduce such mutations into a wild-type viral genome background depends on the purpose of the study. It is possible that by the time core promoter mutations and precore mutation are generated, additional mutations elsewhere in the viral genome are present (depending on the host environment or therapy).

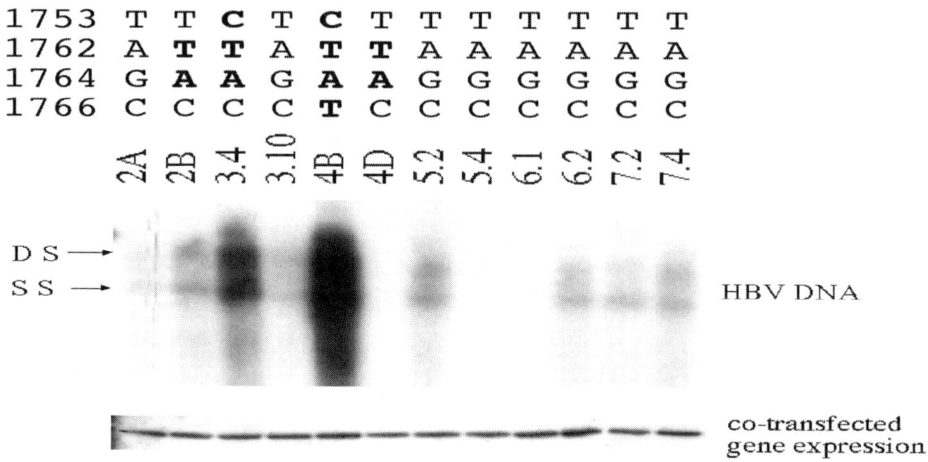

Fig. 3. Replication capacity of naturally occurring core promoter mutants in transfected Huh7 cells. All the HBV clones belong to genotype A and were isolated from HBeAg-positive patients. Sequences at positions 1753, 1762, 1764, and 1766 of the core promoter region are shown (bold face: mutated). Core particles from transfected cells were isolated, and HBV DNA was analyzed by Southern blot (SS: single-stranded DNA; DS: double-stranded linear DNA). Clones 4D, 5.4, and 6.1 failed to replicate as a result of frameshift mutations in the core gene. Clones 4B and 3.4, with 4- and 3-point mutations in the core-promoter region, replicated at a much higher level than did clones with a wild-type core promoter sequence.

These additional mutations may also modify viral replication and protein expression. In this connection, transfection studies of naturally occurring core promoter and precore mutants are more relevant to patient care than the study of such mutations alone. Isolated studies of precore mutation and core-promoter mutations have been performed, although conflicting results were obtained. Finally, the development of cell lines susceptible to HBV infection, without the requirement for cloning and transfection procedures, is urgently needed and should open new avenues in the field of phenotypic studies of HBV mutants.

References

1. Lee, W. M. (1997) Hepatitis B virus infection. *N. Engl. J. Med.* **337**, 1733–1745.
2. Summers, J. and Mason, W. S. (1982) Replication of the genome of a hepatitis B-like virus by reverse transcription of an RNA intermediate. *Cell* **29**, 403–415.
3. Günther, S., Fischer, L., Pult, I., Sterneck, M., and Will, H. (1999) Naturally occurring variants of hepatitis B virus. *Adv. Virus Res.* **52**, 25–137.
4. Stuyver, L., De Gendt, S., Van Geyt, C., et al. (2000) A new genotype of hepatitis B virus: complete genome and phylogenetic relatedness. *J. Gen. Virol.* **81(Pt 1)**, 67–74.
5. Carman, W., Hadziyannis, S., Mc Garvey, M. J., et al. (1989) Mutation preventing formation of hepatitis B e antigen in patients with chronic hepatitis B infection. *Lancet* **2**, 588–591.

6. Tong, S., Li, J., Vivitski, L., and Trépo, C. (1990) Active hepatitis B virus replication in the presence of anti-HBe is associated with viral variants containing an inactive pre-C region. *Virology* **176**, 596–603.
7. Tong, S.P., Diot, C., Gripon, P., Li, J., et al. (1991) In vitro replication competence of a cloned hepatitis B virus variant with a nonsense mutation in the distal pre-C region. *Virology* **181**, 733–737.
8. Tong, S.P., Li, J.S., Vitvitski, L., and Trépo, C. (1992) Replication capacities of natural and artificial precore stop codon mutants of hepatitis B virus: relevance of pregenome encapsidation signal. *Virology* **191**, 237–245.
9. Li, J.-S., Tong, S-P., Wen, Y.-M., Vitvitski, L., Zhang, Q., and Trépo, C. (1993) Hepatitis B virus genotype A rarely circulates as an HBe-minus mutant: possible contribution of a single nucleotide in the precore region. *J. Virol.* **67**, 5402–5410.
10. Tong, S., Li, J., Vitvitski, L., Kay, A., and Trépo, C. (1993) Evidence for a base-paired region of hepatitis B virus pregenome encapsidation signal which influences the patterns of precore mutations abolishing HBe protein expression. *J. Virol.* **67**, 5651–5655.
11. Lok, A., Akarca, U., and Greene, S. (1994) Mutations in the pre-core region of hepatitis B virus serve to enhance the stability of the secondary structure of the pregenome encapsidation signal. *Proc. Natl. Acad. Sci. U S A* **91**, 4077–4081.
12. Bonino, F., Rosina, F., Rizetto, M., et al. (1986) Chronic hepatitis in HBsAg carriers with serum HBV DNA and anti-HBe. *Gastroenterology* **90**, 1268–1273.
13. Brunetto, M., Giarin, M., Oliveri, F., et al. (1991) Wild-type and e antigen-minus hepatitis B viruses and course of chronic hepatitis. *Proc. Natl. Acad. Sci. U S A* **88**, 4186–4190.
14. Okamoto, H., Tsuda, F., Akahane, Y., et al. (1994) Hepatitis B virus with mutations in the core promoter for an e antigen-negative phenotype in carriers with antibody to e antigen. *J. Virol.* **68**, 8102–8110.
15. Chan, H.L., Leung, N.W., Hussain, M., Wong, M.L., and Lok, A.S. (2000) Hepatitis B e antigen-negative chronic hepatitis B in Hong Kong. *Hepatology* **31**, 763–768.
16. Grandjacques, C., Pradat, P., Stuyver, L., et al. (2000) Rapid detection of genotypes and mutations in the pre-core promoter and the pre-core region of hepatitis B virus genome: correlation with viral persistence and disease severity. *J Hepatol.* **33**, 430–439.
17. Lindh, M., Hannoun, C., Dhillon, A.P., Norkrans, G., and Horal, P. (1999) Core promoter mutations and genotypes in relation to viral replication and liver damage in East Asian hepatitis B virus carriers. *J Infect. Dis.* **179**, 775–782.
18. McMillan, J., Bowden, D., Angus, P., McCaughan, G., and Locarnini, S. (1996) Mutations in the hepatitis B virus precore/core gene and core promoter in patients with severe recurrent disease following liver transplantation. *Hepatology* **24**, 1371–1378.
19. Brunetto, M., Giarin, M., Saracco, G., et al. (1993) Hepatitis B virus unable to secrete e antigen and response to interferon in chronic hepatitis B. *Gastroenterology* **105**, 845–850.
20. Lampertico, P., Del Ninno, E., Manzin, A., et al. (1997) A randomized, controlled trial of a 24-month course of interferon alfa 2b in patients with chronic hepatitis B who had hepatitis B virus DNA without hepatitis B e antigen in serum. *Hepatology* **26**, 1621–165.
21. Zhang, X., Zoulim, F., Habersetzer, F., Xiong, S., and Trépo, C. (1996) Analysis of hepatitis B virus genotypes and pre-core region variability during interferon treatment of HBe antigen negative chronic hepatitis B. *J. Med. Virol.* **48**, 8–16.
22. Tassopoulos, N.C., Volpes, R., Pastore, G., et al. (1999) Efficacy of lamivudine in patients with hepatitis B e antigen-negative/hepatitis B virus DNA positive (precore mutant) chronic hepatitis B. *Hepatology* **29**, 889–896.

23. Santantonio, T., Mazzola, M., Iacovazzi, T., Miglietta A., Guastadisegni A., and Pastore, G. (2000) Long-term follow-up of patients with anti-HBe/HBV DNA-positive chronic hepatitis B treated for 12 months with lamivudine. *J. Hepatol.* **32**, 300–306.
24. Pichoud, C., Berby, F., Stuyver, L., Petit, M. A., Trépo, C., and Zoulim, F. (2000) Persistence of viral replication after anti-HBe seroconversion during antiviral therapy for chronic hepatitis B. *J. Hepatol.* **32**, 307–316.
25. Cho, S. W., Hahm, K. B., and Kim, J. H. (2000) Reversion from precore/core promoter mutants to wild-type hepatitis B virus during the course of lamivudine therapy. *Hepatology* **32**, 1163–1169.
26. Lok, A. S., Hussain, M., Cursano, C., et al. (2000) Evolution of hepatitis B virus polymerase gene mutations in hepatitis B e antigen-negative patients receiving lamivudine therapy. *Hepatology* **32)**, 1145–1153.
27. Nafa, S., Ahmed, S., Tavan, D., et al. (2000) Early detection of viral resistance by determination of hepatitis B virus polymerase mutations in patients treated by lamivudine for chronic hepatitis B. *Hepatology* **32**, 1078–1088.
28. Zhou, T., Saputelli, J., Aldrich, C. E., Deslauriers, M., Condreay, L. D., Mason, W. S. (1999) Emergence of drug-resistant populations of woodchuck hepatitis virus in woodchucks treated with the antiviral nucleoside lamivudine. *Antimicrob. Agents Chemother.* **43**, 1947–1954.
29. Argentini, C., La Sorsa, V., Bruni, R., D'Ugo, E., Giuseppetti, R., and Rapicetta, M. (1999) Hepadnavirus evolution and molecular strategy of adaptation in a new host. *J. Gen. Virol.* **80(Pt 3)**, 617–626.
30. Seigneres, B., Pichoud, C., Ahmed, S. S., Hantz, O., Trépo, C., Zoulim, F. (2000) Evolution of hepatitis B virus polymerase gene sequence during famciclovir therapy for chronic hepatitis B. *J. Infect. Dis.* **181**, 1221–1233.
31. Günther, S., Piwon, N., and Will, H. (1998) Wild-type levels of pregenomic RNA and replication but reduced pre-C RNA and e-antigen synthesis of hepatitis B virus with C(1653)->T, A(1762)->T and G(1764)->A mutations in the core promoter. *J. Gen. Virol.* **79**, 375–380.
32. Lamberts, C., Nassal, M., Velhagen, I., Zentgraf, H., and Schroder, C. (1993) Precore mediated inhibition of hepatitis B virus progeny DNA synthesis. *J. Virol.* **67**, 3756–3762.
33. Buckwold, V. E., Xu, Z., Chen, M., Yen, T. S. B., and Ou, J.-H. (1996) Effects of a naturally occurring mutation in the hepatitis B virus basal core promoter on precore gene expression and viral replication. *J. Virol.* **70**, 5845–5851.
34. Scaglioni, P. P., Melegari, M., Wands, J. R. (1997) Posttranscriptional regulation of hepatitis B virus replication by the precore protein. *J. Virol.* **71**, 345–353.
35. Günther, S., Li, B.-C., Miska, S., Kruger, D., Meisel, H., and Will, H. (1995) A novel method for efficient amplification of whole hepatitis B virus genomes permits rapid functional analysis and reveals deletion mutants in immunosuppressed patients. *J. Virol.* **69**, 5437–5444.
36. Pichoud, C., Seignères, B., Wang, Z., Trépo, C., and Zoulim, F. (1999) Transient selection of a hepatitis B virus polymerase gene mutant associated with a decreased replication capacity and famciclovir resistance. *Hepatology* **29**, 230–237.
37. Horwich, A. L., Furtak, K., Pugh, J., and Summers J. (1990) Synthesis of hepadnavirus particles that contain replication-defective duck hepatitis B virus genomes in cultures HuH7 cells. *J. Virol.* **64**, 642–650.
38. Seigneres, B., Aguesse-Germon, S., Pichoud, C., et al. (2001) Duck hepatitis B virus polymerase gene mutants associated with resistance to lamivudine have a decreased replication capacity in vitro and in vivo. *J Hepatol* **341**, 114–122.

24

A *cis/trans* Genetic Test for Pleiotropic Phenotypes Associated with a Frequent Naturally Occurring Mutation at Amino Acid 97 of HBV Core Protein

Chiaho Shih and Ta-Tung Thomas Yuan

1. Introduction

Hepatitis B virus (HBV) is a major human infectious pathogen. Worldwide, there are more than 350 million chronic carriers of HBV. Sequence divergence within the HBV genome is observed during long-term infection of HBV in patients as a result of the low fidelity of HBV reverse transcriptase. The important roles played by naturally occurring HBV variants have been implicated in the development of chronic hepatitis B. However, functional characterization of HBV variants remains difficult because of the lack of *a priori* knowledge to predict the possible abnormality of variants and to choose the relevant functional assay accordingly. This issue is further complicated by the possibility that a mutant phenotype could arise from either the *trans* defect of a mutant protein or the *cis* defect of a mutated genome.

HBV core antigen (HBcAg) is a 22-kDa protein and assumes multiple functions in replication: It is involved in capsid formation *(1)*, encapsidation of pregenomic RNA *(2)*, reverse transcription and DNA elongation *(3)*, import of relaxed circular (RC) DNA into the nucleus *(4)*, and targeting to the endoplasmic reticulum for envelope formation *(5,6)*. A frequent missense mutation of HBcAg, changing from phenylalanine (F) or isoleucine (I) into leucine (L), has been identified at codon 97 in chronically infected patients *(7–26)*. We recently reported that there are two distinct phenotypes, intracellular and extracellular, associated with this frequent 97L mutation *(27,28)*.

In brief, the intracellular phenotype of mutant F97L is the absence of the full-length RC form DNA at the 4.0-kb position (**Fig. 1A**, left panel), which could result from a specific defect in plus-strand DNA synthesis (**Fig. 1A**, middle panel). The extracellular phenotype of mutant F97L is to nonselectively secrete minus-strand DNA genome

From: *Methods in Molecular Medicine, vol. 95: Hepatitis B and D Protocols, volume 1*
Edited by: R. K. Hamatake and J. Y. N. Lau © Humana Press Inc., Totowa, NJ

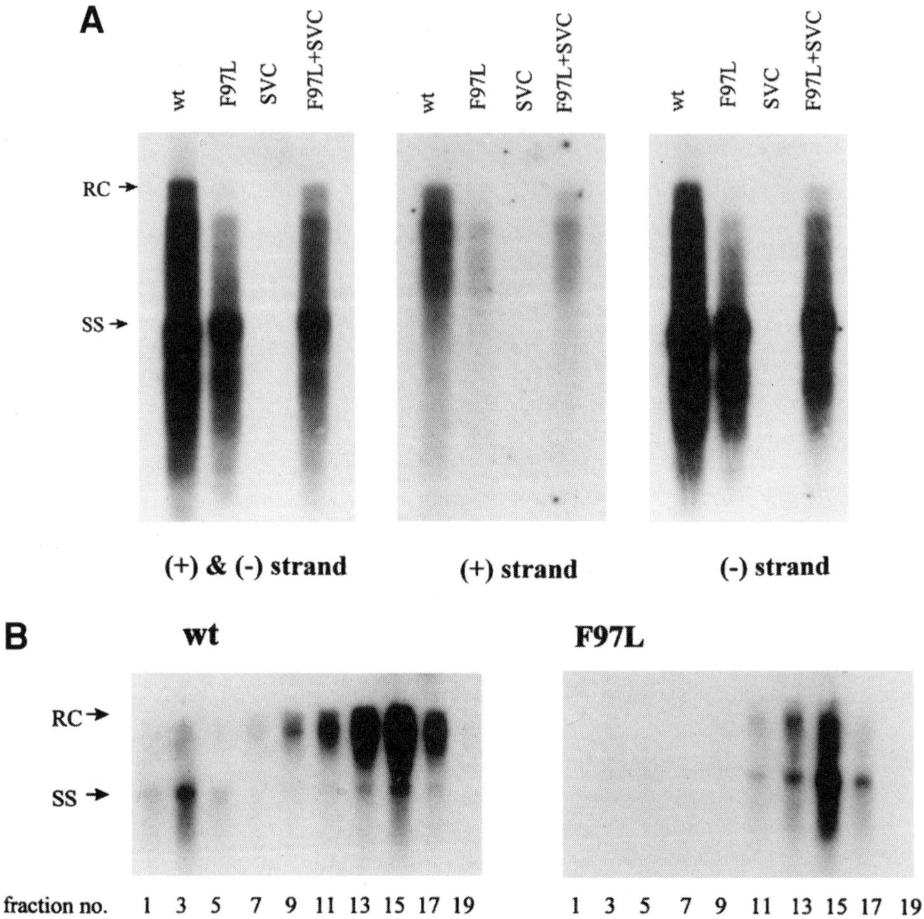

Fig. 1. The intracellular and extracellular phenotypes of mutant F97L. **(A)** The significant decrease of plus-strand and relaxed-circular (RC) DNA synthesis of mutant F97L. Ten micrograms of each plasmid DNA were transfected into Huh7 cells. Core particle–associated DNA was harvested 5 d post-transfection and analyzed by Southern blot analysis. Intracellular HBV DNA was then detected by a 3.1-kb HBV double-strand (ds) DNA probe (Left Panel), a plus-strand–specific riboprobe (Middle Panel), and a minus-strand–specific riboprobe (Right Panel). These three different probes were applied to the same nitrocellulose membrane sequentially. Full-length relaxed-circular form (RC) at the 4.0-kb and single-stranded (SS) DNAs at the 1.5-kb position are indicated by arrows. **(B)** Mutant F97L secretes viral particles containing unexpected immature genome with single-strand HBV DNA in the virion (Dane particle) fractions (1.24 g/cm^3). Conditioned media were collected on the third and fifth days post-transfection. Viral particles were first purified from the media through a 20% sucrose cushion, followed by isopycnic centrifugation in a gradient of 20 to 50% (w/v) cesium chloride. Fractions were separated according to their buoyant density, followed by dialysis and enzyme immunoassay for HBsAg and HBcAg *(27)*. Extracellular HBV DNA in each fraction was analyzed by Southern blot analysis using double-strand–specific 3.1-kb HBV DNA probes.

(immature secretion), which is normally retained intracellularly by wild-type virus **(Fig. 1B)**. The striking difference between wild-type HBV and mutant F97L was the presence of single-strand (SS) viral DNA below the 1.5-kb position in the Dane particle fractions ***(15,16,18,29)*** **(Fig. 1B)**. In contrast, the majority of wild-type HBV DNA in these same density fractions always occurs as the mature RC form above the 1.5-kb position **(Fig. 1B)**. HBV core protein has been hypothesized to serve as a signal transducer that can sense and transmit the signal of genomic DNA maturation inside the core particle to the machinery of envelope formation for secretion ***(30)***. The immature secretion of mutant F97L suggests that such a genome maturation signal, although necessary in the wild-type duck HBV system, is either not required or can be bypassed for human HBV mutants (see detailed discussion in ref. ***27***).

In theory, either a *trans* or *cis* defect (or both) of F97L mutation could contribute to the aforementioned pleiotropic phenotypes. Here, we illustrate a genetic approach to dissect the *trans* and *cis* effects of F97L mutation with regard to the intracellular and extracellular phenotypes of mutant F97L.

1.1. A Complementation Test for the trans Effect of the Mutant F97L Core Protein

1.1.1. The Mutant F97L Core-Protein Product Contributes to the Intracellular Phenotype of Plus-Strand DNA Deficiency

The deficiency in plus-strand viral DNA and RC form synthesis of mutant F97L can be partially rescued by co-transfection with the wild-type core-protein expression plasmid pSVC **(Fig. 1)**. This finding suggests that at least part of the intracellular plus-strand deficiency of mutant F97L is caused by the mutant core protein itself.

To test this hypothesis, a core-protein–defective virus was created by ablating the translational initiation codon AUG of core (p1903, with wild-type sequence for codon 97). The *trans* effect of mutant core protein (pSVC97) on intracellular DNA synthesis was examined by its capability to rescue the core-defective mutant **(Fig. 2A)**. As shown in **Fig. 3A** (middle panel), a reproducible reduction (albeit only twofold or so) in plus-strand DNA synthesis of mutant 1903 rescued with mutant 97L core (pSVC97) was observed when compared with the rescue of mutant 1903 by wild-type core protein (pSVC). Consistent with this difference in plus-strand synthesis (**Fig. 3A**, middle panel), a small and reproducible difference in overall DNA (left panel) and minus-strand DNA synthesis **(Fig. 3A**, right panel) was also observed.

1.1.2. The Core Protein of Mutant F97L is Necessary and Sufficient for the Extracellular Phenotype of Immature Secretion

To determine whether the mutant core protein contributes to the phenotype of immature secretion, we compared the gradient profiles of viruses produced by co-transfection of p1903 plus pSVC or p1903 plus pSVC97. As shown in **Fig. 3B**, mutant core from pSVC97 (lower panel), but not wild-type core from pSVC (middle panel), can reproduce the immature secretion phenotype of mutant F97L. Therefore, mutant F97L core protein alone is necessary and sufficient for immature secretion.

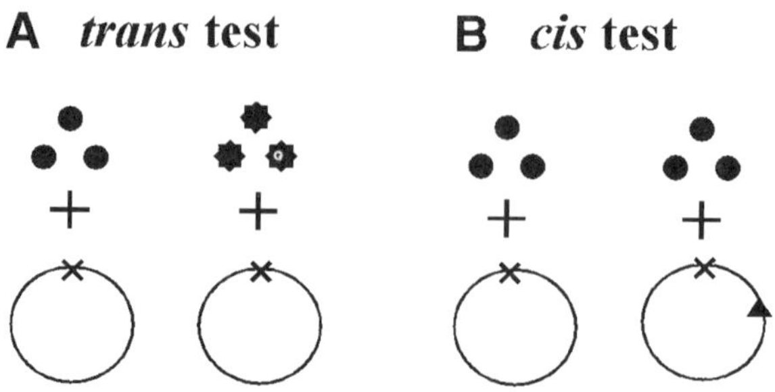

Fig. 2. Cartoon illustrations of the *cis*- and *trans*-genetic test for the mutant F97L phenotypes. **(A)** *trans*-test. Two different core proteins, wild-type (smooth dots) vs mutant (starry dots), were compared side by side for their respective abilities to rescue the same core-defective mutant 1903. **(B)** *cis*-test. The same wild-type core protein was used to rescue two different replication-defective HBV: the core-defective single-mutant 1903 (X symbol) vs the double-mutant 1903/F97L, which contained an additional F97L mutation (triangle symbol).

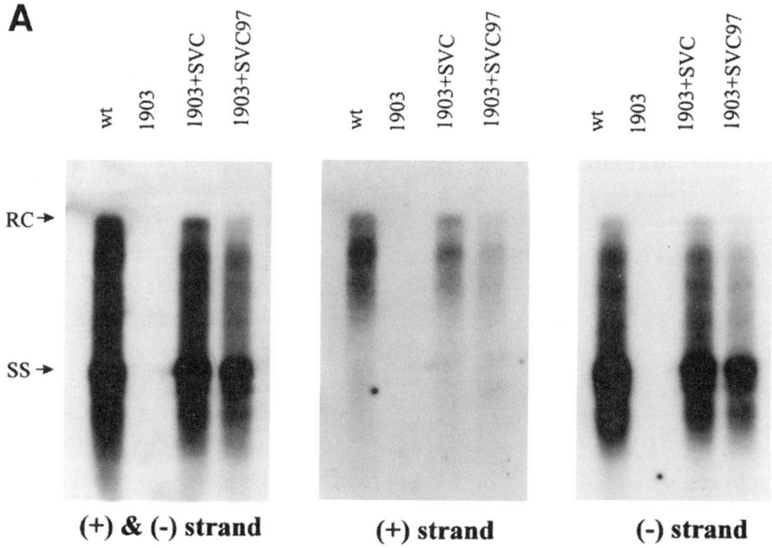

Fig.3. **(A)** A complementation assay for the *trans*-defect of mutant F97L core protein in the intracellular phenotype of plus-strand and RC DNA deficiency. The mutant core protein results in a less than twofold decrease in overall DNA synthesis (Left Panel) as well as a reproducible twofold decrease in plus-strand DNA synthesis (Middle Panel). Specific probes used in each experiment are labeled at the bottom of each panel. **(B)** A complementation assay for the *trans*-defect of mutant F97L core protein in the extracellular phenotype of immature secretion. Co-transfection of the F97L mutant core protein alone is necessary and sufficient to result in the secretion of Dane particles containing excessive immature genome of single-strand DNA.

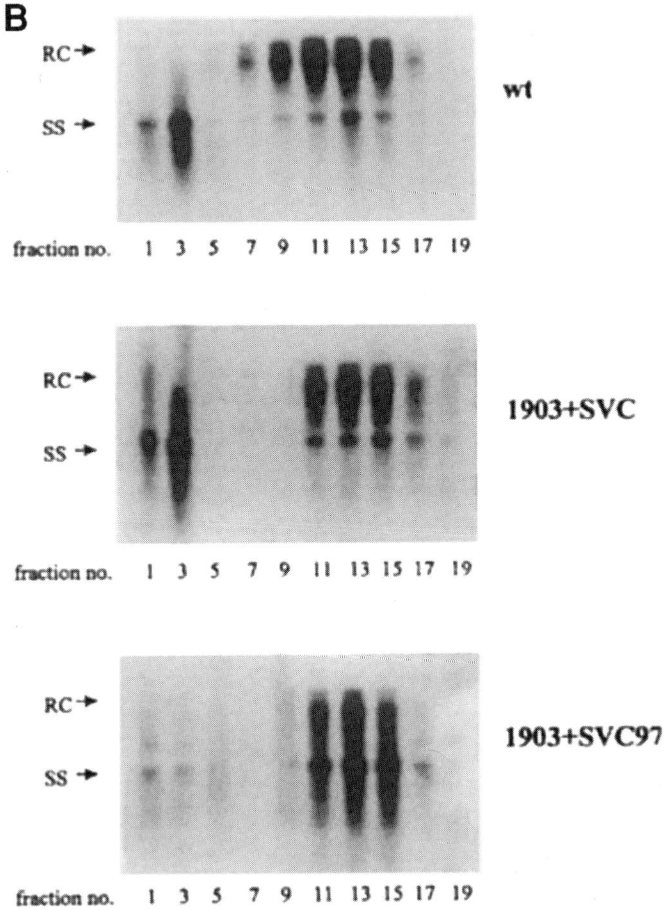

1.2. A Novel Complementation Test for the cis *Effect of Mutation F97L*

Although the *trans* effect of the mutant 97L core protein alone is sufficient for the extracellular phenotype of immature secretion **(Fig. 3B)**, the result in **Fig. 3A** (a two-fold reduction) does not appear to be sufficient to explain the dramatic reduction (five-fold) in the intracellular plus-strand and RC DNA synthesis of mutant F97L observed in **Fig. 1A**. In addition to the *trans* defect of a mutant core protein, another potential consequence of mutation F97L is to create a *cis* defect in the mutant genome.

To examine this possibility, we compared the replication activity between the single mutant 1903 and the double mutant 1903/F97L when these two core-defective mutants were rescued with the same wild-type core protein expressed from pSVC **(Fig. 2B)**. Any difference in their replication activities will be the result of the *cis* effect of the F97L nucleotide change, because the same wild-type core protein was used in both co-transfection experiments. As shown in **Fig. 4**, although the *cis* effect of mutation F97L has only a twofold or so reduction in overall DNA synthesis (left panel), its effect on intracellular plus-strand synthesis in this complementation assay is a decrease of close to 10-fold (middle panel), and its effect on minus-strand synthesis is a decrease of about 2.4-fold (right panel) compared with its wild-type counterpart.

Taken together, these results suggest that the intracellular plus-strand deficiency is in part a result of the *cis* defect of the mutant genome. In addition to its effect on plus-strand synthesis, mutation F97L seems to affect minus-strand synthesis in this experimental setting. Dane particles produced from co-transfecting mutant 1903/F97L plus wild-type core-expression vector pSVC exhibited a gradient profile similar to that of wild-type HBV, albeit at a significantly reduced level, and did not have the immature secretion phenotype (unpublished result). Therefore, although there is some *cis* effect on the intracellular plus-strand DNA level, there is no apparent *cis* effect on the immature secretion phenotype.

Because of the compact size of the HBV genome, it is conceivable that a single mutation could have both *cis* and *trans* effects with consequent pleiotropic phenotypes, as exemplified here by F97L mutation. The genetic approach demonstrated in this chapter can be applied to the study of the biological significance of other mutations in HBV or non-HBV viral systems ***(29,31–33)***.

2. Materials

2.1. Solutions and Buffers

1. 1 *M* Tris-HCl, pH 7.5 and pH 7.4.
2. 5 *M* NaCl.
3. 0.5 *M* ethylenediaminetetraacetic acid (EDTA).
4. TNE, 150 m*M* NaCl, 20 m*M* Tris-HCl, pH 7.4, 1 m*M* EDTA.
5. 10 mg/mL proteinase K.
6. 10% sodium dodecyl sulfate (SDS).
7. 70% and 100% ethanol.
8. Nonidet P-40.
9. 20% and 25% sucrose (w/v) in TNE.
10. 1 *M* $CaCl_2$.
11. 1 *M* $MgCl_2$.
12. 26% polyethylene glycol (molecular weight 8000) (w/v).
13. 20% and 50% (w/v) cesium chloride in TNE.
14. Phenol.
15. Chloroform.
16. α-^{32}P dCTP (3000 Ci/mmol).
17. α-^{32}P UTP (3000 Ci/mmol).
18. dATP, dTTP, dCTP, dGTP.
19. Sephadex G 50.

2.2. Cell Lines and Tissue Culture

The human hepatoma cell line Huh7, which has been shown to be permissive for HBV replication, was used for DNA transfection. All cell lines were maintained in Dul-

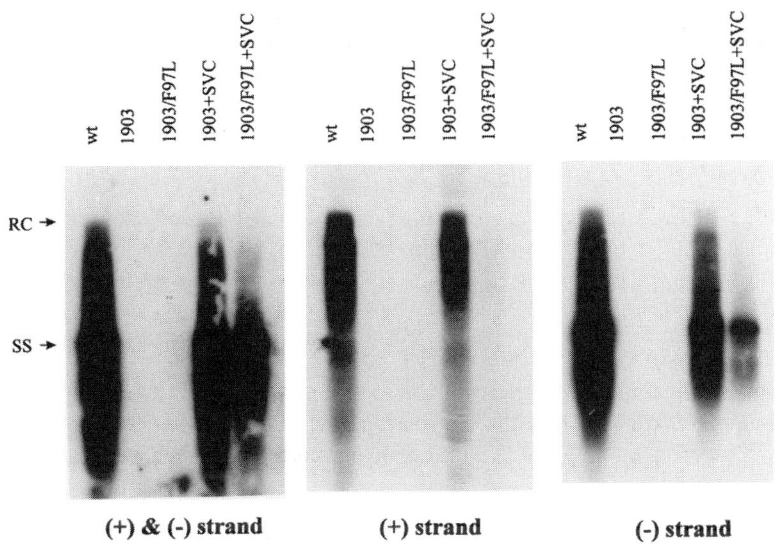

Fig. 4. A complementation assay for the *cis*-defect of the mutant F97L genome in the intracellular phenotype of plus-strand and RC DNA deficiency. Wild-type core protein was used to *trans*-complement both the single mutant 1903 and the double mutant 1903/F97L. The probes used for each blot are shown at the bottom of each panel.

becco's modified Eagle's medium (DMEM) with 10% fetal bovine serum (FBS) at 37°C in the presence of 5.5% CO_2.

2.3. Plasmid Constructs

1. pWT: Described as pSV2NeoHBV2x elsewhere *(34)*, it is a replication vector of wild-type HBV with a tandem dimer configuration.
2. pF97L: Site-directed mutagenesis was performed to introduce specific mutations into the HBV monomer genome, which was subsequently dimerized to mimic the genetic configuration of HBV *(35)*. The oligonucleotide used to create mutation F97L is 5'-GGGCCTAAA GCTCAGGCAACT-3'.
3. p1903: The initiation codon of the core antigen in mutant p1903 was abolished with the oligonucleotide 5'-TTT TGG GGC ATA GAC ATC GAC C-3'.
4. pF97L/1903: Contains double mutations, F97L and 1903.
5. pSVC: Wild-type core-antigen–expression vector under the control of simian virus 40 (SV40) enhancer and early promoter. The cloning strategy of pSVC has been described previously *(35)*.
6. pSVC97: The same protocol for constructing pSVC was used for the construction of pSVC97, using mutant pF97L as a polymerase chain reaction (PCR) DNA template.

3. Methods

3.1. Co-transfections to Analyze cis-/trans Complementation

1. Approximately 2–3 × 10^6 Huh7 or HepG2 cells are seeded in each 10-cm-diameter dish 12–16 h before transfection. Ten micrograms of each plasmid DNA is used as donor DNAs

for calcium phosphate transfection. In each transfection, the total amount of donor DNA is kept constant (35 μg DNA/2–3 × 10^6 cells/10-cm-dish/transfection). Carrier DNA of Huh7 origin is used to adjust the final amount of donor DNA to a total of 35 μg ***(36)***.

2. Donor DNA is removed at approx 6 h post-transfection and cells fed with fresh DMEM containing 10% FBS.

3.2. Preparation of Intracellular Core Particles

1. At 5 d post-transfection, lyse the cells from one 10-cm dish (6 × 10^6 cells) at 37°C (15 min) in 1 mL of buffer containing 10 m*M* Tris-HCl, pH 7.5, 1 m*M* EDTA, 50 m*M* NaCl, 0.25% Nonidet P-40, and 8% sucrose.
2. Spin the lysate in a microcentrifuge for 2 min and transfer the supernatant to another tube.
3. Add 30 U of micrococcal nuclease and 1 U of DNase I to the supernatant (adjusted to 8 m*M* $CaCl_2$ and 6 m*M* $MgCl_2$). Incubate at 37°C for 15 min.
4. Precipitate the crude core particles by adding 330 μL of 26% polyethylene glycol (molecular weight 8000) in 1.5 *M* NaCl and 60 m*M* EDTA.
5. After incubation for 1 h at 4°C, pellet the crude core particle by spinning in a microcentrifuge for 4 min.

3.3. Sedimentation and Fractionation of Secreted Viral Particles

1. Collect conditioned media on d 5 and 7 from 6 × 10^6 cells post-transfection.
2. Clear the medium by centrifugation at 3000 rpm for 30 min at 4°C.
3. Pellet virus particles from the clarified medium through a 16-mL sucrose cushion (20% sucrose in TNE) by spinning at 26,000 rpm for 16 h at 4°C in a Beckman SW28 rotor.
3. Resuspend the pellet in 200 μL of TNE buffer and fractionate the particles by isopycnic centrifugation through a gradient of 20–50% cesium chloride at 35,000 rpm in a Beckman SW41 rotor for 16 h at 4°C. The 20–50% cesium chloride gradient is made from a two-chamber gradient maker. Equal volumes (1.8 mL) of 20% and 50% cesium chloride are mixed by the gradient maker into a centrifuge tube to form a 20–50% gradient (from top to bottom). After centrifugation, fractionated viral particles are collected in a volume of 200 μL per fraction.

3.4. Preparation of Core-Associated DNA

1. Resuspend the core pellet in 100 μL of buffer containing 10 m*M* Tris-HCl, pH 7.5, 8 m*M* $CaCl_2$, and 6 m*M* $MgCl_2$.
2. Remove input plasmid DNA by adding 30 U of micrococcal nuclease and 1 U of DNase I and incubate for 15 min at 37°C.
3. Lyse the core particles by adding 300 μL of lysis buffer containing 25 m*M* Tris-HCl, pH 7.5, 10 m*M* EDTA, and 1% SDS in the presence of proteinase K, at a final concentration of 400 μg/mL. Incubate at 50°C for 1 h.
4. Phenol/chloroform and then ethanol precipitate DNA.

3.5. HBV-Specific Probes for Southern Blot Analyses

3.5.1. Full-Length HBV DNA Probe

1. Excise and purify the full-length 3.1-kb HBV DNA fragment from pSV2ANeoHBV by *Eco*RI digestion.
2. Radiolabel approx 25 ng of the 3.1-kb DNA fragment using a random primed DNA labeling kit (Boehringer Co.) and α-^{32}P-dCTP.
3. Purify the labeled probe by passing through a Sephadex G 50 column.

3.5.2. Plus Strand–Specific Riboprobe

Insert one copy of the HBV monomer genome in the pGEM-4Z vector (Promega Co., WI). Use T7 polymerase and the *Xho*I-linearized pGEM-4Z-HBV DNA as a template for in vitro transcription using α-^{32}P-UTP for labeling.

3.5.3. Minus Strand-Specific Riboprobe

Use SP6 polymerase and *Hind*III-linearized pGEM-4Z HBV DNA as a template for in vitro transcription using α-^{32}P-UTP for labeling.

3.6. DNA Quantitation and Analysis

1. Southern blots using the core-associated DNA from **Subheading 3.4.** and probes from **Subheading 3.5.** are performed using standard procedures and will not be detailed here.
2. The amounts of DNA in replicative intermediates detected with the different probes are quantitated either by phosphorimager analysis or scanning autoradiographs (*see* **Note 1**).

4. Notes

1. The *cis*-effect of the F97L mutation on intracellular plus-strand viral DNA synthesis is a decrease of close to 10-fold when assayed in the experimental setting of complementation (co-transfection) (**Fig. 4**). However, in the experimental setting using a tandem dimer context, the difference in plus-strand DNA synthesis between wild-type virus and mutant F97L is only about four- to five-fold (**Fig. 1**). The discrepancy in the plus-strand DNA deficiency between these two experimental settings remains unclear.

References

1. Birnbaum, F. and M. Nassal. (1990) Hepatitis B virus nucleocapsid assembly: primary structure requirements in the core protein. *J. Virol.* **64**, 3319–3330.
2. Nassal, M. and Schaller, H. (1996) Hepatitis B virus replication—an update. *J. Viral Hepat.* **3**, 217–226.
3. Haton, T., Zhou, S., and Standring, D. N. (1992) RNA- and DNA-binding activities in hepatitis B virus capsid protein: a model for their roles in viral replication. *J. Virol.* **66**, 5232–5241.
4. Tuttleman, J., Pourcel, C., and Summers, J. (1986) Formation of the pool of covalently closed viral DNA in hepadnavirus-infected cells. *Cell* **47**, 451–460.
5. Bruss, V., and Ganem, D. (1991) The role of envelope proteins in hepatitis B virus assembly. *Proc. Natl. Acad. Sci. USA* **88**, 1059–1063.
6. Ou, J.-H. and Rutter, W. J. (1987) Regulation of secretion of the hepatitis B virus major surface antigen by the pre-S1 protein. *J. Virol.* **61**, 782–786.
7. Akarca, U. S. and Lok, A. S. F. (1995) Naturally occurring hepatitis B virus core gene mutations. *Hepatology* **22**, 50–60.
8. Bozkaya, H., Ayola, B., and Lok, A. S. F. (1996) High rate of mutations in the hepatitis B core gene during the immune clearance phase of chronic hepatitis B virus infection. *Hepatology* **24**, 32–37.
9. Chuang, W. L., Omata, M., Ehata, T., Yokosuka, O., Ito, Y., and Ohto, M. (1993) Concentrating missense mutations in core gene of hepatitis B virus. *Dig. Dis. Sci.* **38**, 594–600.
10. Chuang, W. L., Omata, M., Ehata, T., et al. (1993) Precore mutations and core clustering mutations in chronic hepatitis B virus infection. *Gastroenterology* **104**, 263–271.

11. Ehata, T., Omata, M., Yokosuka, O., Hosoda, K., and Ohto, M. (1992) Variations in codons 84–101 in the core nucleotide sequence correlate with hepatocellular injury in chronic hepatitis B virus infection. *J. Clin. Invest.* **89**, 332–338.
12. Ehata, T., Omata, M., Chuang, W. L., et al. (1993) Mutations in core nucleotide sequence of hepatitis B virus correlate with fulminant and severe hepatitis. *J. Clin. Invest.* **91**, 1206–1213.
13. Gotoh, K., Mima, S., Uchida, T., Shikata, T., Yoshizawa, K., Irie, M., and Mizui, M. (1995) Nucleotide sequence of hepatitis B virus isolated from subjects without serum anti-hepatitis B core antibody. *J. Med. Virol.* **46**, 201–206.
14. Gray, A. H., Fang, J. W. S., Davis, G. L., et al. (1997) Variations of hepatitis B virus core gene sequence in Western patients with chronic hepatitis B virus infection. *J. Viral Hepatitis* **4**, 371–378.
15. Gunther, S., Baginski, S., Kissel, H., et al. (1996) Accumulation and persistence of hepatitis B virus core gene deletion mutants in renal transplant patients are associated with end-stage liver disease. *Hepatology* **24**, 751–758.
16. Hosono, S., Tai, P. C., Wang, W., et al. (1995) Core antigen mutations of human hepatitis B virus in hepatomas accumulate in MHC class II-restricted T cell epitopes. *Virology* **212**, 151–162.
17. Hur, G. M., Lee, Y. I., Sun, D. J., Lee, J. H., and Lee, Y. I. (1996) Gradual accumulation of mutations in precore/core region of HBV in patients with chronic active hepatitis: implication of clustering changes in a small region of the HBV core region. *J. Med. Virol.* **48**, 38–46.
18. Karasawa, T., Shirasawa, T., Okawa, Y., et al. (1997) Association between frequency of amino acid changes in core region of hepatitis B virus (HBV) and the presence of precore mutation in Japanese HBV carriers. *J. Gastroenterol.* **32**, 611–622.
19. McMillan, J. S., Bowden, D. S., Angus, P. W., McCaughan, G. W., and Locarnini, S. A. (1996) Mutations in the hepatitis B virus precore/core and core promoter in patients with severe recurrent disease following liver transplantation. *Hepatology* **24**, 1371–1378.
20. Miska, S., Gunther, S., Vassilev, M., Meisel, H., Pape, G., and Will, H. (1993) Heterogeneity of hepatitis B virus C-gene sequences: implications for amplification and sequencing. *J. Heptol.* ***18***, 53–61.
21. Pollicino, T., Campo, S., and Raimondo, G. (1995) PreS and core gene heterogeneity in hepatitis B virus (HBV) genomes isolated from patients with long-lasting HBV chronic infection. *Virology* **208**, 672–677.
22. Pollicino, T. S., Zanetti, A. R., Cacciola, I., et al. (1997) Pre-S2 defective hepatitis B virus infection in patients with fulminant hepatitis. *Hepatology* **26**, 495–499.
23. Rodriguez-Frias, F., Buti, M., Jardi, R., et al. (1995) Hepatitis B virus infection: precore mutants and its relation to viral genotypes and core mutations. *Hepatology* **22**, 1641–1647.
24. Uchida, T., Aye, T. T., Becher, S. O., et al. (1993) Detection of precore/core-mutant hepatitis B virus genome in patients with acute or fulminant hepatitis without serological markers for recent HBV infection. *J. Hepatol.* **18**, 369–372.
25. Uchida, T., Aye, T. T., Shihata, T., et al. (1994) Evolution of the hepatitis B virus gene during chronic infection in seven patients. *J. Med. Virol.* **43**, 148–154.
26. Valliammai, T., Thyagarajan, S. P., Zuckerman, A. J., and Harrison, T. J. (1995) Precore and core mutations in HBV from individuals in India with chronic infection. *J. Med. Virol.* **45**, 321–325.
27. Yuan, T. T., Sahu, G. K., Whitehead, W. E., Greenberg, R., and Shih, C. (1999) The mechanism of an immature secretion phenotype of a highly frequent naturally occurring missense mutation at codon 97 of human hepatitis B virus core antigen. *J. Virol.* **73**, 5731–5740.

28. Yuan, T. T., Tai, P. C., and Shih, C. (1999) Subtype-independent immature secretion and subtype-dependent replication deficiency of a highly frequent, naturally occurring mutation of human hepatitis B virus core antigen. *J. Virol.* **73**, 10122–10128.
29. Le Pogam, S. and Shih, C. (2002) Influence of a putative intermolecular interaction between core and the pre-S1 domain of the large envelope protein on hepatitis B virus secretion. *J. Virol.* **76**, 6510–6517.
30. Summers, J. and Mason, W. S. (1982) Replication of the genome of a hepatitis B-like virus by reverse transcription of an RNA intermediate. *Cell* **29**, 403–415.
31. Le Pogam, S., Yuan, T. T., Sahu, G. K., Chatterjee, S., and Shih, C. (2000) Low-level secretion of human hepatitis B virus virions caused by two independent, naturally occurring mutations (P5T and L60V) in the capsid protein. *J. Virol.* **74**, 9099–9105.
32. Tai, P. C., Suk, F. M., Gerlich, W. H., Neurath, A. R., and Shih C. C. (2002) Hypermodification and immune escape of an internally deleted middle-envelope (M) protein of frequent and predominant hepatitis B virus variants. *Virology* **292**, 44–58.
33. Yuan, T. T. and Shih, C. (2000) A frequent, naturally occurring mutation (P130T) of human hepatitis B virus core antigen is compensatory for immature secretion phenotype of another frequent variant (I97L). *J. Virol.* **74**, 4929–4932.
34. Shih, C., L. Li, S., Roychoudhury, S., and Ho, M. H. (1989) In vitro propagation of human hepatitis B virus in a rat hepatoma cell line. *Proc. Natl. Acad. Sci. USA* **86**, 6323–6327.
35. Roychoudhury, S., Faruqi, A., and Shih, C. (1991) Pregenomic RNA encapsidation analysis of eleven missense and nonsense polymerase mutants of human hepatitis B virus. *J. Virol.* **65**, 3617–3624.
36. Yuan, T.-T., Lin, M. H., Qiu, S. M., and Shih, C. (1998) Functional characterization of naturally-occurring variants of human hepatitis B virus containing the core internal deletion mutation *J. Virol.* **72**, 2168–2176.

25

Studying DHBV Polymerase by In Vitro Transcription and Translation

Jianming Hu

1. Introduction

Duck hepatitis B virus (DHBV), like all other hepadnaviruses, is a retroid virus that bears a small DNA genome and replicates this DNA genome via reverse transcription through an RNA intermediate called pregenomic RNA (pgRNA; *1*). All hepadnaviruses encode a multifunctional polymerase (pol), which is a specialized reverse transcriptase (RT) and plays key roles in several different aspects of the viral life cycle *(2–5)*. Pol has an RNA- and DNA-directed DNA polymerase (i.e., RT) activity that is responsible for DNA genome replication, which also entails its intrinsic RNase H activity responsible for degrading the pgRNA as the pgRNA is being reverse transcribed into the first (minus) strand of the DNA genome. In addition to the RT and RNase H activities, which are shared with retroviral RTs, the hepadnavirus polymerase displays the unique ability to initiate DNA synthesis de novo using pol itself as a protein primer (protein priming) *(6–9)*.

Like its human HBV counterpart, the DHBV polymerase has a domain structure that is reflective of its multiple functions (**Fig. 1A**). The central and C-terminal regions constitute the RT and RNase H domains, which share significant homologies with the corresponding domains of retroviral RTs. By contrast, the N-terminal domain does not share any significant homologies with any other known polypeptides, except among the hepadnavirus polymerases. Separated by a tether (or spacer) from the RT domain, the N-terminal domain bears a specific tyrosine residue (Y96) that acts as the primer for the initiation of RNA-directed DNA synthesis during protein priming and thus is termed the terminal-protein (TP) domain. As a consequence of this unusual protein priming reaction, the 5' end of the viral minus strand DNA becomes covalently linked to the N terminus of the polymerase and remains attached during the entire DNA synthesis process *(10–12)*.

In addition to these essential roles in DNA synthesis, both as a catalytic enzyme and a primer, pol is also essential for packaging of the pgRNA into viral core particles, the

From: *Methods in Molecular Medicine, vol. 95: Hepatitis B and D Protocols, volume 1*
Edited by: R. K. Hamatake and J. Y. N. Lau © Humana Press Inc., Totowa, NJ

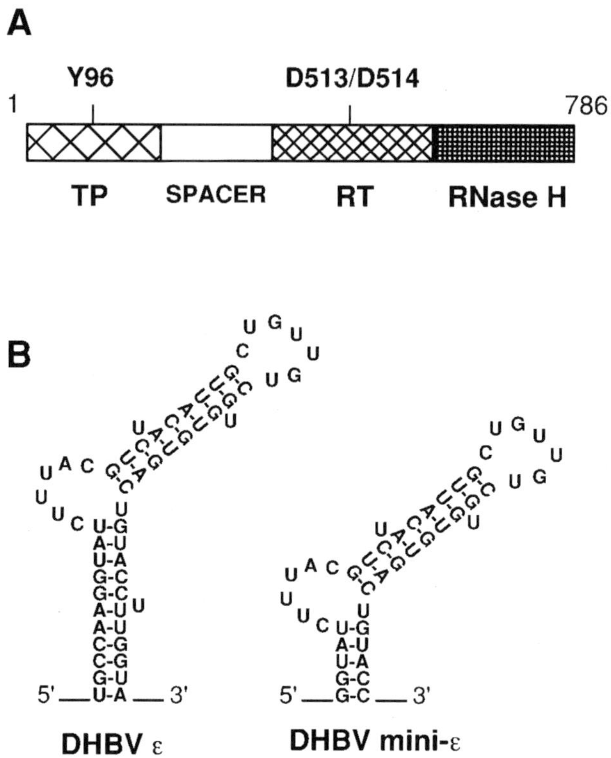

Fig. 1. Domain structure of the DHBV polymerase and the proposed secondary structure of the ϵ RNA. **(A)** The DHBV pol consists of 786 amino-acid residues and can be divided into four structural domains: the N-terminal domain (also called the terminal protein, TP), the central reverse-transcriptase domain (RT), the C-terminal RNase H domain, and a spacer region separating the TP and the RT domains ***(29)***. The RT and RNase H domains share significant homologies with other RTs; the two highly conserved aspartic-acid residues believed to reside in the RT active site are indicated. The N-terminal domain of the DHBV pol does not show any significant homologies to other known polypeptides, except for the corresponding domain of the other hepadnavirus polymerases. The position of the tyrosine residue (Y96) within the TP domain that serves as the primer for initiating viral minus-strand DNA synthesis is indicated. The spacer region is highly divergent among different viral isolates and appears to be dispensable for the known enzymatic functions of pol. **(B)** Secondary structures of the DHBV ϵ RNA (positions 2560–2616) ***(30)***. As proposed initially by Junker-Niepmann et al. ***(15)***, the ϵ RNA features a lower and an upper stem, an apical loop, and an internal bulge. These structural features are conserved among all hepadnavirus ϵ RNAs despite their limited sequence identity ***(24)***. Also shown is the mini-DHBV ϵ, which has the lower portion of the lower stem deleted but remains fully active in pol binding and protein priming ***(26,36)***.

site of viral DNA synthesis ***(13, 14)***. Central to both protein-primed initiation of reverse transcription and the packaging of the pgRNA is the specific interaction between pol and a short RNA signal located at the 5' end of the pgRNA, termed ϵ. Initially identified as the RNA-packaging signal that specifically directs the incorporation of the pgRNA into the nucleocapsids ***(15, 16)***, ϵ also proved to be the origin of reverse transcription. The RNA-packaging process is initiated by binding of pol to ϵ, forming a specific ribonucleoprotein (RNP) complex, which is, in turn, recognized by the assembling capsid proteins, leading to the specific incorporation of both pol and pgRNA into nucleocapsids ***(13,14,17,18)***.

The role of ϵ as the origin of reverse transcription was revealed when it was shown that the pol–ϵ RNP complex formation is a prerequisite for the initiation of protein-primed reverse transcription, and indeed ϵ serves as the template for protein priming ***(18–22)***. All hepadnavirus ϵ RNAs bear two inverted repeat sequences and can fold into a conserved stem-loop structure, with a lower and an upper stem, an apical loop, and an internal bulge ***(15,16,23–25)*** (**Fig. 1B**). As depicted in **Fig. 2**, it is the sequence within the internal bulge of ϵ that serves as the template for the protein-primed initiation of reverse transcription in all hepadnaviruses. The product of protein priming is a three-to-four-nucleotide-long DNA oligomer that is covalently attached to pol via the primer tyrosine residue in the TP domain. Two separate regions of pol, one in the RT domain and the other in the TP domain, are required for the formation of the RNP complex with ϵ and for protein priming ***(18,22,26)***. Interestingly, the entire pol polypeptide, but not any of its known enzymatic activities, is required for pgRNA packaging, perhaps by acting as a scaffold for the assembling nucleocapsids ***(13,14,27)***.

Detailed structural and functional studies on the hepadnavirus polymerase, a most unusual enzyme critical for viral replication, have been, and still are, hampered by the inability to obtain sufficient amounts of a highly purified, enzymatically active pol protein. Although an "endogenous" DNA polymerase activity able to extend the incomplete viral DNA genome in the viral particles could be detected 30 years ago ***(3)***, the polymerase packaged in the viral particles cannot accept exogenous DNA or RNA sequences as templates for DNA synthesis ***(28)***, thus limiting their application for biochemical and genetic studies. Furthermore, efforts to express and purify an enzymatically active pol in recombinant forms have met with only limited success until recently ***(29)***.

A major breakthrough came in 1992, when it was first demonstrated by Wang and Seeger that a functional DHBV pol can be expressed in a rabbit reticulocyte lysate in vitro translation system ***(7)***. The in vitro-expressed polymerase is active in RNP formation with ϵ and in priming DNA synthesis using the ϵ RNA as the authentic template. As a result of its simplicity, the reticulocyte lysate system has proved to be amenable to genetic and biochemical analyses of the DHBV polymerase. Indeed, much of what we know today regarding the mechanisms of RNP formation and protein priming in hepadnaviruses in general, as outlined above, has been obtained by using this simple cell-free system. Here, I provide a detailed description of the cell-free translation system for the expression of the DHBV polymerase and the methods to assay for its protein-priming activity in vitro.

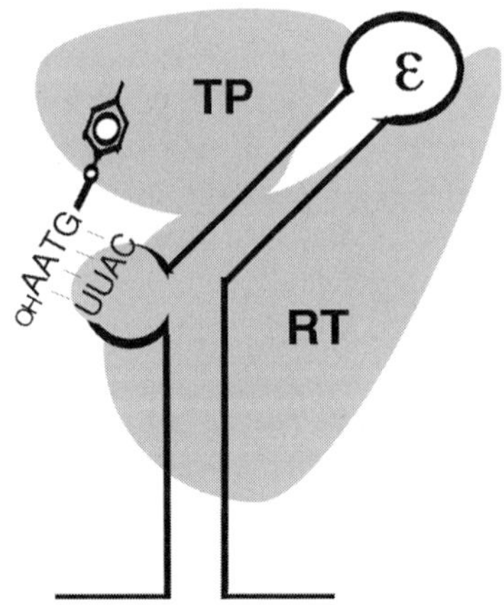

Fig. 2. Protein-priming mechanism of hepadnaviruses. Priming of viral DNA synthesis occurs at the ϵ RNA sequence located near the 5' end of pregenomic RNA, with a specific tyrosine residue within the polymerase polypeptide acting as a primer. As depicted, both the TP domain, where the primer tyrosine resides, and the RT domain, where the polymerase active site resides, are required for this protein-primed initiation of reverse transcription. The template for protein priming is the internal-bulge sequence (5'-UUAC-3' in DHBV) of the ϵ stem-loop structure. The product of protein priming is a four-nucleotide long oligodeoxynucleotide covalently attached to pol through the primer tyrosine residue. In DHBV, the DNA oligomer has the sequence 5'-GTAA-3', with dGMP being the first nucleotide of the viral minus-strand DNA that is attached to pol.

2. Materials

2.1. Plasmids for In Vitro Transcription

1. To make the DHBV pol RNA for in vitro translation, the pol-coding sequence (*see* **Note 1**), starting from the second in frame AUG in the pol open reading frame (ORF) at position 170 of the DHBV genome ***(7,30)***, is cloned into an appropriate in vitro transcription vector (such as pSP65, Promega; pcDNA3, Invitrogen), downstream of the phage promoter (SP6 or T7). Purified phage polymerases are commercially available and are highly specific and efficient for in vitro transcription.
2. In addition to the pol-coding sequence, the coding sequence for the ϵ RNA can also be included downstream of the pol ORF in the same vector (***7,22***). An advantage of such a construction is that one RNA transcribed in vitro can serve as the template for pol translation as well as provide the ϵ RNA template for protein priming (*see* **Note 2**).
3. The ϵ RNA can also be transcribed from a separate DNA template. In that case, the ϵ-coding sequence (**Fig. 1B**) is cloned into an appropriate in vitro transcription vector, as described above.
4. Alternatively, a synthetic DNA template is made by annealing two DNA oligomers: one representing the forward SP6 or T7 promoter sequence and the other representing the antisense promoter sequence fused downstream to the antisense ϵ coding sequence ***(22,26)***.

2.2. Other Reagents

1. Reliable kits for in vitro transcription are available from several commercial sources, such as Ambion and Promega (*see* **Note 3**). We routinely use the Ambion MegaScript Kit, which is designed to make large amounts (up to milligrams) of RNA in vitro. Store the transcription kit at –20°C or below as recommended by the suppliers.
2. Rabbit reticulocyte lysate in vitro translation systems are available from several suppliers, including Promega and Ambion. We routinely use the nuclease-treated rabbit reticulocyte lysate system from Promega, which includes all reagents necessary for in vitro translation. In addition, coupled in vitro transcription and translation systems are also commercially available. We routinely use the TnT rabbit reticulocyte lysate system from Promega, which includes all reagents necessary to conduct protein translation directly from DNA template (*see* below). Store the translation system at –70°C as recommended by the supplier.
3. A modified TMN buffer (50 m*M* Tris-HCl, pH 7.5, 2 m*M* $MgCl_2$, 15 m*M* NaCl) is recommended for the in vitro protein-priming reaction (*see* **Note 4**). For convenience, this buffer is made as a 10X stock and is diluted 10-fold into the protein-priming reaction. Keep the 10X TMN buffer at room temperature in small aliquots. Use RNase-free reagents, including dH_2O.
4. dNTPs (deoxynucleoside triphosphates) stocks (Sigma or Gibco BRL) are suitable for the protein-priming reaction. For convenience, a 10X dNTP stock, containing all dNTPs except that corresponding to the ^{32}P-labeled nucleotide (*see* **Note 5**), at 140 μ*M* each, is made in nuclease-free dH_2O and stored in aliquots at –70°C.
5. ^{32}P-radiolabeled nucleotide, either [α-^{32}P]dGTP, [α-^{32}P]dATP, or [α-^{32}P]TTP, at a specific activity of 400–800 Ci/mmol, is purchased from NEN or Amersham.
6. Translation grade ^{35}S methionine (specific activity, 1200 Ci/mmol) is purchased from NEN or Amersham and stored in small aliquots at –70°C.
7. Nuclease-free dH_2O: Add diethyl pyrocarbonate to dH_2O to a final concentration of 0.1%, shake well, and incubate in a 37°C water bath overnight. Then autoclave for 30 min. Alternatively, nuclease-free dH_2O can be purchased from commercial sources.

3. Methods

3.3. Preparation of DNA Template for In Vitro Transcription

1. DNA template for in vitro transcription is prepared using commercial DNA Miniprep or Maxiprep Kits (e.g., Promega, Qiagen).
2. Before being used for RNA synthesis, the DNA plasmid containing the pol-coding sequence is linearized with a restriction endonuclease downstream of the pol stop codon. Alternatively, to synthesize an RNA containing both the pol-coding sequence and the ε RNA, the plasmid DNA is linearized downstream of the ε-coding sequence.
3. When the ε RNA is to be transcribed from a separate plasmid DNA template, the plasmid is similarly linearized with a restriction endonuclease downstream of the ε coding sequence. For ε RNA synthesis from a synthetic DNA template (DNA oligonucleotide template, *see* **Subheading 2.1.**), the template DNA is already in a linear form.
4. The linearized DNA is then further "cleaned" by digestion with proteinase K (200 μg/mL) in the presence of 0.5% sodium dodecyl sulfate (SDS) for 30 min to 1 h at 37°C, followed by standard phenol/chloroform extraction and ethanol precipitation *(31)* to remove residual amounts of contaminating RNases and other impurities. The purified, linearized DNA is then resuspended in nuclease-free dH_2O.

5. On the other hand, when the DNA template is to be used for coupled in vitro transcription and translation reaction (**Subheading 3.4.**), the plasmid should not be linearized. The DNA is simply treated with proteinase K digestion followed by phenol/chloroform extraction and ethanol precipitation, as described above.

3.2. In Vitro Transcription

1. RNA synthesis using the in vitro transcription kit (such as the MEGAscript kit from Ambion) is carried out according to the procedure recommended by the manufacturer.
2. Following the transcription reaction, remove the DNA template by digestion with RNase-free DNase I and purify the RNA by phenol extraction and ethanol precipitation using standard procedures *(31)*.
3. Following ethanol precipitation, the purified RNA is resuspended in nuclease-free dH_2O. Using the Ambion MEGAscript kit, we routinely obtain 10–100 μg of purified RNA, depending on the size of the transcript, from a standard 20-μL reaction, ready for in vitro translation.
4. If desired, the quality of RNA can be verified by electrophoresis on standard agarose gel (either native or denaturing) under RNase-free conditions and visualized by ethidium bromide staining *(31)*.

3.3. In Vitro Translation

1. In vitro translation reaction in the rabbit reticulocyte lysate system is carried out as recommended by the supplier. We routinely use 2 μL (5–10 μg) of purified RNA obtained from **Subheading 3.2.** in a standard 50-μL reaction.
2. To visualize the translation product, the translation reaction is supplemented with ^{35}S-methionine, according to procedures recommended by the manufacturer.
3. Translation reactions are incubated for 60–90 min at 30°C and stopped by addition of cycloheximide to a final concentration of 50 μg/mL. The concentration of the polymerase in the translation reaction is approximately 1 ng/μL.
4. If the ε RNA is part of the RNA used to translate pol (i.e., *in cis)*, pol will become associated with the ε RNA as it is being translated. When ε is to be added, *in trans*, as a separate RNA, it can be added to the translation reaction before starting the reaction. Again, pol will bind to ε co-translationally. In the latter case, we usually add 1 μL (approx 1 μg) of ε RNA per 50-μL translation. Alternatively, the ε RNA can be added later during the protein priming reaction (*see* **Subheading 3.5.**).

3.4. One-Step Coupled In Vitro Transcription and Translation

To express pol using a coupled in vitro transcription and translation system, circular plasmid DNA template is used. We routinely use the TnT rabbit reticulocyte lysate system from Promega for this purpose. Here, transcription and translation are carried out in one step; as the pol RNA is being transcribed from the DNA template, the RNA is, in turn, being translated to the protein, all in one reaction step. Significantly higher (5- to 10-fold) amounts of pol protein may be obtained using the TnT system, as compared with the conventional translation system described above.

3.5. In Vitro Protein Priming

1. To 5 μL of the reticulocyte lysate translation reaction containing the polymerase, the following components are added to initiate the protein-priming reaction: 1 μL 10X TMN, 1 μL

10X dNTP mix (minus dGTP), 2.5 µL nuclease-free dH_2O, and 0.5 µL of [α-^{32}P]dGTP. When another [α-^{32}P]dNTP (dATP or TTP) is used, the corresponding unlabeled dNTP is omitted from the 10X dNTP mix.

2. As discussed earlier, the ε RNA can be added to the protein-priming reaction, following in vitro translation, if it is not already present, in *cis*, on the RNA used to translate pol or added in *trans* during translation (*see* **Note 6**). For a 10-µL priming reaction, we routinely add 0.2 µL (approx 200 ng) ε RNA obtained from in vitro transcription (**Subheading 3.2.**).
3. The priming reaction is incubated at 30°C for 30 min, and the reaction products are resolved by electrophoresis on an SDS/10% polyacrylamide gel using standard procedures *(31)*.
4. An aliquot of the in vitro pol translation reaction supplemented with ^{35}S-methionine can also be resolved to visualize the translation product.
5. As shown in **Fig. 3,** translation of an in vitro transcript encoding the DHBV pol fused to a 6X histidine tag *(9)* in the reticulocyte lysate produces a major protein product with an apparent molecular weight of approx 90 kDa (lane 1), which is in good agreement with the expected size of 90.5 kDa calculated from the predicted amino-acid sequence (785 amino-acid residues of the polymerase plus the six-histidine tag). Incubation of the in vitro-expressed polymerase in a solution that includes [α-^{32}P]dGTP leads to the incorporation of the ^{32}P label into the polymerase polypeptide as the labeled dGMP residue is covalently attached to pol (**Fig. 3,** lane 2). As discussed earlier, the ^{32}P-labeled pol represents the main product of the in vitro protein-priming reaction, i.e., a four-nucleotide long DNA oligomer with the sequence 5'-GTAA-3' covalently linked to the polymerase (via tyrosine 96 of the TP domain), with the template for DNA synthesis being the internal bulge sequence (5'-UUAC-3') of the ε RNA (*see* **Note 7**).

4. Notes

1. RNA leader sequences that stimulate translation, such as the bromo mosaic virus leader, can be added upstream of the pol ORF to enhance pol expression in vitro *(9)*. Also, affinity tags such as six histidine residues or the hemagglutinin or c-myc epitope can be fused to either terminus of pol or inserted into the spacer region; they do not affect pol functions but can facilitate pol purification and detection *(9,26)*.
2. As long as the minimal ε sequence (as defined in **Fig. 1B**) is present, some additional flanking RNA sequences do not appear to affect the folding and function of ε in protein priming in vitro. In fact, long RNAs, such as the full-length pgRNA, or RNA containing the ε sequence downstream of the pol-coding sequence, can be used as a functional ε RNA template for protein priming in vitro *(7)*.
3. All reagents for in vitro transcription, except the phage polymerase, can also be easily made in the lab. One precaution is that RNase-free reagents must be used.
4. The original TMN buffer contained 10 m*M* $MgCl_2$ *(7)*. We subsequently found that this relatively high concentration of $MgCl_2$ inhibits pol–ε interaction (but not protein priming per se) such that the protein-priming activity of the in vitro translated pol is dramatically decreased when the TMN buffer and ε RNA are added at the same time to the priming reaction following in vitro translation. Lowering the $MgCl_2$ concentration to 2 m*M* alleviates this problem *(29, 32)*.
5. As can be predicted from the template sequence at the internal bulge of the ε stem loop (UUAC, with no GMP residue), use of [α-^{32}P]dCTP as the labeled nucleotide does not lead to significant labeling of pol during protein priming *(7)*.
6. As discussed earlier, ε RNA can be present *in cis* on the RNA template coding for pol or added *in trans* as a separate RNA, either during or after the completion of the in vitro trans-

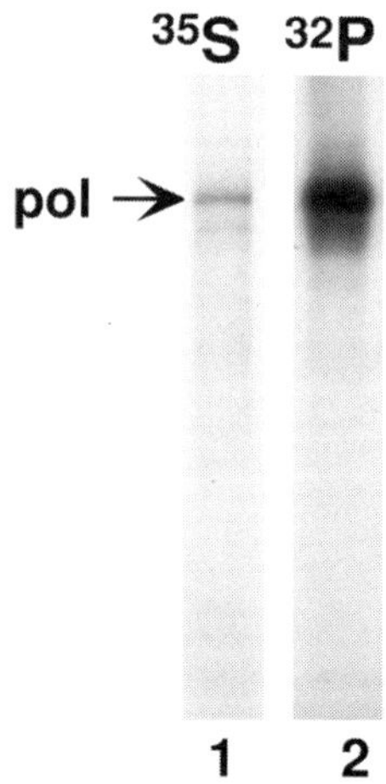

Fig. 3. Protein-priming activity of DHBV polymerase expressed in the reticulocyte-lysate in vitro translation system. Lane 1 shows the protein products obtained from an in vitro translation reaction in the rabbit reticulocyte lysate in the presence of ^{35}S methionine, using an in vitro transcribed RNA template encoding the DHBV pol fused to a 6X histidine tag at its N terminus. Lane 2 shows the products of an in vitro protein-priming reaction, whereby the in vitro translated polymerase was incubated with an in vitro transcribed DHBV ϵ RNA in the presence of [α-^{32}P]dGTP and unlabeled dATP, TTP, and dCTP. The translation and priming-reaction products were then resolved on an SDS/10% polyacrylamide gel, and an autoradiograph of the dried gel is shown. The full-length ^{35}S-(lane 1) or ^{32}P-labeled (lane 2) polymerase polypeptide is indicated by an arrow.

lation reaction. The protein-priming activity of pol increases as a function of the concentration of ϵ and is optimal at a final concentration of approx 1 μ*M* *(22)*.

7. The realization that the ϵ RNA can be provided *in trans* led to the development of convenient in vitro assays to directly detect the interaction between pol and ϵ. In one case, pol is incubated with ^{32}P-labeled ϵ RNA to allow RNP-complex formation, which is then immunoprecipitated using antibodies against epitope tags on pol. The labeled, coprecipitated ϵ RNA is then detected by polyacrylamide gel electrophoresis and autoradiography *(22,26)*. Alternatively, biotinylated ϵ RNA is synthesized by in vitro transcription in the presence of biotinylated ribonucleotides and incubated with ^{35}S-labeled pol. The biotinylated ϵ RNA and the pol–ϵ RNP complex are then isolated by avidin affinity beads, and the labeled pol in the RNP complex is detected by SDS/polyacrylamide gel electrophoresis and autoradiography (*18*). The apparent K_d for the pol–ϵ interaction has been estimated to be in the range of 8–26 n*M* (**18,22**). A small fraction of the nascent DNA strands formed during protein priming is further elongated in the in vitro reaction and ranges in length from 100–500 nucleotides *(7)*. When an RNA template containing the pol ORF plus the additional downstream pgRNA sequence was used to express pol in the reticulocyte lysate, it was found that during the DNA synthesis reaction, approx 10% of the protein-priming product (pol–dGTAA) was further extended either *in situ* or after template switching to a pgRNA site (the "acceptor" site) called DR1, situated between the end

of the pol-coding sequence and ϵ. This discovery, together with additional experiments carried out in cell cultures with complete viral DNA synthesis, led to the current model for minus-strand DNA–template switching during hepadnavirus reverse transcription, whereby the nascent minus-strand DNA–pol complex formed during protein priming at ϵ is translocated, across 3 kb of RNA sequence, to DR1 before DNA-strand elongation continues ***(7,21)***.

The in vitro pol translation/protein-priming system has proved to be useful for the identification of factors that can inhibit or activate the reaction. All available evidence indicates that pol adopts a different conformation during the protein-priming reaction and displays differential sensitivity to inhibitory agents, as compared with that adopted by pol during the subsequent DNA-elongation reaction. For example, inhibitors such as the pyrophosphate analog foscarnet and most nucleoside analogs, known to inhibit the elongation reaction, have little or no effect on the priming reaction ***(7,33)***. Furthermore, the in vitro expression system was also instrumental in the discovery that specific cellular factors are essential for pol to interact with ϵ and to carry out protein priming, most likely by helping to establish a pol conformation competent for ϵ binding. One of the initial clues suggesting that cellular factors present in the translation reaction may be important for pol function came from the observation that the in vitro-synthesized pol is present in high-molecular-weight complexes with cellular proteins in the reticulocyte lysate ***(32)***. In addition, it was found that pol translated in the wheat-germ extract is not active in ϵ binding or protein priming and furthermore can be activated by adding the reticulocyte lysate ***(32)***. Subsequent work led to the conclusion that the molecular chaperone, the heat-shock protein 90 (Hsp90) and its cofactors are associated with pol and are required to establish a pol conformation competent for ϵ binding and protein priming ***(26,32,34,35)***.

References

1. Summers, J. and Mason., W. S. (1982) Replication of the genome of a hepatitis B-like virus by reverse transcription of an RNA intermediate. *Cell* **29**, 403–415.
2. Chang, L. J., Hirsch, R. C., Ganem, D., and Varmus, H. E. (1990) Effects of insertional and point mutations on the functions of the duck hepatitis B virus polymerase. *J. Virol.* **64**, 5553–5558.
3. Kaplan, P. M., Greenman, R. L., Gerin, J. L., Purcell, R. H., and Robinson, W. S. (1973) DNA polymerase associated with human hepatitis B antigen. *J. Virol.* **12**, 995–1005.
4. Radziwill, G., Tucker, W., and Schaller, H. (1990) Mutational analysis of the hepatitis B virus P gene product: domain structure and RNase H activity. *J. Virol.* **64**, 613–620.
5. Toh, H., Hayashida, H., and Miyata, T. (1983) Sequence homology between retroviral reverse transcriptase and putative polymerases of hepatitis B virus and cauliflower mosaic virus. *Nature* **305**, 827–829.
6. Lanford, R. E., Notvall, L., and Beames, B. (1995) Nucleotide priming and reverse transcriptase activity of hepatitis B virus polymerase expressed in insect cells. *J. Virol.* **69**, 4431–4439.
7. Wang, G. H. and Seeger, C. (1992) The reverse transcriptase of hepatitis B virus acts as a protein primer for viral DNA synthesis. *Cell* **71**, 663–670.
8. Weber, M., Bronsema, V., Bartos, H., Bosserhoff, A., Bartenschlager, R., and Schaller, H. (1994) Hepadnavirus P protein utilizes a tyrosine residue in the TP domain to prime reverse transcription. *J. Virol.* **68**, 2994–2999.
9. Zoulim, F. and Seeger, C. (1994) Reverse transcription in hepatitis B viruses is primed by a tyrosine residue of the polymerase. *J. Virol.* **68**, 6–13.

10. Bartenschlager, R. and Schaller, H. (1988) The amino-terminal domain of the hepadnaviral P-gene encodes the terminal protein (genome-linked protein) believed to prime reverse transcription. *EMBO J.* **7**, 4185–4192.
11. Gerlich, W. and Robinson, W. S. (1980) Hepatitis B virus contains protein covalently attached to the 5' terminus of its complete DNA strand. *Cell* **21**, 801–809.
12. Molnar-Kimber, K. L., Summers, J., Taylor, J. M., and Mason, W. S. (1983) Protein covalently bound to minus-strand DNA intermediates of duck hepatitis B virus. *J. Virol.* **45**, 165–172.
13. Bartenschlager, R., Junker-Niepmann, M., and Schaller, H. (1990) The P gene product of hepatitis B virus is required as a structural component for genomic RNA encapsidation. *J. Virol.* **64**, 5324–5332.
14. Hirsch, R. C., Lavine, J. E., Chang, L. J., Varmus, H. E., and Ganem, D. (1990) Polymerase gene products of hepatitis B viruses are required for genomic RNA packaging as well as for reverse transcription. *Nature* **344**, 552–555.
15. Junker-Niepmann, M., Bartenschlager, R., and Schaller, H. (1990) A short cis-acting sequence is required for hepatitis B virus pregenome encapsidation and sufficient for packaging of foreign RNA. *EMBO J.* **9**, 3389–3396.
16. Pollack, J. R. and Ganem, D. (1993) An RNA stem-loop structure directs hepatitis B virus genomic RNA encapsidation. *J. Virol.* **67**, 3254–3263.
17. Bartenschlager, R. and Schaller, H. (1992) Hepadnaviral assembly is initiated by polymerase binding to the encapsidation signal in the viral RNA genome. *EMBO J.* **11**, 3413–3420.
18. Pollack, J. R. and Ganem, D. (1994) Site-specific RNA binding by a hepatitis B virus reverse transcriptase initiates two distinct reactions: RNA packaging and DNA synthesis. *J. Virol.* **68**, 5579–5587.
19. Fallows, D. A. and Goff, S. P. (1995) Mutations in the epsilon sequences of human hepatitis B virus affect both RNA encapsidation and reverse transcription. *J. Virol.* **69**, 3067–3073.
20. Tavis, J. E., Perri, S., and Ganem, D. (1994) Hepadnavirus reverse transcription initiates within the stem-loop of the RNA packaging signal and employs a novel strand transfer. *J. Virol.* **68**, 3536–3543.
21. Wang, G. H. and Seeger, C. (1993) Novel mechanism for reverse transcription in hepatitis B viruses. *J. Virol.* **67**, 6507–6512
22. Wang, G. H., Zoulim, F., Leber, E. H., Kitson, J., and Seeger, C. (1994) Role of RNA in enzymatic activity of the reverse transcriptase of hepatitis B viruses. *J. Virol.* **68**, 8437–8442.
23. Beck, J., Bartos, H., and Nassal, M. (1997) Experimental confirmation of a hepatitis B virus (HBV) ε-like bulge-and-loop structure in avian HBV RNA encapsidation signals. *Virology* **227**, 500–504.
24. Hu, J. and Seeger, C. (1997) RNA signals that control DNA replication in hepadnaviruses. *Semin. Virol.* **8**, 205–211.
25. Knaus, T. and Nassal, M. (1993) The encapsidation signal on the hepatitis B virus RNA pregenome forms a stem-loop structure that is critical for its function. *Nucl. Acids Res.* **21**, 3967–3975.
26. Hu, J. and Anselmo, D. (2000) In vitro reconstitution of a functional duck hepatitis B virus reverse transcriptase: posttranslational activation by Hsp90. *J. Virol.* **74**, 11,447–11,455.
27. Chen, Y., Robinson, W. S., and Marion, P. L. (1994) Selected mutations of the duck hepatitis B virus P gene RNase H domain affect both RNA packaging and priming of minus-strand DNA synthesis. *J. Virol.* **68**, 5232–5238.
28. Radziwill, G., Zentgraf, H., Schaller, H., and Bosch, V. (1988) The duck hepatitis B virus DNA polymerase is tightly associated with the viral core structure and unable to switch to an exogenous template. *Virology* **163**, 123–132.

29. Hu, J. and Seeger, C. (1996) Expression and characterization of hepadnavirus reverse transcriptases. *Methods Enzymol.* **275**, 195–208.
30. Mandart, E., Kay, A., and Galibert, F. (1984) Nucleotide sequence of a cloned duck hepatitis B virus genome: comparison with woodchuck and human hepatitis B virus sequences. *J. Virol.* **49**, 782–792.
31. Sambrook, J., Fritsch, E. F., and Maniatis, T. (1989) *Molecular Cloning: A Laboratory Manual*, 2nd ed, Cold Spring Harbor Laboratory, Cold Spring Harbor, NY.
32. Hu, J. and Seeger, C. (1996) Hsp90 is required for the activity of a hepatitis B virus reverse transcriptase. *Proc. Natl. Acad. Sci. USA* **93**, 1060–1064.
33. Staschke, K. A. and Colacino, J. M. (1994) Priming of duck hepatitis B virus reverse transcription in vitro: Premature termination of primer DNA induced by the 5'-triphosphate of fialuridine. *J. Virol.* **68**, 8265–8269.
34. Hu, J., Toft, D., Anselmo, D., and Wang, X. (2002) In vitro reconstitution of functional hepadnavirus reverse transcriptase with cellular chaperone proteins. *J. Virol.* **76**, 269–279.
35. Hu, J., Toft, D. O., and Seeger, C. (1997) Hepadnavirus assembly and reverse transcription require a multi-component chaperone complex which is incorporated into nucleocapsids. *EMBO J.* **16**, 59–68.
36. Beck, J. and Nassal, M. (1996) A sensitive procedure for mapping the boundaries of RNA elements binding in vitro translated proteins defines a minimal hepatitis B virus encapsidation signal. *Nucl. Acids Res.* **24**, 4364–4366.

26

Expression and Purification of Functional Hepatitis B Virus Polymerase in the Baculovirus Insect Cell System

Lisa Lott, Lena Notvall, and Robert E. Lanford

1. Introduction

Hepatitis B virus (HBV) is the human member in the family *Hepadnaviridae*. Several bird and rodent hepadnaviruses have been isolated, including duck *(1)*, heron *(2)*, woodchuck *(3)*, ground squirrel *(4)*, and Arctic ground squirrel HBVs *(5)*. A primate hepadnavirus has recently been isolated from a New World monkey and was designated woolly monkey HBV *(6)*. Approximately 5–10% of HBV infected adults and almost all infected newborns become chronically infected. Chronic carriers of HBV may have an asymptomatic infection for decades and yet still develop liver cirrhosis or hepatocellular carcinoma. More than 350 million chronic carriers of HBV exist worldwide. Despite a vaccine and several efficacious antivirals, current antiviral therapy does not result in viral clearance. The purification of the HBV polymerase (pol) and experimental in vitro assays for pol are useful for the evaluation of antivirals that may inhibit HBV replication.

In the HBV replication cycle, a pregenomic RNA molecule serves as the mRNA for core and pol. During HBV replication, an ϵ stem-loop structure on the pregenomic RNA molecule (pgRNA) functions as an encapsidation signal and is also the sequence to which pol binds to initiate a protein-primed reverse transcription reaction (nucleotide priming) *(7–10)*. In nucleotide priming, pol becomes covalently bound to the first nucleotide in minus-strand DNA through a phosphodiester bond with a tyrosine residue at amino-acid 63 in the TP (terminal protein) domain of pol *(11)*. Reverse transcription and DNA replication take place within the capsid particle.

A sequence in the bulge of the 5' copy of the ϵ stem-loop structure serves as the template for the addition of the first four nucleotides in minus-strand DNA *(8,9)*. The primed Pol complex is then translocated to a complementary sequence in the 3' end of pgRNA, termed direct repeat 1 (DR1) *(12–18)*. The RNaseH activity of pol

From: *Methods in Molecular Medicine, vol. 95: Hepatitis B and D Protocols, volume 1*
Edited by: R. K. Hamatake and J. Y. N. Lau © Humana Press Inc., Totowa, NJ

degrades pgRNA concurrently with minus-strand DNA synthesis with the exception of 12 to 18 nucleotides at the 5' end of pgRNA that function as a primer for plus-strand DNA synthesis ***(19)***. When minus-strand DNA synthesis has reached the 5' end of pgRNA, the short oligoribonucleotide is then translocated to a sequence near the 5' end of minus-strand DNA, termed direct repeat 2 (DR2) for initiation of plus-strand DNA synthesis ***(14,15,18)***. A final-strand transfer occurs from the 5' to the 3' end of minus-strand DNA, resulting in a noncovalently closed, circularized genome. Plus-strand DNA replication is halted before completion, leaving a single-stranded gap, and yields partially double-stranded, relaxed circular DNA (rcDNA).

The expression of HBV pol utilizing the recombinant baculovirus system in insect cells has proved useful in overcoming the historical difficulty of obtaining an ample quantity of pol from other expression systems or natural sources. The overexpression of pol in insect cells provides sufficient pol for purification as well as for performance of in vitro polymerase assays. As discussed in this chapter, purification of pol is performed by affinity chromatography utilizing a 10 amino-acid FLAG epitope fused to the amino terminus of pol ***(20)***. Pol is purified on M2 monoclonal-antibody columns that recognize an epitope in the FLAG sequence. Although only a small fraction of the total pol purified from insect cells is active, the significant quantity of pol synthesized utilizing the recombinant baculovirus system and the method of purification nonetheless allow for a substantial purification of functional pol ***(20)***.

The nucleotide priming reaction, or polymerase assay, is used to examine the protein priming step in DNA replication and may be performed in the absence of the core protein ***(20–23)***. In an in vitro priming reaction, pol is covalently attached to labeled nucleotides extending from 100 to 500 nucleotides by elongation of the primed product in minus-strand DNA synthesis by reverse transcription ***(20)***. For this analysis, a pol construct was utilized containing a 3' extension of the DR1 and the ϵ stem-loop sequence (FPL–pol) that was engineered downstream of the pol open reading frame, as previously described ***(20)***. By primer extension analysis, the 5' end of minus-strand DNA was mapped to the DR1 site of pol mRNA. In this instance, pol may be priming from the 3' copy of the ϵ stem-loop sequence followed by a translocation to DR1. However, full-length pol expressed in insect cells will prime in the absence of an ϵ stem-loop structure, suggesting that in this system, pol may be priming from an endogenous insect-cell RNA or a cryptic site on pol mRNA when ϵ is not present ***(20)***.

Alternatively, conducting endogenous polymerase reactions with core and pol expressed in insect cells offers the benefit of analyzing DNA replication as influenced by the environment of the capsid particle. Previous reports utilized baculovirus expression vectors to demonstrate a protein–protein interaction between core and pol ***(24)***. Core–pol interaction requires concomitant expression of the proteins within the same cells. Therefore, the core–pol endogenous polymerase assay is performed following coinfection of insect cells with baculoviruses expressing core and pol within the same flask. Prior to the reaction, immunoprecipitation is performed with anticore antibodies to collect core particles. As a result, this method allows for the detection of DNA that is synthesized only by those pol molecules that are packaged or associated with the core particle.

2. Materials

2.1. Insect-Cell Cultivation and Baculovirus Infection

1. The SF9 cell line is maintained in TMN-FH medium *(25)* consisting of Grace's antherea medium (JRH Biosciences) supplemented with 3.3 g/L yeastolate, 3.3 g/L lactalbumin hydrolysate, 5% fetal bovine serum (FBS), and 0.1% Pluronic F68 (Gibco/BRL). Following infections of adherent cultures in flasks, the insect-cell medium was changed to Grace's medium supplemented with 2% FBS. Following infections maintained in spinner flasks, the medium was changed to Grace's medium supplemented with 2% FBS, 0.1% Pluronic F68, and 50 μg/mL gentamicin.
2. Insect cells are maintained in 250-mL or 500-mL spinner flasks (Bellco).
3. Forma Scientific Incubator (model 3919) maintained at 27°C by refrigeration.
4. Nonheating magnetic stirplate (Bellco, model 7760).
5. Culture flasks for adherent insect cell cultures: 25-cm^2 flasks, 75-cm^2 flasks, or 150-cm^2 flasks (Corning Science Products).
6. Phosphonoformic acid (PFA) (150 m*M* stock solution) (Sigma).
7. Disposable conical centrifuge tubes (Corning).

2.2 Preparation of Affinity Column for Pol Purification

1. Anti-FLAG M2 agarose gel affinity beads (Sigma).
2. Glass Econo-column (Bio-Rad; 1.5 × 15 cm).
3. TN buffer: 100 m*M* Tris-HCl, 30 m*M* NaCl, pH 7.5.
4. Pretreatment elution buffer: 0.1 *M* glycine, pH 3.0.
5. Pretreatment neutralization buffer: 1 *M* Tris base.

2.3. Pol Purification

1. PEB: PBS containing 0.5% NP40, 10% glycerol.
2. Proteinase inhibitors: For extraction of pol, adjust PEB to contain a final concentration of 100 μ*M* leupeptin (Sigma), 1 m*M* Pefabloc (Boehringer-Mannheim), 10 μ*M* aprotinin (Sigma), 10 μg of pepstatin per mL (Boehringer-Mannheim), and 1 m*M* ethylenediaminete-traacetic acid (EDTA; Sigma).
3. RNAse inhibitor: 50 U/mL final concentration in PEB (Eppendorf).
4. Dithiothreitol (DTT): 5 m*M* final concentration in PEB.
5. TNG: 100 m*M* Tris HCl, pH 7.5, 30 m*M* NaCl, 10% glycerol.
6. TNG + 1 *M* NaCl.
7. Elution buffer: 0.1 *M* glycine, pH 3.0, containing 10% glycerol.
8. Neutralization buffer: 25 μL 1 *M* Tris-HCl, pH 7.5, 25 μL 1 *M* Tris base, 8 μL nuclease-free water, 5 μL 1 *M* DTT. Prepare at least 1 mL of mixture in ratio as described above.

2.4. In Vitro Nucleotide Priming Assay (Polymerase Assay)

1. Purified polymerase (approx 0.1 to 0.2 μg of purified protein or 10 μL of peak fraction from pol purification). Purified pol is in a mixture composed of neutralization and elution buffer adjusted to contain 0.2 % Triton, 5 m*M* DTT, and 50 U/mL RNasin (*see* **Subheading 3.3., steps 15–19**).
2. $MgCl_2$ (10 m*M* final concentration).
3. Unlabeled deoxyribonucleoside triphosphates (–TdNTPs) (100 μ*M* final concentration).
4. TTP (α-^{32}P; 3000 Ci/mmol; NEN) (5 μCi per reaction).

2.5. Core–Pol Endogenous Polymerase Assay

1. Baculoviruses expressing pol and core (8 PFU pol virus/cell and 2 PFU core virus/cell).
2. PEB: PBS containing 0.5% NP40, 10% glycerol.
3. Anticore antibodies (hyperimmune rabbit antibody produced against core particles purified from baculovirus infected in insect cells).
4. Protein-A beads (Repligen).
5. Endogenous polymerase (EP) buffer: 50 m*M* Tris-HCl, pH 7.4, 75 m*M* NH_4Cl, 1 m*M* EDTA, pH 8, 20 m*M* $MgCl_2$, 0.1 m*M* 2-mercaptoethanol, 0.5% Tween-20.
6. Unlabeled –TdNTPs (100 μ*M* final concentration).
7. TTP (α-^{32}P; 3000 Ci/mmol; NEN) (10 μCi per reaction).
8. Micrococcal nuclease (MCN) buffer: 10 m*M* Tris-HCl, pH 8.0, 3 m*M* $CaCl_2$.
9. Micrococcal nuclease (0.15 U/μL; USB).
10. TENS: 20 m*M* Tris-HCl, 20 m*M* NaCl, 20 m*M* EDTA, 1% SDS.
11. EGTA: 250 m*M* stock solution (Sigma).
12. Proteinase K: 10 mg/mL stock solution (Gibco/BRL).

3. Methods

3.1. Insect-Cell Cultivation and Baculovirus Infection

1. Insect cells to be used in infections are normally maintained in 250-mL spinner flasks with no more than a 150-mL volume for aeration. Insect cells to be used for purification are expanded to 500-mL spinner flasks using no more than a 250-mL volume to allow for aeration.
2. Insect cells are maintained in a refrigerated incubator at 27°C, spinning on a nonheating magnetic stirrer at 100 rpm.
3. For infection in spinner flasks, a volume of 750-mL SF9 cells are grown to a cell density of between 2 and 3×10^6 cells/mL.
4. Pour cells for spinner flask infection into sterile 250-mL disposable conical centrifuge tubes and pellet cells at 100*g* for 10 min at room temperature.
5. Remove all medium from centrifuge tube and suspend each cell pellet in 25 mL of virus stock. Then transfer infected cell suspension back to spinner flask.
6. Incubate infected cell culture in spinner flask for 1 h at 27°C.
7. Add 225 mL Grace's medium supplemented with 2% FBS, 0.1% F68, and 50 mg/mL gentamicin to infected cell suspension in spinner flask.
8. Incubate infected cell culture in spinner flask at 27°C for 48 h prior to purification.
9. For infection of adherent insect cell cultures in flasks, seed insect cells approx 24 h prior to infection at a density of 4.0×10^5 cells/25-cm^2 flask, 1.0×10^7 cells/75-cm^2 flask, or 2.0×10^7 cells/150-cm^2 flask. Incubate overnight at 27°C.
10. Infect or coinfect insect cells with baculovirus constructs at a multiplicity of 5 to 10 pfu/cell.
11. Remove the culture medium from infected flasks and add undiluted virus stock to each flask (1 mL per infection in a 75-cm^2 flask).
12. Incubate the cultures for 1 h at 27°C.
13. Add Grace's medium supplemented with 2% FBS to the infected cells to bring the total volume in a 75-cm^2 flask to 10 mL.
14. Incubate cultures for 48 h at 27°C prior to harvest.

3.2. Preparation of Affinity Column for Pol Purification

1. Add anti-FLAG M2 agarose gel affinity beads to a 15-mL conical tube. (The beads are provided as a 50% slurry, so add twice the volume of packed beads needed.)

2. Pellet beads at 250*g* for 1 min.
3. Wash beads once with TN buffer.
4. Pretreat the beads by adding 5 mL of the pretreatment elution buffer and gently shake by hand for 1 min.
5. Neutralize the glycine by adding 125 μL of the pretreatment neutralization buffer to the beads.
6. Wash the beads twice with TN buffer and pack the prepared anti-FLAG M2 agarose gel affinity beads into the column.

3.3. Pol Purification

1. Prior to pol purification, *see* **Subheading 3.1.** for insect-cell preparation and infection.
2. Pour cell suspension into 250-mL conical centrifuge tubes and cool on ice.
3. Pellet cells at 100 *g* for 10 min (+4°C).
4. Discard supernatant carefully without disturbing the loose cell pellet.
5. Wash cell pellet twice with cold, sterile phosphate-buffered saline (PBS) (200 mL per wash). Pellet at 100*g* for 10 min (+4°C) between each wash.
6. Extract each cell pellet with 5-mL PEB containing 5 m*M* DTT, 50 U RNasin per mL, and a final concentration of proteinase inhibitors as follows: 100 μ*M* leupeptin, 1 m*M* Pefabloc, 10 μ*M* aprotinin, 10 μg of pepstatin per mL, and 1 m*M* EDTA.
7. Incubate on ice for 20 min and vortex frequently.
8. Clarify at 2000*g* for 20 min (4°C).
9. Clarify supernatant a second time at 31,000*g* for 20 min (4°C).
10. Pass extract over prepared FLAG M2 affinity column at 1 mL/min by collecting flowthrough and passing back over column continuously for 2–3 h.
11. Save 1 mL of final flowthrough for determination of unbound pol by Western blot analysis.
12. Wash column with 20 mL TNG at 1 mL/min (first wash).
13. Wash column with 20 mL TNG + 1 *M* NaCl (second wash).
14. Wash column with 20 mL TNG (third wash).
15. Elute pol from column in 5-mL elution buffer at 1 mL/min. Follow by washing column with 10 mL of PBS.
16. Collect 15 fractions (1 mL each) into tubes containing 67 μL neutralization buffer.
17. Read OD of each fraction at 280 n*M* (blank with a solution containing 67 μL neutralization buffer in 1 mL elution buffer).
18. Pool fractions with the highest ODs (usually three fractions).
19. Add 8 μL of 25% Triton and 50 U RNasin per 1 mL of pooled fractions.
20. Aliquot and freeze at –70°C.

3.4. In Vitro Nucleotide Priming Assay (Polymerase Assay)

1. Following purification, pol is in a mixture equivalent to the elution neutralization buffer, as described in **Subheading 2.4.** (*see* **Note 1**). Nucleotide priming assays are performed with 10 μL of purified polymerase (approx 0.1–0.2 μg of purified protein) in a reaction mixture adjusted to contain a final concentration of 10 m*M* $MgCl_2$, 100 μ*M* unlabeled –TdNTPs, and 5 μCi α-^{32}P-TTP.
2. Priming reactions are typically conducted at 30°C for 30 min.
3. To detect further elongation of the primed product, reactions are conducted at 37°C for up to 6 h.
4. Adding PFA to the reaction mixture at a final concentration of 1.0 m*M* will block elongation but not priming (*see* **Fig. 1**).

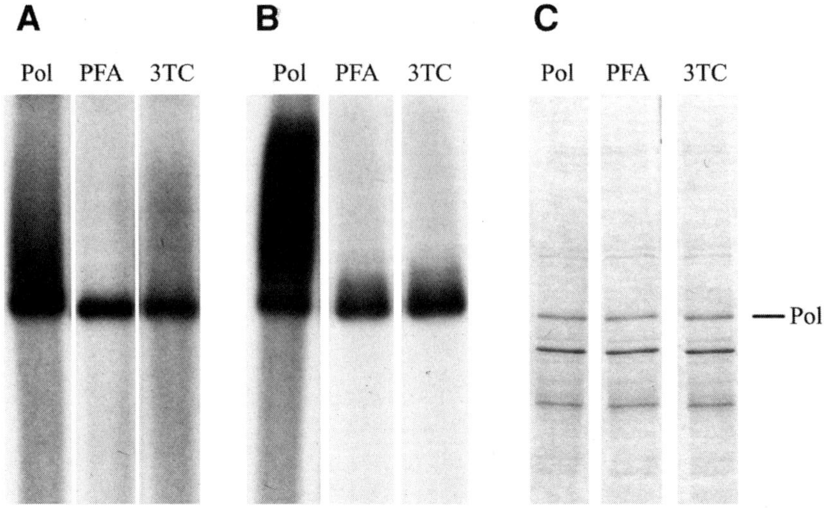

Fig. 1. Analysis of purified pol. **(A)** Immunoaffinity-purified pol was examined in an in vitro nucleotide priming assay. Purified polymerase was incubated in elution-neutralization buffer adjusted to contain a final concentration of 10 m*M* $MgCl_2$, 100 μ*M* unlabeled –TdNTPs, and 5 μCi α-^{32}P-TTP at 30°C for 30 min or **(B)** at 37°C for 2 h to detect further elongation of the primed product. Lanes: pol, purified pol with no treatment. PFA, purified pol with 1.0 m*M* PFA added to the reaction as a control to block elongation but not priming. 3TC, purified pol with 100 μ*M* 3TC triphosphate added to the reaction as a chain terminator to block elongation of the primed product. The products of the priming assay were analyzed by SDS-PAGE and autoradiography. **(C)** Coomassie blue staining of the gel in **(B)** to illustrate purified pol.

5. Phosphatidyl-2',3'-dideoxy-3'-thiacytidine (3TC) is a synthetic cytosine analog. Adding 3TC triphosphate to the nucleotide priming reaction at a final concentration of as low as 10 μ*M* will cause chain termination and block elongation of the primed product (*see* **Fig. 1**).
6. Terminate the reaction with sodium dodecyl sulfate (SDS) gel electrophoresis sample buffer and analyze by SDS-PAGE (polyacrylamide gel electrophoresis) and autoradiography.

3.5. Core–Pol Endogenous Polymerase Assay

1. Infect insect cells with baculoviruses expressing pol at 8 PFU/cell and core at 2 PFU/cell (*see* **Notes 2** and **3**).
2. Extract cells in PEB.
3. Immunoprecipitate core particles with 10 μL of anticore antibodies bound to 25 μL protein-A beads for 24 h at 4°C.
4. Wash beads two times with EP buffer.
5. Adjust pelleted beads to contain a final concentration of 100 μ*M* –TdNTPs and 10 μCi α-^{32}P-TTP in a 50-μL reaction in EP buffer.
6. Incubate at 37°C for 6 h.
7. Wash beads three times with PEB. (Pellet between washes at 900*g* for 1 min at room temperature) (*see* **Note 4**).

8. Add 100 μL MCN buffer.
9. Add 10 μL of 0.15 U/μL micrococcal nuclease.
10. Incubate at 37°C for 30 min.
11. Stop reaction with 2 μL of 250 m*M* EGTA.
12. Pellet beads and discard supernatant.
13. Add 200 μL TENS to beads.
14. Vortex and incubate at room temperature for 10 min.
15. Pellet in a microcentrifuge for 10 min and remove supernatant to new tube (discard beads).
16. Add proteinase K (10 μL of 10 mg/mL) to supernatant for 2 h at 65°C.
17. Perform phenol chloroform extraction/ethanol precipitation.
18. Perform agarose gel electrophoresis (1% agarose gel at 80 V for 1 h 20 min).
19. Fix gel by gently shaking in 7% trichloroacetic acid.
21. Wash agarose gel in water.
21. Dry gel for 2 h at 65°C and analyze by autoradiography.

4. Notes

1. Nucleotide priming reactions may be conducted following immunoprecipitation with anti-FLAG M2 antibodies while pol is still bound to the affinity beads. The beads are suspended in TNM (100 m*M* Tris-HCl, pH 7.5, 30 m*M* NaCl, 10 m*M* $MgCl_2$) in a 50-μL reaction adjusted to contain a final concentration of 100 μ*M*-unlabeled –TdNTPs and 5 μCi α-^{32}P-TTP.
2. The core protein is more stable and expresses better than HBV pol in the baculovirus insect-cell system. Therefore, to obtain the best core–Pol ratio in coinfections, adjust PFUs to account for this difference. Insect cells should be infected with baculoviruses expressing pol at 8 PFU/cell and core at 2 PFU/cell.
3. The addition of PFA at a final concentration of 1.5 m*M* to the insect cells following infection and 24 h post-infection will enhance the core–pol endogenous polymerase assay. Adding PFA to the infected insect cells temporarily blocks elongation by pol. PFA is washed away after harvest, and used in this way serves to block elongation of the DNA until the time that the reaction is conducted.
4. Following the core–pol endogenous polymerase assay, an alternative method of analysis may be performed by washing beads three times with PEB, adding 50 μL SDS gel electrophoresis buffer to each sample, and conducting SDS-PAGE analysis. The pol protein is labeled by the covalent attachment of radiolabeled nucleotides. Dry gel and analyze by autoradiography (*see* **Fig. 2A,** Lane 3).

Acknowledgments

This work was supported by grant CA53246 and PS1 RR13986 from the National Institutes of Health.

References

1. Mason, W. S., Seal, G., and Summers, J. (1980) Virus of Pekin ducks with structural and biological relatedness to human hepatitis B virus. *J. Virol.* **36**, 829–836.
2. Sprengel, R., Kaleta, E. F., and Will, H. (1988) Isolation and characterization of a hepatitis B virus endemic in herons. *J. Virol.* **62**, 3832–3839.
3. Summers, J., Smolec, J. M., and Snyder, R. (1978) A virus similar to human hepatitis B virus associated with hepatitis and hepatoma in woodchucks. *Proc. Natl. Acad. Sci. USA* **75**, 4533–4537.

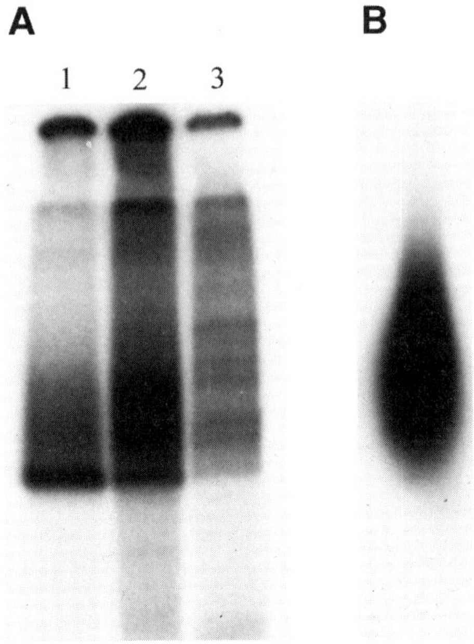

Fig. 2. Functional analysis of pol by nucleotide priming and endogenous polymerase assays. **(A)** Lanes 1 and 2: Insect cells were infected with baculoviruses expressing pol. Immunoprecipitation was performed with anti-FLAG M2 agarose gel–affinity beads, followed by in vitro priming assays. Nucleotide-priming reactions were conducted with polymerase bound to anti-FLAG M2 beads suspended in TNM (100 m*M* Tris-HCl [pH = 7.5], 30 m*M* NaCl, 10 m*M* $MgCl_2$) in a 50 µL reaction adjusted to contain a final concentration of 100 µ*M* unlabeled –TdNTPs and 10 µCi α-^{32}P-TTP. Priming reactions were conducted at (Lane 1) 30°C for 30 min or (Lane 2) 37°C for 6 h. Lane 3: Insect cells were infected with baculoviruses expressing pol and core. Immunoprecipitation was performed with anticore antibodies on protein-A beads followed by an endogenous polymerase reaction. The reaction was conducted on protein-A beads in EP buffer adjusted to contain a final concentration of 100 µ*M* –TdNTPs and 10 µCi α-^{32}P TTP at 37°C for 6 h. The products of the priming assays and endogenous polymerase assay were analyzed by SDS-PAGE and autoradiography. **(B)** The products of a core–pol endogenous polymerase assay (as described in **A**, Lane 3) were subjected to treatment with micrococcal nuclease and proteinase K, followed by phenol–chloroform extraction and analyzed by agarose gel electrophoresis.

4. Marion, P. L., Oshiro, L. S., Regnery, D. C., Scullard, G. H., and Robinson, W. S. (1980) A virus in Beechey ground squirrels that is related to hepatitis B virus of humans. *Proc. Natl. Acad. Sci. USA* **77**, 2941–2945.
5. Testut, P., Renard, C.-A., Terradillos, O., et al. (1996) A new hepadnavirus endemic in artic ground squirrels in Alaska. *J. Virol.* **70**, 4210–4219.
6. Lanford, R. E., Chavez, D., Brasky, K. M., Burns, R. B., III, and Rico-Hesse, R. (1998) Isolation of a hepadnavirus from the woolly monkey, a New World primate. *Proc. Natl. Acad. Sci. USA* **95**, 5757–5761.

7. Bartenschlager, R., Junker-Niepmann, M., and Schaller, H. (1990) The P gene product of hepatitis B virus is required as a structural component for genomic RNA encapsidation. *J. Virol.* **64**, 5324–5332.
8. Tavis, J. E., Perri, S., and Ganem, D. (1994) Hepadnavirus reverse transcription initiates within the stem-loop of the RNA packaging signal and employs a novel strand transfer. *J. Virol.* **68**, 3536–3543.
9. Wang, G.-H. and Seeger, C. (1993) Novel mechanism for reverse transcription in hepatitis B viruses. *J. Virol.* **67**, 6507–6512.
10. Pollack, J. R. and Ganem, D. (1993). An RNA stem-loop structure directs hepatitis B virus genomic RNA encapsidation. *J. Virol.* **67**, 3254–3263.
11. Lanford, R. E., Notvall, L., Lee, H., and Beames, B. (1997) Transcomplementation of nucleotide priming and reverse transcription between independently expressed TP and RT domains of the hepatitis B virus reverse transcriptase. *J. Virol.* **71**, 2996–3004.
12. Condreay, L. D., Wu, T.-T., Aldrich, C. E., et al. (1992) Replication of DHBV genomes with mutations at the sites of initiation of minus- and plus-strand DNA synthesis. *Virology* **188**, 208–216.
13. Lien, J., Petcu, D. J., Aldrich, C. E., and Mason, W. S. (1987) Initiation and termination of duck hepatitis B virus DNA synthesis during virus maturation. *J. Virol.* **61**, 3832–3840.
14. Molnar-Kimber, K. L., Summers, J. W., and Mason, W. S. (1984) Mapping of the cohesive overlap of duck hepatitis B virus DNA and of the site of initiation of reverse transcription. *J. Virol.* **51**, 181–191.
15. Seeger, C., Ganem, D., and Varmus, H. E. (1986) Biochemical and genetic evidence for the hepatitis B virus replication strategy. *Science* **232**, 477–484.
16. Seeger, C. and Maragos, J. (1990) Identification and characterization of the woodchuck hepatitis virus origin of DNA replication. *J. Virol.* **64**, 16–23.
17. Seeger, C. and Maragos, J. (1991) Identification of a signal necessary for initiation of reverse transcription of the hepadnavirus genome. *J. Virol.* **65**, 5190–5195.
18. Will, H., Reiser, W., Weimer, T., et al., (1987). Replication strategy of human hepatitis B virus. *J. Virol.* **61**, 904–911.
19. Lien, J.-M., Aldrich, C. E., and Mason, W. S. (1986). Evidence that a capped oligoribonucleotide is the primer for duck hepatitis B virus plus-strand DNA synthesis. *J. Virol.* **57**, 229–236.
20. Lanford, R. E., Notvall, L., and Beames, B. (1995) Nucleotide priming and reverse transcriptase activity of hepatitis B virus polymerase expressed in insect cells. *J. Virol.* **69**, 4431–4439.
21. Seifer, M. and Standring, D. N. (1993) Recombinant human hepatitis B virus reverse transcriptase is active in the absence of the nucleocapsid or the viral replication origin, DR1. *J. Virol.* **67**, 4513–4520.
22. Tavis, J. E. and Ganem, D. (1993) Expression of functional hepatitis B virus polymerase in yeast reveals it to be the sole viral protein required for correct initiation of reverse transcription. *Proc. Natl. Acad. Sci. USA* **90**, 4107–4111.
23. Wang, G. H., Zoulim, F., Leber, E. H., Kitson, J., and Seeger, C. (1994) Role of RNA in enzymatic activity of the reverse transcriptase of hepatitis B viruses. *J. Virol.* **68**, 8437–8442.
24. Lott, L., Beames, B., Notvall, L., and Lanford, R. E. (2000) Interaction between hepatitis B virus core protein and reverse transcriptase. *J. Virol.* **74**, 11479–11489.
25. Summers, M. D. and Smith, G. E. (1987) A manual of methods for baculovirus vectors and insect cell culture procedures. *Tex. Agric. Exp. Stn. Bull. 1555* 1–48, plus appendix.

27

Localization of Duck Hepatitis B Virus Polymerase Within Cells

Ermei Yao and John E. Tavis

1. Introduction

Hepadnaviruses are small, DNA-containing viruses that replicate by reverse transcription *(1)*. They have a lipid envelope surrounding an icosahedral protein core particle, whose shell is composed of a single viral protein, the core protein. Within the core particle, the viral reverse transcriptase (polymerase) is covalently linked to the double-stranded viral genome.

The polymerase has two roles in the formation of virions. The first role is structural, as the polymerase must bind to a stem-loop epsilon (ϵ) at the 5' end of the RNA form of the viral genome (the pregenomic RNA) to form the ribonucleoprotein complex that is encapsidated into a nascent core particle *(2–4)*. If this complex does not form, neither the polymerase nor pregenomic RNA is encapsidated. The second role of the polymerase is enzymatic, because the polymerase synthesizes the viral DNA. ϵ is essential for the enzymatic role of the polymerase for two reasons: Binding of ϵ to the polymerase promotes the maturation of the polymerase to an enzymatically active form *(5,6)* and ϵ is the origin of reverse transcription *(7–10)*.

The hepadnaviral polymerase contains four domains (**Fig. 1**; *11,12)*. The terminal protein and spacer domains are unique to the hepadnaviral polymerases. The terminal-protein domain contains the tyrosine residue that primes DNA synthesis and covalently links the polymerase to the viral DNA *(13,14)*. The spacer domain has no known function other than to link the terminal protein to the rest of the molecule. The reverse transcriptase and RNase H domains contain the two known enzymatic active sites. These latter two domains are related to the corresponding domains of the polymerases from retroviruses and other retroelements *(15–17)*.

The polymerase has been difficult to detect because of a lack of adequate antibodies. Polyclonal antibodies have been generated to fragments of the HBV or duck HBV (DHBV) polymerase, but they were of limited sensitivity *(18–21)*. Polymerase has also

From: *Methods in Molecular Medicine, vol. 95: Hepatitis B and D Protocols, volume 1*
Edited by: R. K. Hamatake and J. Y. N. Lau © Humana Press Inc., Totowa, NJ

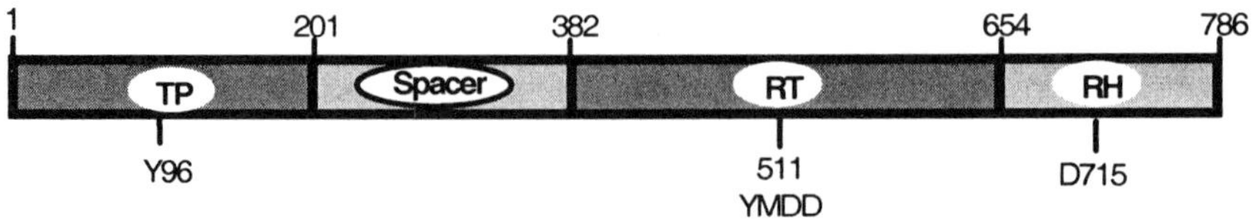

Fig. 1. Domain structure of the hepadnaviral polymerase. Amino-acid numbers of the domain boundaries for DHBV are indicated. TP, terminal-protein domain; Spacer, spacer domain; RT, reverse-transcriptase domain; RH, RNase H domain; Y96, tyrosine 96 that forms the covalent linkage to DNA. YMDD, a key motif of the RT active site; D715, aspartic acid 715, a key residue of the RNase H active site.

been detected by addition of a protein kinase A recognition site followed by in vitro phosphorylation with [γ-^{32}P]ATP *(21,22)* or activity gel analysis *(18, 23–25)*. However, a newer generation of antibodies has been made that is more sensitive. Six monoclonal antibodies against HBV polymerase exist that detect recombinant HBV polymerase in Western analysis, immunoprecipitation, and immunofluorescence, but detection of HBV polymerase from viral cores has not been reported *(26)*. We raised 10 monoclonal antibodies and a rabbit polyclonal antibody against a histidine-tagged fragment of the DHBV polymerase expressed in *Escherichia coli* (DTP3'His; amino acids 1–207, comprising the terminal protein domain; **27**). The techniques described here all employ either the polyclonal antibody or one of the monoclonal antibodies, mAb9.

By Western analysis, mAb9 can detect DHBV polymerase encapsidated in core particles from transfected LMH cells and from infected duck liver tissue at its predicted mass of 89 kDa. Intracellular core particles were partially purified from transfected LMH cells by sucrose gradient centrifugation *(6)*; the extracts were denatured in Laemmli buffer, resolved by sodium dodecyl sulfate–polyacrylamide gel electrophoresis (SDS-PAGE), and detected by Western analysis with mAb9 **(Fig. 2)**. Detection of polymerase was enhanced by removing the viral DNA prior to electrophoresis (Lanes 2 and 3), as expected for a chimeric DNA-protein molecule. Polymerase detected without nuclease digestion (Lane 2) represents molecules that have not initiated DNA synthesis or that have synthesized only small amounts of DNA because polymerase molecules linked to large DNA strands migrate slowly *(22)* and do not transfer well from gels. Core particles from cells transfected with the encapsidation-deficient DHBV(ϵ-Loop5,6) genome lacked polymerase (Lane 4), as would be expected given that the polymerase and pregenomic RNA are encapsidated together as a ribonucleoprotein complex *(2–4)*. This experiment demonstrates that mAb9 can detect the low levels of polymerase in core particles and that it is specific for polymerase, because the large majority of the protein in these extracts is cellular, yet the monoclonal antibodies recognize only polymerase.

DHBV polymerase can also be detected directly from cell lysates by Western analysis. Polymerase detected in this manner is more complex structurally than is encapsidated polymerase. In LMH cells, the full-length 89 kDa form is found, but additional species of approx 80 kDa and 55–60 kDa are also frequently observed **(Fig. 2**, Lane 5).

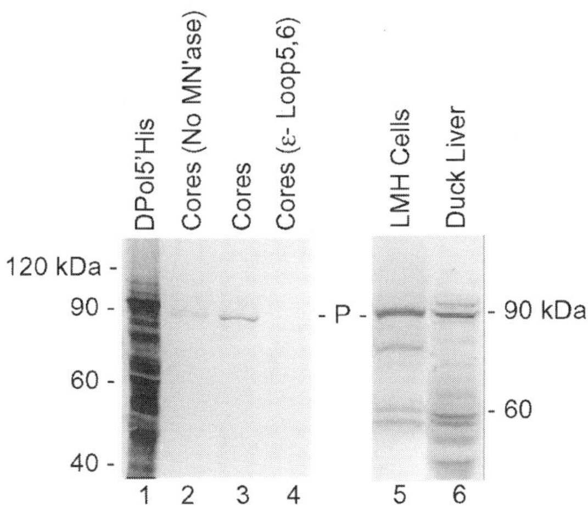

Fig. 2. Polymerase from viral cores and cells. Encapsidated polymerase (Left). Intracellular core particles were partially purified from transfected LMH cells (Lanes 2–4), resolved by electrophoresis, and the polymerase was detected by Western analysis with mAb9. Core particles in Lanes 3 and 4 were permeabilized and treated with micrococcal nuclease to remove covalently attached DNA. Lane 1 contains unpurified recombinant polymerase, Lanes 2 and 3 contain wild-type DHBV core particles, and Lane 4 contains core particles from cells transfected with the encapsidation-deficient mutant DHBV(Loop5,6). Nonencapsidated polymerase (Right). LMH cells transfected with D1.5G or infected liver were lysed in RIPA buffer, and the polymerase was detected by Western analysis with mAb9 (Lanes 5 and 6). (A similar figure originally appeared in ref. *27*.)

The smaller species are probably cleavage products of unknown origin. The 89-kDa polymerase species in LMH cells can be resolved into a doublet, and only the smaller of the doublet is found in core particles *(27)*. The 89-kDa doublet and the smaller polymerase forms are also found in infected liver, although the proportion of the smaller fragments can vary (Lane 6). An additional cluster of forms is found in infected liver, migrating approx 8 kDa heavier than the 89-kDa doublet (Lane 6).

Most of the polymerase detected by Western analysis of cell lysates and liver tissue is outside of core particles (**Fig. 2**, Lanes 5 and 6; ***27***). This was shown by transfecting LMH cells with an overlength DHBV expression vector and 3 d later lysing the cells and immunoprecipitating the lysates with antipolymerase and anticore antibodies. The immunoprecipitates were analyzed by Western analysis for the polymerase and core proteins (**Fig. 3**). A small amount of polymerase was found in the anticore immunoprecipitates, as expected because polymerase is encapsidated into core particles (Lane 1). Surprisingly, much more polymerase was found in the antipolymerase immunoprecipitates (Lane 2). These samples did not contain core particles because core protein was absent (Lane 2), and hence the polymerase in these samples represented an unsuspected nonencapsidated form of polymerase. Nonencapsidated polymerase was also found at

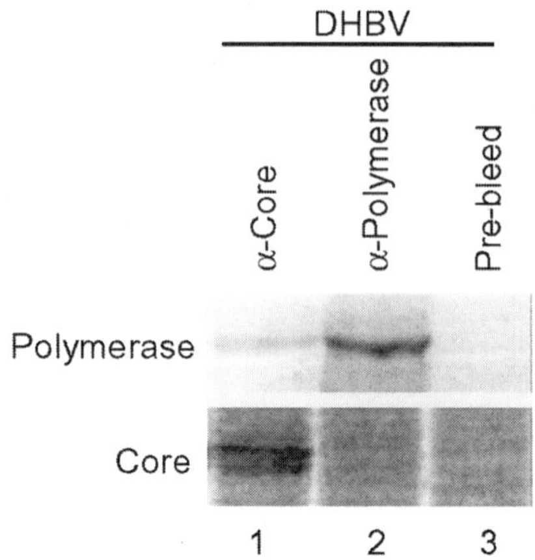

Fig. 3. Immunoprecipitation of encapsidated and nonencapsidated DHBV polymerase. LMH cells were transfected with D1.5G, the cells were lysed, and equal portions were immunoprecipitated with anticore, antipolymerase, or preimmune antibodies. Core and polymerase proteins were detected by Western analysis. (A similar figure originally appeared in ref. *27*.)

high levels in infected duck liver by immunoprecipitation and Western analysis (**Fig. 2**, Lane 6), indicating that nonencapsidated polymerase is not an artifact of cell culture.

The intracellular distribution of the nonencapsidated polymerase was assessed by immunofluorescence of transfected LMH cells with mAb9. Under standard microscopy, the nonencapsidated polymerase was readily detectable in the cytoplasm of transfected LMH cells in an uneven pattern (**Fig. 4**, Panel A), whereas polymerase was not detected when cells transfected with DHBV were stained with an irrelevant mAb (Panel C) or when nontransfected cells were stained with mAb9 (Panel D). Expression of the polymerase under direction of the cytomegalovirus (CMV) immediate early promoter in the absence of the pregenomic RNA or core protein (Panel B) yielded the same staining pattern as was found in cells replicating the virus, but the signal was brighter. When analyzed by confocal immunofluorescence microscopy, the polymerase was found in a grainy pattern **(Fig. 5)** that only partially overlapped that of the core protein *(27)*.

Encapsidated polymerase and nonencapsidated polymerase have different physical properties that affect their detection by standard techniques. Encapsidated polymerase is covalently linked to DNA, which makes it run slowly in SDS-PAGE and difficult to transfer to membranes for Western analysis. Permeabilizing the core particles by brief treatment at pH 2.5 *(28)* and digesting the covalently linked DNA with nuclease facilitate detection of the encapsidated polymerase (**Fig. 2**, Lanes 2 and 3). In contrast, the nonencapsidated polymerase is not linked to DNA and is probably not enzymatically active (data not shown). Rather, it is noncovalently bound to multiple

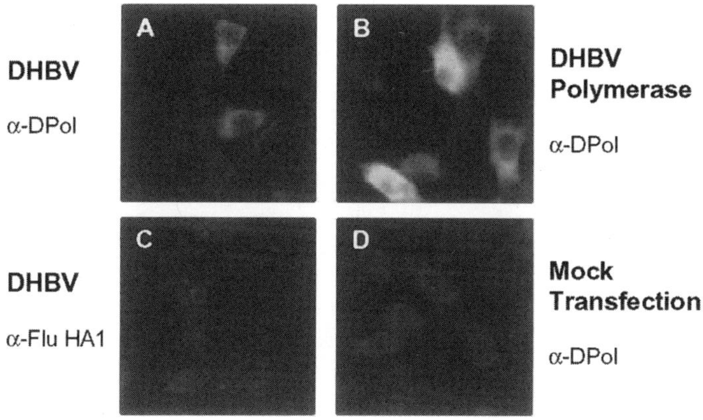

Fig. 4. Immunofluorescent detection of the DHBV polymerase. LMH cells were transfected with D1.5G (Panels A and C) or pCMV–DPol (Panel B) or were mock transfected (Panel C). Cells were fixed and stained with mAb9 (Panels A, B, and D) or monoclonal antibody 12CA5 specific for the influenza virus HA protein followed by fluorescein-labeled antimouse IgG antibody. (A similar figure originally appeared in ref. *27*.)

cytoplasmic structures, necessitating the use of high levels of detergent to extract it from cells *(27)*.

The advantage of the methods described here is that the polymerase can be directly observed within cells or directly detected from cellular extracts, eliminating the need for reporter-gene surrogates. The procedures are sensitive enough to detect the polymerase in cells without overexpression, permitting analysis of polymerase under physiological conditions from cells actively producing virus.

2. Materials

2.1. Viruses, Cells, and Plasmids

1. Viruses: DHBV strain 3 *(29)* was used in all experiments.
2. Cells: LMH cells are a chicken hepatoma cell line *(30)*.
3. Plasmids: D1.5G is a plasmid containing 1.5 copies of the viral genome cloned into pBS(–) (Stratagene). When transfected into LMH cells, D1.5G directs production of infectious DHBV; D1.5G and its derivatives were used whenever transfections employing the complete DHBV genome were performed. DHBV(ϵ-Loop5,6) contains mutations in the 5' copy of the coding sequences for ε that block encapsidation *(31)*. pCMV-DPol contains DHBV nt 170–3021 cloned downstream of the CMV promoter in pCDNA3.1–Zeo+ (Invitrogen). pCMV-DPol expresses polymerase containing a P2A mutation resulting from optimization of the polymerase Kozak sequence *(32)*. pDTP3' His contains DHBV nt 170–791 cloned into the *NdeI-Eco*RI sites of pRSET-C (Invitrogen); this plasmid directs production of DHBV polymerase amino acids 1–207 followed by LGHHHHHH.

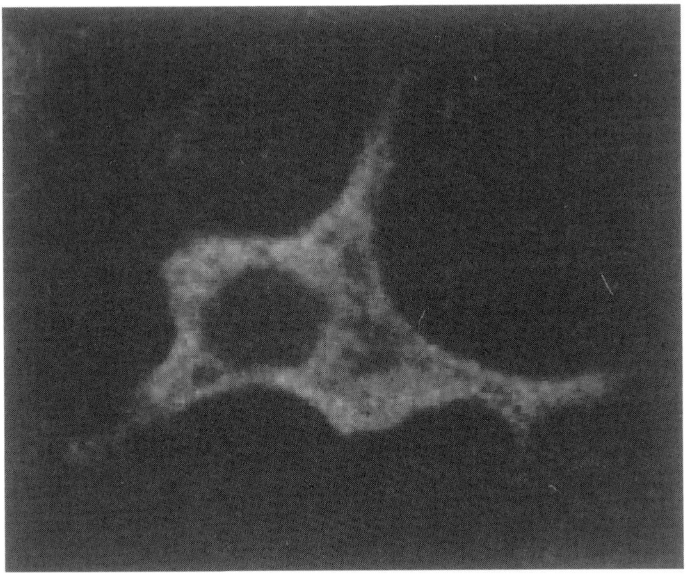

Fig. 5. Confocal image of DHBV polymerase in LMH cells. LMH cells were transfected with D1.5G, the cells were fixed 3 d later, and the polymerase was detected by confocal immunofluorescence microscopy of cells stained with mAb9 and fluorescein-labeled antimouse IgG antibody. (The image previously appeared in ref. ***27***.)

4. DHBV core particles: Core particles were isolated from cytoplasmic lysates of transfected LMH cells by lysis in 0.25% NP40/8% sucrose and sucrose sedimentation as described ***(6)***.

2.2. Solutions

1. RIPA (radioimmunoprecipitation assay buffer): 20 m*M* Tris-HCl, pH 7.2, 1% sodium deoxycholate (SDC), 1% Triton X-100, 0.1% SDS, 150 m*M* NaCl. Dissolve 5 g SDC in 400 mL distilled H_2O, add 5 mL Triton X-100, 5 mL 10% SDS, 10 mL 1 *M* Tris-HCl, pH 7.2, and 15 mL 5 *M* NaCl. Mix well. Bring the volume to 500 mL. Stable at 4°C for 1–3 mo.
2. 10X CAPS: Dissolve 22.13 g CAPS (3-[cyclohexylamino]-1-propanesulfonic acid) (Midwest Scientific) in 900 mL distilled H_2O, adjust pH to 11.0, bring the volume to 1 L with distilled H_2O. Store at 4°C. Dilute to 1X with distilled H_2O before use.
3. 10X TBST: 10 m*M* Tris-HCl, pH 8.0, 150 m*M* NaCl, 0.05% Tween-20 (Midwest Scientific). Dissolve 87.6 g NaCl in 500 mL distilled H_2O, add 100 mL 1 *M* Tris-HCl, pH 8.0, and 5 mL Tween-20. Bring the volume to 1 L with distilled H_2O. Store at 4°C.
4. 1X TBST/2% NFDM: Dissolve 20 g nonfat dry milk in 1000 mL 1X TBST. Make a fresh stock for each use.
5. AP buffer: 100 m*M* Tris-HCl, pH 9.5, 100 m*M* NaCl, 5 m*M* $MgCl_2$. Dissolve 12.11 g Tris-HCl and 5.84 g NaCl in 900 mL distilled H_2O, adjust pH to 9.5, add 5 mL 1 *M* $MgCl_2$, bring the volume to 1 L with distilled H_2O. Store at 4°C. Warm to room temperature before use.
6. 5X Laemmli buffer: 10% SDS, 20% glycerol, 125 m*M* Tris-HCl, pH 6.8, 0.1% bromophenol blue, 10% 2-mercaptoethanol. Mix 1 g SDS, 2 mL glycerol, 1.25 mL 1 *M* Tris-HCl, pH 6.8,

and 0.01 g bromophenol blue. Add distilled H_2O to 9 mL, warm the mixture gently, rock until dissolved, and then add 1 mL 2-mercaptoethanol. Store at –20°C. Solution is stable at 4°C for up to 1 mo in a tightly closed vial.

7. 200 m*M* phenylmethylsulfonyl fluoride (PMSF) (Sigma): Dissolve 0.7 g PMSF in 10 mL ethanol, mix well, warm at 37°C to dissolve faster. Store at –20°C. Every time before using it, incubate at 37°C until PMSF is completely dissolved. Caution: PMSF is toxic; be careful when handling it and wear mask and gloves.
8. 2 μg/μL aprotinin: Dissolve 20 mg aprotinin (Roche) in 10 mL distilled H_2O, aliquot to 0.5 mL/tube. Store at –20°C.
9. 1 μg/μL leupeptin: Dissolve 10 mg leupeptin (Roche) in 10 mL distilled H_2O, aliquot to 0.5 mL/tube. Store at –20°C.
10. 3.7% paraformaldehyde: Dissolve 18.5 g paraformaldehyde (Fisher) in 400 mL PBS, bring the volume to 500 mL with PBS. Store at 4°C.
11. PBS: Dissolve 8 g NaCl, 0.2 g KCl, 1.44 g $Na_2HPO_4 \cdot 7H_2O$, 0.24 g KH_2PO_4 in 900 mL distilled H_2O, adjust pH to 7.4, bring the volume to 1 L. Store at room temperature.
12. PBS/1% BSA (bovine serum albumin)/2% FBS (fetal bovine serum): PBS containing 1% BSA and 2% FBS (w/v).
13. DAPI: 4,6-diamidino-2-phenylindole (Sigma). 1 μg/μL in methanol.

2.3. Biological Reagents

1. Tissue culture medium: LMH cells are maintained in DMEM/F12 (Dulbecco's modified Eagle's medium-F12 medium; Mediatech) with 10% FBS, 2 m*M* glutamine, and 50 U penicillin and 50 U streptomycin for every 100 mL of medium.
2. Transfection reagent: FuGENE 6 (Roche). Store at –20°C.
3. Antibodies: Monoclonal antibody 9 (mAb9) is against DTP3 His, amino acids 1–207 of the DHBV polymerase terminal-protein domain. Rabbit polyclonal antipolymerase antibody R_2B_2 is also against DTP3 His. The titers of these antibodies were empirically determined by immunoprecipitating nonencapsidated polymerase from D1.5G-transfected LMH cell lysates. The secondary antibody for Western analysis is anti-mouse IgG-alkaline phosphatase conjugate (Promega). Secondary antibodies for immunofluorescence are anti-mouse IgG (whole molecule)–fluorescein (ICN/Cappel) and anti-rabbit IgG (whole molecule)–fluorescein (ICN/Cappel). All antibody working stocks are freshly prepared.
4. Protein G plus/protein A agarose (Oncogene Research Products): Immobilized protein A and protein G on beaded agarose in PBS with 0.1% sodium azide. Store at 4°C.
5. Prestained molecular weight marker: Benchmark™ Prestained Protein Ladder (GibcoBRL). Mix 5 μL marker with 10 μL 2X Laemmli buffer to be used as both size and gel orientation marker.
6. Fluoromount G (Southern Biotechnology Associates).
7. Antifade agent (*p*-phenylenediamine, Sigma).

2.4. Equipment and Other Supplies

1. Immobilon P membrane (Millipore).
2. Loose-pestle Dounce homogenizer.
3. Glass cover slips 18 mm^2 (Corning).
4. Cover glass-staining outfit (Coors).
5. High-quality microscope slides (Special Select Micro Slides; VWR Scientific).
6. Olympus fluorescence microscope with attached digital SPOT camera.

7. Bio-Rad MRC 1024 confocal system attached to a Nikon Optiphot microscope.
8. Vertical Mini-Gel Sequencing Kit (CBS Scientific) for running SDS-PAGE gels.
9. Mini-Electrophoretic Blotting System (CBS) for transferring protein from mini gels.

3. Methods

3.1. Preparation of Cell Lysates for Western Analysis or Immunoprecipitation of the Polymerase

3.1.1. Transfecting LMH Cells with FuGENE 6 (*see* **Note 1**)

1. Plate LMH cells at 1.2×10^6 per 60-mm plate the day before transfection (*see* **Note 2**).
2. The next day, change the cell growth medium 1–2 h before the transfection; then prepare DNA/FuGENE 6 complexes.
3. For a 60-mm plate, aliquot 300 μL DMEM/F12 without FBS to a polypropylene microcentrifuge tube, aliquot 13.5 μL FuGENE 6 into the DMEM/F12 (do not touch the plastic wall with undiluted FuGENE 6), and vortex for 10 s. Incubate the mixture at room temperature for 5 min.
4. Aliquot DNA to another microcentrifuge tube, add FuGENE 6 and medium mixture into it dropwise, and then vortex for 10 s.
5. Incubate the mixture at room temperature for 15 min.
6. Finally, vortex the solution again for 10 s and add mixture to cells, swirling the plate to mix. One 60-mm plate is sufficient to detect the polymerase by Western analysis or immunoprecipitation. Let the cells grow for 1–5 d, depending on the experiment.

3.1.2. Preparation of Cell Lysates (*see* **Note 3**)

1. Aspirate the growth medium carefully and wash once with cold PBS. Do not disturb the cells.
2. For a 60-mm plate, add 0.5–1 mL 0.75X or 1X RIPA with 10 μL 200 m*M* PMSF, 2 μL 2 μg/μL aprotinin, and 2 μL 1 μg/μL leupeptin per mL, and let the plate sit on ice for 10 min, rocking it occasionally to make sure the buffer covers the cells (*see* **Note 4**).
3. Scrape the cell lysate into a 1-mL microcentrifuge tube
4. Clarify the lysate at 13,000 *g* in microcentrifuge at 4°C for 10 min. Save the supernatant (*see* **Note 5**). Use the lysate immediately or store it at –75°C until ready to use.

3.2. Western Analysis of Nonencapsidated Polymerase in Transfected LMH Cells (see Note 1)

1. Mix 10 μL 2.5X Laemmli buffer with 10 μL cell lysate, boil 4 min, and let it cool on ice. Load 16 μL on 7.5% SDS–polyacrylamide mini gel, and run the gel until bromophenol blue reaches the bottom of the plates. Load a lane of prestained molecular weight marker as a size marker and to orient the gel.
2. Electrophorese and transfer sample to Immobilon P membrane using standard conditions. We use 10% methanol/1X CAPS buffer as transfer buffer, and perform transfer in the Mini-Electrophoretic Blotting System. Typically, we use 1.3 L 10% methanol/1X CAPS buffer and transfer at 200 mA constant current for 1.5 h.
3. Develop the Western blot with any standard chromogenic, chemiluminescent, or radioactive method preferred. In our experiments, we use 1X TBST/2% NFDM as blocking buffer. For the primary antibody (mAb9), we perform a 1:500 dilution, and the incubation time is 3–4 h or overnight (*see* **Note 7**). For the secondary antibody, we perform a 1:8000 dilution for the anti-mouse IgGs, and the incubation time is also 3–4 h or overnight. The membrane developing buffer is AP buffer for BCIP/NBT Color Substrate (Promega).

3.3. Immunoprecipitation of Nonencapsidated Polymerase from Cell Lysates

1. Lysates from transfected LMH cells are prepared as in **Subheading 3.1.2.** (*see* **Note 8**).
2. Bind primary antibody to protein G plus/protein A agarose (*see* **Note 9**). Put 1 mL 0.75X RIPA in a 1.5-mL microcentrifuge tube, add 40 µL protein G plus/protein A agarose, spin down, remove supernatant, add 300 µL 0.75X RIPA and 18 µL R_2B_2 polyclonal antibody, rock at 4°C for 3–4 h or overnight. After binding, wash the protein G plus/protein A agarose twice with 1 mL 0.75X RIPA.
3. Add 950 µL cell lysates to the antibody–protein G plus–agarose complex, and rock at 4°C for 4 h or overnight. Wash immunocomplex four times with 1 mL 0.75X RIPA (*see* **Note 10**).
4. Release the polymerase with Laemmli buffer. Add 35 µL 2X Laemmli buffer, mix the mixture well, boil for 4 min, put on ice until cold, spin down the protein G-plus agarose, and save the supernatant. The supernatant can then be analyzed by Western analysis as in **Subheading 3.2.** or stored at –75°C until ready to use (*see* **Note 11**).

3.4. Immunofluorescent Detection of the Polymerase

1. Plate LMH cells on sterile 18-mm square glass cover slips in 60-mm tissue culture dishes and transfect the cells as described in **Subheading 3.1.1.**
2. One to three days later, fix and permeabilize the cells directly in the tissue-culture plates. Rinse the plates three times with room temperature PBS, incubate at room temperature with 3.7% paraformaldehyde in PBS for 10 min, then in methanol containing 1 µg/µL DAPI at –20°C for 6 min, and finally in methanol at –20°C for 2 min. Rinse cells with room temperature PBS three times and store in PBS. Staining is best if performed immediately, but the fixed cells can be stored at 4°C for up to 1 wk.
3. Block cells: Place the cover slips on a moist filter paper disk in a Petri plate, cover them with 75 µL PBS containing 2% BSA and 2% FBS, and incubate at 37°C/5% CO_2 for 30–60 min. Remove the blocking solution by picking the slips up with forceps and gently draining the solution onto a Kimwipe. Do not touch the cells to the Kimwipe.
4. Primary antibody: Return the slip to the Petri plate, cover with 75 µL primary antibody solution in PBS containing 2% BSA and 2% FBS, and incubate at 37°C/5% CO_2 for 60–90 min. The antibody dilution is empirical; we typically use 50- to 200-fold dilution of mAb9 supernatant or 100- to 500-fold dilution of R_2B_2 polyclonal serum (*see* **Note 11**).
5. Wash the cells: Drain the antibody solution as in **step 3**, transfer the cover slips to a cover glass-staining outfit, then immerse in room temperature PBS once for 1 min and twice for 5 min, changing the PBS each time. Remove the cover slips from the holder, drain the excess PBS, and return the cover slips to the Petri plate.
6. Secondary antibody: Cover the cover slips with 75 µL secondary antibody solution in PBS containing 2% BSA and 2% FBS, and incubate at 37°C/5% CO_2 for 45–60 min. The secondary antibody must be fluorescently labeled and react with the primary antibody. We typically use anti-mouse IgG (whole molecule)-fluorescein antibodies at 100-fold dilution with mAb9, and anti-rabbit IgG (whole molecule)-fluorescein at 100-fold dilution for polyclonal sera.
7. Wash and mount cells: Wash cells as in **step 5**, adding two immersions in distilled water for 30 s each after the last PBS rinse. Drain the excess water from the slips; allow them to air-dry until they are slightly damp but do not allow them to dry completely. Mount the cover slips cell-side down on high-quality microscope slides with 15 µL Flouromount G containing suf-

ficient antifade agent to faintly color the Fluoromount G. Do not use too much antifade because sensitivity will drop. Seal the edges of the cover slip with clear fingernail polish.

8. Observe cells with fluorescent microscopy at 100- to 1000-fold magnification (*see* **Note 12**). The polymerase will appear as a heterogeneously distributed protein in the cytoplasm of successfully transfected cells (**Figs. 4** and **5**). The intensity of the polymerase signal can vary greatly between cells, and cells with the brightest staining frequently have distorted nuclei visible in the DAPI channel. The stained cover slips can be stored at 4°C for up to a month, but image quality declines with time.

4. Notes

4.1. Preparation of Cell Lysates for Western Analysis or Immunoprecipitation of the Polymerase

1. FuGENE 6 is very good for transfecting LMH cells. In our hands, the efficiency is greatly improved compared with $CaPO_4$ precipitation or Lipofectin (Life Technology).
2. Low cell confluence and even distribution of the cells on the plate are *critical* for high transfection efficiency. We normally plate 1.2×10^6 cells for a 60-mm plate the day before transfection; the next day, the plate is less than 60–70% confluent.
3. Duck liver lysates can be prepared by homogenizing liver in 1X RIPA (5% w/v) plus PMSF/aprotinin/leupeptin (in the same concentrations as for making LMH cell lysates) with a loose-pestle Dounce homogenizer on ice for 10 min and then clarifying the lysates as in **Subheading 3.1.2.** for LMH cells. Liver lysates can be analyzed by either Western analysis or immunoprecipitation.
4. The polymerase is readily detected from whole-cell lysates when the cells are disrupted with a harsh buffer (RIPA), but it is not detectable when cells are lysed with CPLB (core preparation lysis buffer: 10 m*M* Tris-HCl pH 7.5, 1 m*M* ethylenediaminetetraacetic acid [EDTA], 0.25% NP40, 50 m*M* NaCl, 8% sucrose), the mild buffer used to make cytoplasmic extracts from which cytoplasmic core particles are isolated.
5. When clarifying the lysates, the pellet should be solid enough for easy separation from the supernatant. Cell pellets are firmer in 0.75X RIPA, and extraction of the polymerase in 0.75X RIPA is as good as in 1X RIPA.

4.2. Western Analysis of Nonencapsidated Polymerase in Transfected LMH Cells

6. When performing Western analysis for the DHBV core particle–encapsidated polymerase, dissolve the core-particle extract from one 100-mm plate in 100-μL buffer, and use 5–10 μL. Permeabilize 5 μL of core suspension by adding 1 μL 300 m*M* glycine, pH 2.5, and incubate at room temperature for 30 s, then add 1 μL 600 m*M* Tris-HCl, pH 8.0 *(28)*. Digest the nucleic acids by adding 1 μL 100 m*M* $CaCl^2$ and 1 μL 5U/μL micrococcal nuclease (Roche), and incubate at 37ºC for 20 min. Stop the reaction by adding 1 μL 150 m*M* EGTA and 2.5 μL 5X Laemmli buffer. Resolve polymerase on 7.5% SDS-PAGE gel and detect the polymerase by Western analysis as in **Subheading 3.2.** Permeabilizing the viral cores is important for successfully detecting encapsidated polymerase because many polymerase molecules in core particles are attached to large viral DNAs, which makes the polymerase difficult to resolve on SDS-PAGE gel and difficult to transfer from gel to membrane.
7. When performing Western analysis for core protein from cell lysates, the procedures are the same as for analyzing the cell lysates for nonencapsidated polymerase, except that the gel is 10% acrylamide and the primary antibody is an anticore antibody.

4.3. Immunoprecipitation of Nonencapsidated Polymerase from Cell Lysates

8. The nonencapsidated polymerase can be detected by metabolic labeling of transfected LMH cells and then immunoprecipitating the polymerase from the lysates. The cells are labeled 1–3 d after the transfection, depending on the experiment. Wash the cells twice with 5 mL of DMEM (without cystine and methionine; GibcoBRL) without FBS, glutamine, penicillin, or streptomycin; add 1–2 mL of labeling mix, which is DMEM (without cystine and methionine) containing 125 μCi Easy Tag Express-[^{35}S] Protein Labeling Mix (New England Nuclear) per mL of medium; the concentrations of FBS, glutamine, penicillin, and streptomycin are the same as for regular cell maintenance. Incubate the cells at 37ºC with 5% CO_2 for 15 min to overnight, depending on the experiment. Cell lysates are prepared as in **Subheading 3.1.2. Important**: Easy Tag Express-[^{35}S] Protein Labeling Mix is radioactive, so be careful when handling it.
9. The protein G plus/protein A agarose can be substituted by *Staphylococcus aureus* (StaphA, Sigma) cells. StaphA cells give a higher background, but they are less expensive. If StaphA cells are substituted, use 30 μL of 10% (w/v) StaphA cells for each immunoprecipitation sample; the other steps are the same as for using protein G plus/protein A agarose. When washing the immunocomplex, it is critical to suspend StaphA cells well to achieve clean results. When releasing protein from StaphA cells, suspend StaphA cells well to get high and consistent yields. Protein A/G agarose is more expensive than StaphA cells, and because the pellet is not firm when centrifuged, washing immunocomplex and releasing protein must be performed carefully to avoid losing sample.
10. The same procedure can be used to immunoprecipitate core protein, except the immunocomplexes are washed with 1X RIPA instead of 0.75X RIPA to reduce background.

4.4. Immunofluorescent Detection of the Polymerase

11. Dual-channel immunofluorescence can be performed. Use primary antibodies of different species (e.g., mouse and rabbit) simultaneously in the initial incubation and the appropriate secondary antibodies coupled to different fluorescent tags in the secondary incubation (fluorescein and rhodamine work well together). The antibody dilutions are empirical but typically are no different for dual-channel staining than for single-channel staining. Be sure to run appropriate controls to exclude crossreaction between the primary and secondary antibodies.
12. Confocal immunofluorescence can be performed with no changes to the staining procedures.

References

1. Ganem, D. and Schneider, R. J. (2001) Hepadnaviridae: the viruses and their replication. *In*: Knipe, D. M. Howley, P. M. Griffen, D. E. et al. (eds.), *Fields Virology*, 4th ed., vol 2, Lippencott Williams & Wilkins, Philadelphia, PA, 2923–2969.
2. Bartenschlager, R., Junker-Niepmann, M., and Schaller, H. (1990) The P gene product of hepatitis B virus is required as a structural component for genomic RNA encapsidation. *J. Virol.* **64**, 5324–5332.
3. Junker-Niepmann, M., Bartenschlager, R., and Schaller, H. (1990) A short cis-acting sequence is required for hepatitis B virus pregenome encapsidation and sufficient for packaging of foreign RNA. *EMBO J.* **9**, 3389–3396.
4. Hirsch, R. C., Lavine, J. E. Chang, L. J. Varmus, H. E. and Ganem, D. (1990) Polymerase gene products of hepatitis B viruses are required for genomic RNA packaging as well as for reverse transcription. *Nature* **344**, 552–555.

5. Tavis, J. E. and Ganem, D. (1996) Evidence for the activation of the hepatitis B virus polymerase by binding of its RNA template. *J. Virol.* **70**, 5741–5750.
6. Tavis, J. E., Massey, B., and Gong, Y. (1998) The duck hepatitis B virus polymerase is activated by its RNA packaging signal, epsilon. *J. Virol.* **72**, 5789–5796.
7. Wang, G.-H. and Seeger, C. (1993) Novel mechanism for reverse transcription in hepatitis B viruses. *J. Virol.* **67**, 6507–6512.
8. Tavis, J. E., Perri, S., and Ganem, D. (1994) Hepadnavirus reverse transcription initiates within the stem-loop of the RNA packaging signal and employs a novel strand transfer. *J. Virol.* **68**, 3536–3543.
9. Tavis, J. E. and Ganem, D. (1995) RNA sequences controlling the initiation and transfer of duck hepatitis B virus minus-strand DNA. *J. Virol.* **69**, 4283–4291.
10. Nassal, M. and Rieger, A. (1996) A bulged region of the hepatitis B virus RNA encapsidation signal contains the replication origin for discontinuous first-strand DNA synthesis. *J. Virol.* **70**, 2764–2773.
11. Chang, L.-J., Hirsch, R. C., Ganem, D., and Varmus, H. E. (1990) Effects of insertional and point mutations on the functions of the duck hepatitis B virus polymerase. *J. Virol.* **64**, 5553–5558.
12. Radziwill, G., Tucker, W., and Schaller, H. (1990) Mutational analysis of the hepatitis B virus P gene product: domain structure and RNase H activity. *J. Virol.* **64**, 613–620.
13. Zoulim, F. and Seeger, C. (1994) Reverse transcription in hepatitis B viruses is primed by a tyrosine residue of the polymerase. *J. Virol.* **68**, 6–13.
14. Weber, M., Bronsema, V., Bartos, H., Bosserhoff, A., Bartenschlager, R., and Schaller, H. (1994) Hepadnavirus P protein utilizes a tyrosine residue in the TP domain to prime reverse transcription. *J. Virol.* **68**, 2994–2999.
15. McClure, M. A. (1993) Evolutionary history of reverse transcriptase. *In*: Skalka, A. M. and Goff, S. P. (eds.), *Reverse Transcriptase,* Cold Spring Harbor Laboratory Press, Cold Spring Harbor, NY, 425–444.
16. Poch, O., Sauvaget, I., Delarue, M., and Tordo, N. (1989) Identification of four conserved motifs among the RNA-dependent polymerase encoding elements. *EMBO J.* **8**, 3867–3874.
17. Li, M. D., Bronson, D. L., Lemke, T. D., and Faras, A. J. (1995) Phylogenetic analyses of 55 retroelements on the basis of the nucleotide and product amino acid sequences of the pol gene. *Mol. Biol. Evol.* **12**, 657–670.
18. Bavand, M., Feitelson, M., and Laub, O. (1989) The hepatitis B virus-associated reverse transcriptase is encoded by the viral pol gene. *J. Virol.* **63**, 1019–1021.
19. Mack, D. H., Bloch, W., Nath, N., and Sninsky, J. J. (1988) Hepatitis B virus particles contain a polypeptide encoded by the largest open reading frame: a putative reverse transcriptase. *J. Virol.* **62**, 4786–4790.
20. Bartenschlager, R. and Schaller, H. (1988) The amino-terminal domain of the hepadnaviral P-gene encodes the terminal protein (genome-linked protein) believed to prime reverse transcription. *EMBO J.* **7**, 4185–4192.
21. Huang, H.-L., Jeng, K.-S., Hu, C.-P., Tsai, C.-H., Lo, S. J., and Chang, C. (2000) Identification and characterization of a structural protein of hepatitis B virus: a polymerase and surface fusion protein encoded by a spliced RNA. *Virology* **275**, 398–410.
22. Bartenschlager, R., Kuhn, C., and Schaller, H. (1992) Expression of the P-protein of the human hepatitis B virus in a vaccinia virus system and detection of the nucleocapsid-associated P-gene product by radiolabelling at newly introduced phosphorylation sites. *Nucl. Acids Res.* **20**, 195–202.
23. Oberhaus, S. M. and Newbold, J. E. (1996) Preparations of duck hepatitis B virions contain multiple DNA polymerase activities. *Virology* **226**, 132–134.

24. Oberhaus, S. M. and Newbold, J. E. (1993) Detection of DNA polymerase activities associated with purified duck hepatitis B virus core particles by using an activity gel assay. *J. Virol.* **67**, 6558–6566.
25. Bavand, M. R. and Laub, O. (1988) Two proteins with reverse transcriptase activities associated with hepatitis B virus-like particles. *J. Virol.* **62**, 626–628.
26. zu Putlitz, J., Lanford, R. E., Carlson, R. I., Notvall, L., De la Monte, S. M. and Wands, J. R. (1999) Properties of monoclonal antibodies directed against hepatitis B virus polymerase protein. *J. Virol.* **73**, 4188–4196.
27. Yao, E., Gong, Y., Chen, N., and Tavis, J. E. (2000) The majority of duck hepatitis B virus reverse transcriptase in cells is nonencapsidated and is bound to a cytoplasmic structure. *J. Virol.* **74**, 8648–8657.
28. Radziwill, G., Zentgraf, H., Schaller, H., and Bosch, V. (1988) The duck hepatitis B virus DNA polymerase is tightly associated with the viral core structure and unable to switch to an exogenous template. *Virology* **163**, 123–132.
29. Sprengel, R., Kuhn, C., Will, H., and Schaller, H. (1985) Comparative sequence analysis of duck and human hepatitis B virus genomes. *J. Med. Virol.* **15**, 323–333.
30. Condreay, L. D., Aldrich, C. E., Coates, L., Mason, W. S., and Wu, T.-T. (1990) Efficient duck hepatitis B virus production by an avian liver tumor cell line. *J. Virol.* **64**, 3249–3258.
31. Pollack, J. R. and Ganem, D. (1994) Site-specific RNA binding by a hepatitis B virus reverse transcriptase initiates two distinct reactions: RNA packaging and DNA synthesis. *J. Virol.* **68**, 5579–5587.
32. Kozak, M. (1991) Structural features in eukaryotic mRNAs that modulate the initiation of translation. *J. Biol. Chem.* **266**, 19,867–19,870.

28

Endogenous Polymerase Assay for the Analysis of Hepatitis B Virus in Transgenic Mice

Zhenming Xu and Jing-hsiung Ou

1. Introduction

Hepatitis B virus (HBV) is a human pathogen that can cause severe liver diseases. This virus has a high liver tropism and is often found in large quantities in the sera of patients with HBV. HBV is enveloped and has three related envelope proteins. These envelope proteins are collectively called the surface antigens. The virus also contains a core particle inside the envelope. This core particle packages the viral genomic DNA, which is a circular, partially double-stranded DNA molecule slightly larger than 3 kb. The major protein constituent of the core particle is the core protein. The core protein mRNA, also known as the pregenomic RNA (pgRNA), is larger than the genome size, with a terminal redundancy of about 200 nucleotides. In addition to the core protein, this RNA also codes for the viral DNA polymerase, which is also a reverse transcriptase *(1)*.

After its synthesis, the core protein packages the pgRNA and the viral DNA polymerase to form the core particle. This pgRNA is then converted to the minus-strand DNA by the reverse-transcriptase activity of the viral DNA polymerase. The terminal-protein (TP) domain of the DNA polymerase serves as the primer for the minus-strand DNA synthesis and is covalently linked to its 5' end *(2–5)*.

During the reverse transcription, the pgRNA is degraded by the RNase H activity of the viral DNA polymerase. A short RNA fragment derived from the 5' end of the degraded pgRNA then serves as the primer to initiate the plus-strand DNA synthesis *(6,7)*. This RNA primer may prime near the 3' end of the minus-strand DNA to initiate the synthesis of a double-stranded linear (DL) form of the viral genome or prime near the 5' end of the minus strand for the synthesis of a short plus strand, which then switches template to the 3' end of the minus strand to continue the DNA synthesis to form the relaxed circular (RC) form of the viral genome *(8–10)* (**Fig. 1**). The function of the DL form of the viral genome is unclear and may represent a nonfunctional byproduct of DNA synthesis. In contrast, the RC form is the mature viral genome.

From: *Methods in Molecular Medicine, vol. 95: Hepatitis B and D Protocols, volume 1*
Edited by: R. K. Hamatake and J. Y. N. Lau © Humana Press Inc., Totowa, NJ

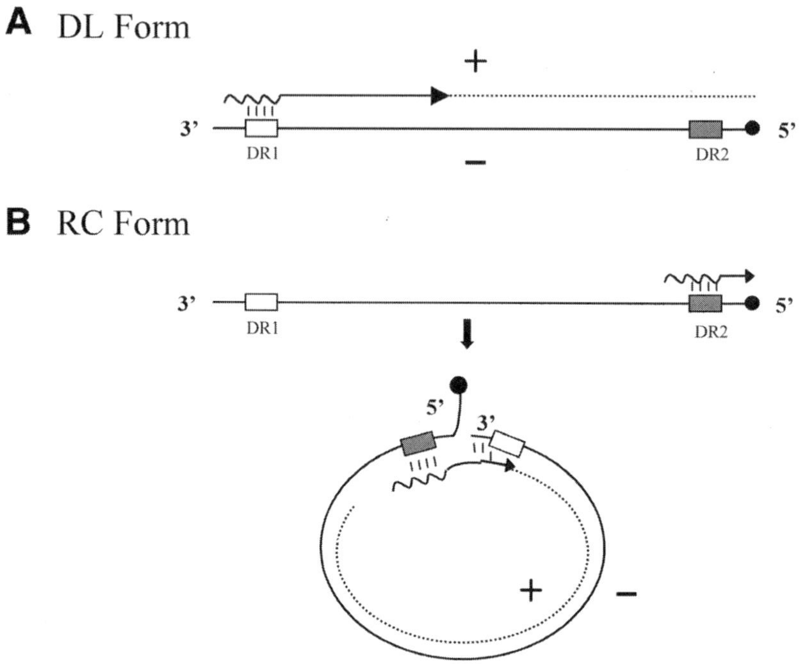

Fig. 1. Illustration of HBV DNA synthesis. "+," the plus-strand DNA; "–," the minus-strand DNA. The solid circle at the 5' end of the minus-strand DNA indicates the terminal protein (TP). After the synthesis of the minus strand, the 5' end of the pgRNA will serve as the primer. **(A)** Binding of the RNA primer to the DR1 sequence located near the 3' end of the minus strand. This will lead to the synthesis of the DL form of the viral genome. **(B)** Binding of the RNA primer to the DR2 sequence located near the 5' end of the minus strand. This will lead to the synthesis of a small plus-strand DNA fragment, which will then switch template to the 3' end of the minus strand using the terminal repeat of the minus strand to synthesize the RC form of the viral genome.

During the synthesis of the plus-strand DNA, the viral core particle will interact with the surface antigens that have already been inserted in the membrane of the endoplasmic reticulum (ER). This interaction results in the budding of the core particle into the ER lumen. HBV acquires its envelope through this budding process and is eventually secreted from the infected hepatocytes to initiate a new round of infection ***(11, 12)***. The partially double-stranded HBV genomic DNA is presumably the result of premature envelopment prior to the completion of plus-strand DNA synthesis. This unique feature of the HBV genome and the co-packaging of the viral DNA polymerase render it possible to perform the "endogenous polymerase assay" ***(13,14)***.

In this assay, HBV virions in the serum are treated with a nonionic detergent for the removal of the envelope. The nucleotides are then provided so that the viral DNA polymerase in the core particle can resume DNA synthesis to fill in the single-stranded gap of the viral genome. This process will result in the production of the full-length DL form and the RC form of the viral DNA. If the nucleotides are radiolabeled with ^{32}P, the resulting viral DNA will also be labeled and can be easily detected on a gel by autoradiography. This endogenous polymerase assay (EPA) is a highly sensitive and quantitative assay for analyzing the HBV virions.

The research with HBV has been hampered by the lack of a convenient laboratory animal host. Although the research with the related duck hepatitis B virus (DHBV), woodchuck hepatitis B virus (WHV), and ground squirrel hepatitis B virus (GSHV) using their respective animal hosts has generated many important results for understanding HBV ***(15–21)***, DHBV is only distantly related to HBV, and WHV and GSHV rely on expensive animal hosts for their replication and are difficult to study. In recent years, transgenic mice carrying an HBV transgene slightly larger than the HBV genome have been produced ***(22)***. These mice can produce high circulating titers of HBV and have become a convenient alternative for studying the replication and pathogenesis of HBV ***(23–25)***. We have produced these transgenic mice in our laboratory and successfully used the EPA to identify the transgenic mice that produced HBV (*26*).

In this chapter, we will describe the EPA procedures for the analysis of the HBV particles in the mouse serum. However, the same procedures can also be used to analyze the HBV particles in the patient sera.

2. Materials

1. Transgenic mice were produced at the Transgenic Mouse Core Facility at the University of Southern California Norris Cancer Center. wtTg05 and wtTg08 are two independent mouse lines that contain the wild-type HBV genome of the adw2 subtype (*see* **Note 1**).
2. Rodents Restraining Cage (VWR, cat. no. 10718-020).
3. Infrared lamp (Home Depot).
4. 1 *M* Tris-HCl, pH 8.0, stock solution: dissolve 12.1 g Tris(hydroxymethyl) aminomethane (Fisher, cat. no. BP152-1) in approx 70 mL deionized H_2O; adjust pH to 8.0 with concentrated HCl; bring volume to 100 mL with deionized H_2O and autoclave. Store at room temperature. 1 *M* Tris-HCl, pH 7.0, is prepared the same way except that the pH is adjusted to 7.0.
5. 1 *M* NH_4Cl: Dissolve 5.35 g NH_4Cl (Fisher, cat. no. A661-500) in deionized H_2O to make a 100-mL solution.
6. 0.2 *M* $MgCl_2$: Dissolve 3.96 g $MgCl_2$ (Fisher, cat. no. M87-500) in deionized H_2O to make a 100-mL solution.
7. 4 *M* NH_4OAc: dissolve 30.8 g NH_4OAc (EM, cat. no. 1220-3) in deionized H_2O for a 100-mL solution.
8. 10 *N* NaOH: Dissolve 40 g NaOH (Fisher, cat. no. BP359-500) in deionized H_2O to make a 100-mL solution. Store in a plastic bottle.
9. 0.5 *M* ethylenediaminetetraacetic acid (EDTA, pH 8.0): dissolve 93.06 g disodium EDTA (Fisher, cat. no. S311-500) in 400 mL deionized H_2O, use 10 *N* NaOH to adjust pH to 8.0, add deionized H_2O to a final volume of 500 mL.
10. EPA buffer (per 100 mL): 50 m*M* Tris-HCl, pH 7.0 (5 mL 1 *M* Tris-HCl, pH 7.0), 40 m*M* NH_4Cl (4 mL 1 *M* NH_4Cl), 20 m*M* $MgCl_2$ (10 mL 0.2 *M* $MgCl_2$), 1% Nonidet P-40 (NP40) (Sigma, cat. no. I-3021; 1 mL) (*see* **Note 2**), 0.3% β-mercaptoethanol (Fisher, cat. no. 03446-100; 0.3 mL) (*see* **Note 3**).
11. The dNTP mixture. 1 m*M* each of dATP, dTTP, and dGTP in deionized H_2O (diluted from the 100 m*M* stock solutions, Amersham, cat. no. 27-2035-01).

12. α-^{32}P dCTP: 10 mCi/mL, >3000 Ci/mmol (ICN, cat. no. 33004X).
13. 5 m*M* dCTP solution in H_2O (diluted from the 100 m*M* stock solution, Amersham, cat. no. 27-2035-01).
14. 50 m*M* EDTA: Diluted from the 0.5 *M* EDTA stock solution.
15. 10% sodium dodecyl sulfate (SDS; Fisher, cat. no. BP 166-500).
16. Diethylpyrocarbonate treated H_2O: Fresh diethylpyrocarbonate (Sigma, cat. no. D5758) was added to H_2O to a final concentration of 0.1%. The water was then autoclaved for 1 h.
17. 10 mg/mL tRNA stock solution: Dissolve tRNA powder (Sigma, cat. no. R8759) in diethylpyrocarbonate-treated deionized H_2O.
18. 10 mg/mL proteinase K, freshly prepared: Dissolve proteinase K powder (Gibco, cat. no. 25530-031) in deionized H_2O.
19. Phenol: Saturate 100 mL phenol (Fisher, cat. no. BP226-100) with 10 mL 1 *M* Tris-HCl, pH 8.0, and 90 mL deionized H_2O.
20. Chloroform/isoamyl alcohol: Mix 24 parts of chloroform (Fisher, cat. no. BP1145-1) with 1 part of isoamyl alcohol (Fisher, cat. no. A393-4).
21. Ethanol: 100%, 70% (Gold Shield Chemical Co.).
22. TE: 10 m*M* Tris-HCl and 1 m*M* EDTA. Add 10 mL 1 *M* Tris-HCl, pH 8.0, and 2 mL 0.5 *M* EDTA to H_2O to a final volume of 1 L.
23. 1X TAE buffer: 40 m*M* Tris-acetate and 1 m*M* EDTA, pH 7.5–7.8. For 1 L, dissolve 4.84 g Tris base in deionized H_2O and add 1.15 mL glacial acetic acid (Fisher, cat. no. A38^{SL}-212) and 2 mL 0.5 *M* EDTA.
24. Agarose gel: Add 1 g agarose (Life Technologies, cat. no. 15510-027) into 100 mL 1X TAE buffer, heat in a microwave oven until agarose is dissolved, and store in a 56°C oven.
25. 20 mg/mL ethidium bromide (EtBr) stock solution: Dissolve 1 g EtBr (Sigma, cat. no. E-8751) in 50 mL deionized H_2O. Wrap in aluminum foil to avoid light.
26. SpeedVac (Savant).
27. Gel dryer (Bio-Rad).
28. Phosphorimager screen and scanner (Amersham).

3. Methods

3.1. Serum Collection from the Transgenic Mice

1. Place the mice under the infrared lamp for 15 min to warm them up.
2. Put a mouse inside the rodent restrainer with the tail sticking outside the restrainer.
3. Lift the tail upward and make a small incision with a clean razor blade.
4. Allow the blood to drip into an Eppendorf tube. Collect approximately 100 μL blood.
5. Allow the blood to coagulate. Microfuge at the maximum speed for 5 min and collect the supernatant (serum) (*see* **Note 4**).
6. Store the serum in small aliquots at –80°C (*see* **Note 5**).

3.2. The Endogenous Polymerase Assay

1. Mix the following: 39 μL EPA buffer, 5 μL 1 m*M* dNTP mixture, 5 μL α-^{32}P dCTP, and 1 μL mouse serum (*see* **Notes 6 and 7**).
2. Incubate the reaction mixture at 37°C for 2 h.
3. Add 1 μL 5 m*M* dCTP and continue the reaction at 37°C for another hour (*see* **Note 8**).
4. Add 7 μL 10% SDS, 3.5 μL 50 m*M* EDTA, 3.5 μL 10 mg/mL proteinase K (*see* **Note 9**), and 5 μL 10 mg/mL tRNA carrier (*see* **Note 10**).
5. Incubate the reaction at 56°C for 2 h.

6. Add an equal volume of phenol, vortex well, add another volume of chloroform/isoamyl alcohol, vortex again. Centrifuge in a microfuge for 2 min to separate the aqueous phase and the organic phase. Transfer the aqueous phase to a new Eppendorf tube. Repeat the extraction process one more time.
7. Add 70 µL 4 *M* NH_4OAc and 280 µL 100% ethanol to the aqueous phase, mix well, sit at 4°C for 10 min (*see* **Note 11**).
8. Microfuge for 5 min at room temperature and discard the supernatant.
9. Resuspend the pellet in 50 µL autoclaved H_2O, add 50 µL 4*M* NH_4OAc and 200 µL 100% ethanol, mix well, and sit at 4°C for 10 min to allow the nucleic acid to precipitate.
10. Microfuge for 5 min and discard the supernatant.
11. Rinse the pellet with 70% ethanol and dry the pellet in a Savant SpeedVac.
12. Resuspend the pellet in 10 µL TE (*see* **Note 12**).
13. Subject the sample to electrophoresis in a 1% agarose minigel in TAE (*see* **Note 13**).
14. Stain the agarose gel with 1 µg/mL EtBr and photograph the gel.
15. Dry the gel in a gel dryer. Expose the gel to a Phosphorimager screen overnight.
16. Quantify the DL and RC forms of the HBV genome.
17. A representative result is shown in **Fig. 2.**

4. Notes

1. The EPA can also be used for quantitative analysis. We have been able to follow the changes of the viral titers in our transgenic mice over their life span. There is a declining trend in the circulating viral titer as the mouse grows older.
2. NP40 has been discontinued by Sigma. Igepal CA-630 (Sigma, cat. no. I3021), which is chemically identical to NP40, has been used.
3. The inclusion of NP40 in the EPA buffer is for the removal of the viral envelope. This is essential to make the nucleotides accessible to the polymerase packaged in the core particle. If NP40 is not included in the buffer, the EPA with the transgenic mouse serum will generate a negative result. This observation indicates that the HBV DNA signals that we detected in the mouse serum were derived from the virions and not from the core particles released from the hepatocytes **(Fig. 2)**. In contrast, the EPA generated positive signals with the sera isolated from patients with HBV in our previous studies regardless of whether NP40 was included in the reaction or not. This observation indicates that a large amount of free core particles were present in the patients' sera. These core particles were presumably released from the injured hepatocytes.
4. As the EPA is simple and sensitive, it is a useful technique to screen for HBV transgenic mice that produce circulating HBV virions.
5. Sera can be stored at –80°C for years without any apparent effect on the EPA reactions. Freezing and thawing also do not seem to affect the EPA reactions.
6. Although the procedures described above are for analyzing the serum obtained from the HBV transgenic mouse, the same procedures work equally well for the sera obtained from patients with HBV.
7. The EPA can also be used to determine the HBV titers in the cell-culture media. To conduct such an experiment, immunoprecipitation with the antisurface antigen antibody is performed prior to the EPA to concentrate HBV virions. For example, 10 mL of the incubation medium of the 2.2.15 cell line, which secretes HBV virions, was incubated with 1 µL antisurface antibody at 4°C overnight, followed by the addition of 10 µL Protein G Sepharose (Amersham, cat. no. 17-0886-01) and a further incubation at 4°C for 1h. After centrifugation in a

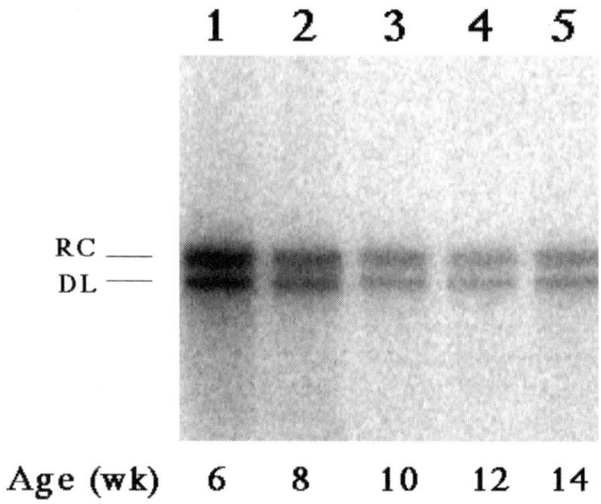

Fig.2. The endogenous polymerase assay (EPA) of the sera of a transgenic mouse. The mouse sera were collected from the mouse tail when the mouse was 6, 8, 10, 12, and 14 wk old. One microliter of the serum of each time point was then analyzed by the EPA. The locations of the DL form and the RC form of the HBV genome are indicated.

microfuge for 2 min, the immunoprecipitates were resuspended in 40 μL EPA buffer. The NP40 in the EPA buffer solubilized the viral envelope and released the core particles. After centrifugation in a microfuge for 5 min, the supernatant, which contained the HBV core particles, was recovered. As described above, 5 μL of dNTP mixture and 5μL α-^{32}P dCTP were then added to the supernatant to perform EPA.

8. The chase of the EPA reaction with 1 μL 5 m*M* dCTP for an additional hour is to allow the completion of plus-strand DNA synthesis.
9. Proteinase K is used to break the core particle and to remove the TP covalently linked to the 5' end of the minus-strand DNA. Without the proteinase K treatment, the viral DNA will be extracted by phenol into the organic phase to generate negative results.
10. The tRNA added during the proteinase K digestion plays dual roles: one in to serve as a carrier to precipitate the viral DNA and the other is to serve as an internal control for quantifying the recovery efficiency following the ethanol precipitations.
11. The use of 4 *M* NH_4OAc in ethanol precipitation helps the removal of unincorporated nucleotides.
12. Final EPA products can be stored at –80°C for up to 1 wk before being analyzed with gel electrophoresis. These DNA samples can also be digested with restriction enzymes for further analysis.
13. The EPA analyzes the synthesis of only the plus strand of the HBV genomic DNA. This plus strand can also be analyzed with an alkaline agarose gel. In this case, the DNA sample after the EPA reaction is heated at 56°C for 5 min in the sample buffer containing 50 m*M* NaOH, 1 m*M* EDTA, and 3% Ficoll (Sigma, cat. no. F-9378) before electrophoresis in a 1% agarose gel containing 1 m*M* NaOH and 1 m*M* EDTA. The running buffer used for the gel electrophoresis is the same as the gel buffer. Because alkaline agarose gels cannot be stained with EtBr, a nondenaturing TAE gel should also be run in parallel to determine the recovery efficiency of the viral DNA following ethanol precipitation. The autoradi-

ograms of such single-stranded DNA analysis usually reveal a major DNA band co-migrating with the 3.2-K b molecular marker. This DNA band presumably is the full-length positive strand.

References

1. Ganem, D. and Schneider, R. (2001) Hepadnaviridae: the viruses and their replication. In (Knipe, D.M. and Howley, P.M. (eds.), *Fields Virology* Lippincott-Raven Publishers, Philadelphia, PA,. 2923–2970.
2. Bartenschlager, R. and Schaller, H. (1988) The amino-terminal domain of the hepadnaviral P-gene encodes the terminal protein (genome-linked protein) believed to prime reverse transcription. *EMBO J.* **7**, 4185–4192.
3. Wang, G.H. and Seeger, C. (1992) The reverse transcriptase of hepatitis B virus acts as a protein primer for viral DNA synthesis. *Cell* **71**, 663–670.
4. Weber, M., Bronsema, V., Bartos, H., Bosserhoff, A., Bartenschlager, R., and Schaller, H. (1994) Hepadnavirus P protein utilizes a tyrosine residue in the TP domain to prime reverse transcription. *J. Virol.* **68**, 2994–2999.
5. Zoulim, F. and Seeger, C. (1994) Reverse transcription in hepatitis B viruses is primed by a tyrosine residue of the polymerase. *J. Virol.* **68**, 6–13.
6. Lien, J.M., Aldrich, C.E., and Mason, W.S. (1986) Evidence that a capped oligoribonucleotide is the primer for duck hepatitis B virus plus-strand DNA synthesis. *J. Virol.* **57**, 229–236.
7. Loeb, D.D., Hirsch, R.C., and Ganem, D. (1991) Sequence-independent RNA cleavages generate the primers for plus strand DNA synthesis in hepatitis B viruses: implications for other reverse transcribing elements. *EMBO J* **10**, 3533–3540.
8. Seeger, C., Ganem, D., and Varmus, H.E. (1986) Biochemical and genetic evidence for the hepatitis B virus replication strategy. *Science* **232**, 477–484.
9. Lien, J.M., Petcu, D.J., Aldrich, C.E., and Mason, W.S. (1987) Initiation and termination of duck hepatitis B virus DNA synthesis during virus maturation. *J. Virol.* **61**, 3832–3840.
10. Will, H., Reiser, W., Weimer, T., et al. (1987) Replication strategy of human hepatitis B virus. *J. Virol.* **61**, 904–911.
11. Bruss, V. and Ganem, D. (1991) The role of envelope proteins in hepatitis B virus assembly. *Proc. Natl. Acad. Sci. USA* **88**, 1059–1063.
12. Ganem, D. (1991) Assembly of hepadnaviral virions and subviral particles. *Curr. Top. Microbiol. Immunol.* **168**, 61–83.
13. Landers, T.A., Greenberg, H.B., and Robinson, W.S. (1977) Structure of hepatitis B Dane particle DNA and nature of the endogenous DNA polymerase reaction. *J. Virol.* **23**, 368–376.
14. Miller, R.H., Marion, P.L., and Robinson, W.S. (1984) Hepatitis B viral DNA-RNA hybrid molecules in particles from infected liver are converted to viral DNA molecules during an endogenous DNA polymerase reaction. *Virology* **139**, 64–72.
15. Zhang, Y.Y. and Summers, J. (1999) Enrichment of a precore-minus mutant of duck hepatitis B virus in experimental mixed infections. *J. Virol.* **73**, 3616–3622.
16. Yang, W. and Summers, J. (1998) Infection of ducklings with virus particles containing linear double-stranded duck hepatitis B virus DNA: illegitimate replication and reversion. *J. Virol.* **72**, 8710–8717.
17. Yang, W., Mason, W.S., and Summers, J. (1996) Covalently closed circular viral DNA formed from two types of linear DNA in woodchuck hepatitis virus-infected liver. *J. Virol.* **70**, 4567–4575.
18. Zoulim, F., Saputelli, J., and Seeger, C. (1994) Woodchuck hepatitis virus X protein is required for viral infection in vivo. *J. Virol.* **68**, 2026–2030.

19. Chen, H. S., Kaneko, S., Girones, R., et al.(1993) The woodchuck hepatitis virus X gene is important for establishment of virus infection in woodchucks. *J. Virol.* **67**, 1218–1226.
20. Transy, C., Fourel, G., Robinson, W. S., Tiollais, P., Marion, P. L., and Buendia, M. A. (1992) Frequent amplification of c-myc in ground squirrel liver tumors associated with past or ongoing infection with a hepadnavirus. *Proc. Natl. Acad. Sci. USA* **89**, 3874–3878.
21. Cullen, J. M. and Marion, P. L. (1996) Non-neoplastic liver disease associated with chronic ground squirrel hepatitis virus infection. *Hepatology* **23**, 1324–1329.
22. Guidotti, L. G., Matzke, B., Schaller, H., and Chisari, F. V. (1995) High-level hepatitis B virus replication in transgenic mice. *J. Virol.* **69**, 6158–6169.
23. Raney, A. K., Eggers, C. M., Kline, E. F., et al. (2001) Nuclear covalently closed circular viral genomic DNA in the liver of hepatocyte nuclear factor 1 alpha-null hepatitis B virus transgenic mice. *J. Virol.* **75**, 2900–2911.
24. Wieland, S. F., Guidotti, L. G., and Chisari, F. V. (2000) Intrahepatic induction of alpha/beta interferon eliminates viral RNA-containing capsids in hepatitis B virus transgenic mice. *J. Virol.* **74**, 4165–4173.
25. Kakimi, K., Guidotti, L. G., Koezuka, Y., and Chisari, F. V. (2000) Natural killer T cell activation inhibits hepatitis B virus replication in vivo. *J. Exp. Med.* **192**, 921–30.
26. Xu, Z., Yen, T. S. B., Wu, L., Madden, C. R., Tan, W., Slagle, B. L. and Ou, J.-H. (2002) Enhancement of hepatitis B virus replication by its X protein in transgenic mice. *J. Virol.* **76**, 2579–2584.

29

Transcriptional Control of Hepatitis B Virus

Anneke K. Raney

1. Introduction

Hepatitis B virus (HBV) transcriptional regulation has been extensively studied in vitro by transient transfection using the activity of a reporter molecule as the readout for transcriptional activity ***(1–5)***. Several reporter molecules, such as chloramphenicol acetyl transferase (CAT), β-galactosidase (β-gal), and luciferase (LUC), have been used for this purpose. Because of the sensitivity and ease of the assay system, LUC has become the reporter molecule most widely used. Alternatively, the levels of HBV transcripts themselves can also be measured in cell-culture systems, and, in recent years, several groups have analyzed HBV transcription in this manner ***(6,7)***. With the introduction of HBV transgenic mice, in vivo analyses of HBV transcription have allowed the application of our in vitro knowledge to the more physiologically relevant and complex environment of the liver ***(8)***. Using transcription factor knock-out mice crossed with the HBV transgenic mice, or administering compounds to the HBV transgenic mice, the effects on transcription in the context of viral replication in the liver can be assessed ***(9,10)***. This chapter will cover transcriptional analysis in in vitro systems, but the methods used for the analysis of RNA will be applicable to the in vivo system. The 3.2-kb HBV DNA genome encodes four transcripts of 3.5, 2.4, 2.1, and 0.7 kb, from which are translated the HBcore/HBe and polymerase polypeptides, the large surface antigen, the middle and major surface-antigen polypeptides, and the X-gene polypeptide, respectively. The small HBV genome lends itself to the molecular manipulation necessary to study the regulation of synthesis of the viral transcripts. Transcriptional analysis in cell culture has shown that the levels of the 3.5-, 2.4-, 2.1-, and 0.7-kb transcripts are regulated by the nucleocapsid, large surface antigen, major surface antigen, and X-gene promoters, respectively, as well as by the two viral enhancers ***(4,11)***. In the absence of an infectious cell-culture system, the majority of the in vitro transcriptional analysis has been performed by transient transfection of plasmids containing portions of the viral DNA genome into cell lines. Several types of cell lines have been used to study the liver-specific aspects of HBV transcriptional regulation. They include, but are not lim-

From: *Methods in Molecular Medicine, vol. 95: Hepatitis B and D Protocols, volume 1*
Edited by: R. K. Hamatake and J. Y. N. Lau © Humana Press Inc., Totowa, NJ

ited to, the differentiated human hepatoblastoma cell lines HepG2 ***(12)*** and Huh7 ***(13)***, the dedifferentiated HepG2.1 cell line ***(2)***, the human nonhepatoma cell line, HeLaS3 ***(14)***, and the mouse fibroblast line, NIH3T3. Similar analyses have been conducted in the duck HBV (DHBV) system, transfecting DHBV DNA into HepG2, Huh7, or the chicken hepatoma cell line, LMH ***(15–18)***. Some in vitro transcriptional studies with woodchuck and ground squirrel hepatitis viruses have also been performed ***(19,20)***.

The methods used to study transcriptional control of HBV employ many standard molecular biology techniques. The details of plasmid construction will depend on the region of the genome under study and the type of reporter molecule or endogenous RNA used to measure transcriptional activity. The type of cell line chosen will depend on the specific intent of the study. To determine the regions of the genome important for transcriptional activity, one should start with a cell line that mimics as closely as possible the cell type in which the virus naturally replicates. The differentiated hepatoblastoma cell lines most widely used are HepG2 and Huh7. Results may vary from one cell line to another and presumably reflect the differences in transcription-factor levels, cell-growth characteristics, and general physiological state of each cell line. To determine which functional transcriptional elements may be involved in the liver-specific expression of HBV transcripts, dedifferentiated hepatoblastoma cell lines, such as HepG2.1, nonhepatoma cell lines such as HeLaS3, or mouse fibroblast NIH3T3, have been used in comparison with the differentiated hepatoma cell lines. The nondifferentiated or nonhepatoma cell lines are particularly useful for studying the effect of ectopic expression of liver-enriched transcription factors on the activity of transcriptional regulatory elements.

Transient transfection analysis using reporter molecules as the measure of transcriptional activity has permitted the identification of the major transcriptional regulatory elements that comprise the enhancers and promoters of the HBV genome and the transcription factors that interact with these elements. Starting with the full-length genome, a 5' deletion analysis enables one to map regions of the genome that mediate transcriptional activity. Mutational analyses of the genome help to define the functional elements and their relative roles in the regulation of transcription. Construction of plasmids containing a defined functional element upstream of a minimal promoter will allow one to determine whether transcriptional activity can be mediated through this element. Cotransfection of expression vectors containing the cDNA for a transcription factor can demonstrate the ability of a particular transcription factor to mediate its effects through isolated regulatory elements. Additional assays such as electrophoretic mobility shift analysis (EMSA) and DNase I footprinting are used to demonstrate direct DNA–protein interactions. Either purified proteins or nuclear extracts from tissues, cell lines, or cells transfected to express known transcription factors can be used in these assays to determine the binding specificities of the promoter or enhancer regions.

Transient transfection analysis of constructs containing 1.2 or 1.3 copies of the HBV genome allow one to measure the levels of HBV transcripts in vitro in the context of viral replication. Plasmids containing 1.3 genomes, similar to the construct used for the HBV transgenic mouse model, have been used because the four viral transcripts are synthesized under the control of the HBV-regulatory elements ***(6,8)***. The effects of exogenous expression of transcription factors or the addition of transcriptional regulators on the steady-state levels of HBV RNAs can be measured by Northern hybridization or RNase protection analyses.

I will describe the basic methods for in vitro transcriptional analysis by transient transfection of luciferase reporter-molecule plasmids. They will include the transfection protocol, lysis of the transfected cells, and the assays to detect the reporter-molecule activity. The method for transient transfection using HBV genome–plasmid constructs to measure the HBV transcripts is essentially the same, so only the differences from the reporter-molecule transfection protocol will be detailed. The preparation of HBV RNA from transfected cells and the analysis of the RNA by ribonuclease protection will be described. Although Northern filter hybridization is also an important tool for the analysis of transcriptional control, the methodology is well known ***(21)*** and will not be presented in this chapter.

2. Materials

2.1. Reporter Molecule Analysis

2.1.1. Luciferase Transfections

1. Cesium-chloride–purified luciferase plasmid containing the HBV genome or portion of the genome upstream of the LUC open reading frame (ORF) (*see* **Note 1**). The HBV DNA should include the sequences immediately 5' to the ATG of the gene of interest to contain as much of the regulatory sequence as possible (*see* **Note 2**). Promoterless luciferase vectors appropriate for inserting HBV-regulatory elements are available from several companies (*see* **Note 3**).
2. Expression vector containing the cDNA of a transcription factor of interest under the control of a strong promoter, such as the cytomegalovirus (CMV) immediate early promoter, the simian virus 40 (SV40) promoter, or a retrovirus long terminal repeat (LTR).
3. Internal control plasmid containing a second reporter molecule, such as β-galactosidase or *Renilla* luciferase, under the control of a promoter that should not be responsive to the experimental treatment being tested, such as the CMV or SV40 promoters. pCMVβ directs the expression of the *Escherichia coli* β-galactosidase gene using the CMV immediate early promoter (Clontech Laboratories, Palo Alto, CA).
4. The human hepatoma cell lines Huh7, HepG2, and HepG2.1 and the mouse NIH3T3 fibroblast cell line are grown in RPMI-1640 medium (Invitrogen) and 10% fetal bovine serum (FBS) at 37°C in 5% CO_2/air. The $CaPO_4$ transfection is performed in Dulbecco's modified Eagle's medium (DMEM; Invitrogen).
5. Supplement 500 mL of media with: 5 mL HEPES buffer, 1 *M* solution; 5 mL nonessential amino acids, 10 m*M* solution; 5 mL penicillin–streptomycin, 5000 U penicillin/5000 μg streptomycin solution; 5 mL L-glutamine, 200 m*M* solution, and 55 mL FBS (all available from Invitrogen).
6. A 0.25 % solution of trypsin–ethylenediaminetetraacetic acid (EDTA; Invitrogen) is used to harvest cells for passage.
7. Tissue-culture–treated six-well plates are used for transfection. Larger flasks may be used to carry the cells.
8. Calcium phosphate buffers: 2 *M* $CaCl_2$, filtered through 0.2 μm filter; 2X HeBs (0.273 *M* NaCl, 0.01 *M* KCl, 1.5 mM Na_2HPO_4, 42 m*M* HEPES, pH 7.08), filtered through 0.2-μm filter (*see* **Note 4**).

9. Glycerol shock buffer: 10 m*M* HEPES, pH 7.6, 140 m*M* NaCl, 15% glycerol filtered through 0.2-μm filter.

2.1.2. Cell Lysis for Luciferase and β-Galactosidase Assays

1. Phosphate-buffered saline (PBS; Invitrogen).
2. Galactolight™ Lysis Solution (Tropix, Bedford, MA): 0.1 *M* phosphate buffer, pH 7.8, 0.2 % Triton X-100. Store at 4°C.

2.1.3. Luciferase Assay

1. D-Luciferin, potassium salt (BD Pharmingen). Dilute to 1 m*M* in water. Store at –20°C.
2. Luminometer: Any model with an automatic injector function.
3. Luminometer cuvets: 12 × 75, clear polystyrene.
4. Luciferase assay buffer: 0.1 *M* phosphate buffer, pH 7.8 (titrate 0.1 *M* KH_2PO_4 and 0.1 *M* K_2HPO_4 to pH 7.8), 0.015 *M* $MgSO_4$, 5 m*M* adenosine triphosphate (ATP) 1 m*M* dithiotreitol (DTT). Make this fresh each time.

2.1.4. β-Galactosidase Assay

1. Galacton™ substrate (Tropix, Bedford, MA) diluted 1:100 in Galacton™ reaction buffer diluent. Both solutions are stored at 4°C.
2. Galacto™ accelerator (Tropix, Bedford, MA).

2.2. Viral RNA Analysis (see Note 8)

2.2.1. HBV DNA Transfections

1. The materials required for these transfections are the same as for the luciferase transfections (**Subheading 2.1.1.**) except for the plasmid DNA and the size of the tissue-culture plate.
2. The transfections are performed in 10-cm tissue-culture dishes (Corning/Costar or B-D Falcon).
3. A cesium-chloride–purified plasmid containing HBV sequences (subtype ayw) 1072–3182/1–1990 in a pUC 13 vector will provide the template for the transcription of all of the HBV RNAs. The same internal control plasmids and transcription factor expression vectors used in the reporter-molecule analysis may be used for this analysis.

2.2.2. Cell Lysis for RNA Analysis (see **Note 9**)

1. 17 × 100 mm polypropylene culture tubes (B-D Falcon cat. no. 2059), microcentrifuge tubes.
2. GTC solution: 25 m*M* sodium citrate, pH 7.0 (made from citric acid, trisodium salt; Sigma), 4 *M* guanidinium isothiocyanate (Fluka), 0.5% (v/v) sarcosyl (Sigma), 0.1 *M* 2-mercaptoethanol (Sigma); (*see* **Note 10**).
3. 2 *M* sodium acetate, pH 4.0.
4. Saturated phenol, pH 6.6 (Ambion, Austin, TX).
5. Chloroform-isoamyl alcohol (49:1); (both available from Sigma).
6. Isopropanol, ethanol (Sigma).
7. 10 m*M* Tris-HCl, pH 8.0, 5 m*M* EDTA containing 1% sodium dodecyl sulfate (SDS).

2.2.3. Ribonuclease Protection Analysis

1. Linearized plasmid containing HBV sequences adjacent to the T3 or T7 binding site so that transcription by T3 or T7 RNA polymerase produces an RNA complementary to the HBV plus strand (has the minus-strand sequence) (*see* **Note 13**).

2. Ambion Maxiscript™ Kit for the synthesis of radiolabeled RNA probes.
3. Radiolabeled UTP (α-^{32}P-UTP, 100 µCi at 3000 Ci/mmol, 10 mCi/mL). It is important to obtain high-quality α-^{32}P-UTP. Dupont NEN is a good source.
4. 0.5 *M* EDTA, pH 8.0.
5. Tris-saturated phenol/chloroform/isoamyl alcohol solution (50:48:2).
6. Proteinase K (Roche), 20 mg/mL solution.
7. 1-kb Plus DNA Ladder (Invitrogen).
8. DNA Polymerase Large Fragment (Klenow) (NEB).
9. α-^{32}P-dATP (50 µCi at 3000 Ci/mmol, 10 mCi/mL) (ICN Biomedicals).
10. STE: 10 m*M* Tris-HCl, pH 8.0, 1 m*M* EDTA, 150 m*M* NaCl.
11. 6% acrylamide–7 *M* urea-sequencing gel.
12. 0.5X TBE.
13. Whatman 3MM filter paper.

3. Methods

3.1. Reporter Molecule Analysis

3.1.1. Luciferase Transfections

1. Split cells the day before transfection to obtain 30–50% confluency for the next day, seeding approx 3×10^5 cells/well in a six-well plate.
2. Change media on cells 2–4 h before transfection. DMEM, not RPMI, must be used for $CaPO_4$–DNA precipitation (*see* **Note 5**).
3. Use 5 µg reporter plasmid, 0.25 µg internal control plasmid, and 0.5 µg transcription factor expression vector, when appropriate, for six-well plates. For a negative control, transfect an equivalent amount of vector containing the reporter molecule cDNA without upstream regulatory elements, such as pGL3-Basic. Similarly, transfect with a promoterless internal control reporter molecule to generate a negative control for the internal control reporter molecule assay. If a transcription factor co-transfection is being performed, be sure to transfect each reporter molecule construct with the empty transcription factor expression vector. Dispense DNAs into microcentrifuge tube. Adjust volume to 37 µL with sterile TE.
4. In tissue culture hood, add 463 µL sterile 0.272 *M* $CaCl_2$ to DNA. Prepare the 0.272 *M* $CaCl_2$ by adding 63 µL 2 M $CaCl_2$ to 400 µL sterile water.
5. In a sterile 12×75 tube (B-D Falcon cat. no. 2063), add 0.5 mL sterile 2X HeBs buffer.
6. Add DNA sample to the tube containing 2X HeBs buffer, two drops at a time, vortexing at a low speed setting (approx 5) between each addition.
7. Incubate 15–30 min at room temperature to form precipitate.
8. Add 1 mL mixture to each well of cells containing 2 mL DMEM. Mix well. Check for precipitate among cells.
9. Glycerol shock 4–6 h later: Aspirate media/ DNA precipitate from plate. Add 1 mL glycerol solution. Swirl. Incubate at 37° C for 2 min. Aspirate glycerol from plate. Wash plate with 2 mL media. Aspirate. Add 2 mL culture media per well (return to RPMI-1640 if that is the appropriate medium for the cells).
10. Incubate 40–48 h in 37°C 5% CO_2, then lyse cells for reporter-molecule assays.

3.1.2. Cell Lysis for Luciferase and β-Galactosidase Assays

The methods described here for cell lysis and performance of the LUC and β-galactosidase assays are simple, relatively low-cost methods for the needs of a basic research lab. Complete assay systems including lysis buffers and detection systems are available from various companies (*see* **Note 3**). Many of these systems provide higher sensitivity and a luminescent signal with a long half-life, permitting the analysis of many samples over a longer period. The choice will depend largely on personal preference as well as the necessary throughput and sensitivity levels. Numerous luminometers are available on the market, including plate readers as well as single-tube readers. The assay described below involves automatic injection of the substrate, necessitating a luminometer with an injector function. One should determine which assay system is compatible with the detection equipment available to the laboratory.

1. Remove supernatant from the plate by aspirating.
2. Wash wells with 1 mL PBS. Aspirate PBS, making sure to remove all residual volume.
3. Add 150 μL Galactolight Lysis Solution.
4. Incubate 2–3 min at room temperature, shaking occasionally to cover surface.
5. Loosen cell layer by tapping plate against hand.
6. Resuspend cells by pipetting and transfer 150 μL cell suspension to a microcentrifuge tube.
7. Centrifuge for 5 min at 20,000*g* in a microcentrifuge to clarify lysate.
8. Transfer lysate to a fresh microcentrifuge tube.
9. Store at 4°C if the assays will be run the same day. Otherwise, store at-20°C.

3.1.3. Luciferase Assay

1. Warm 1 m*M* luciferin to room temperature.
2. Add 100 μL cell extract to 100 μL assay buffer in luminometer cuvets (*see* **Note 6**).
3. Read light output for 10 s with automatic injection of 100 μL 1 m*M* luciferin.
4. Read assay buffer alone for luminometer background and a negative cell extract for assay background (*see* **Note 7**).

3.1.4. β-Galactosidase Assay

1. Add 5 μL cell extract to 70 μL Galacton reaction buffer in luminometer cuvet (*see* **Note 6**).
2. Incubate 15–60 min at room temperature.
3. Read light output for 10 s with manual or automatic addition of 100 μL Galacto accelerator. The timing is not as critical as with the luciferase assay, so automatic injection is not absolutely necessary.
4. Read the reaction buffer alone as a luminometer background control and a negative cell extract as an assay background sample (*see* **Note 7**).

3.1.5. Data Analysis

1. Subtract the background light units, which is the reading from the negative-control cell extract, from the light units of the experimental samples (for both the LUC and β-galactosidase assays).
2. Normalize the samples for transfection efficiency by dividing the LUC value by the β-galactosidase value for each sample.
3. Compare the relative activities of the normalized values. Generally, the activity of a full-length wild-type construct is designated as 1 (or 100%), and the activities of the deletion or mutation constructs are compared with the "parent" construct. Similarly, if transcription factor expression factors are co-transfected, the activities from the reporter molecules in the presence of transcription factor expression are compared with the activities in the absence of the transcription factor.

3.2. Viral RNA Analysis (see Note 8)

3.2.1. HBV DNA Transfections

1. Follow the protocol as described in **Subheading 3.1.1.** with the following changes: In **step 1**, seed approx 1×10^6 cells/10-cm dish. In **step 3**, use 10 μg HBV DNA plasmid, 0.75 μg internal-control plasmid, and 1.5 μg transcription factor expression vector, when appropriate, to make the 1-mL $CaPO_4$-DNA precipitate. Transfect in 10-cm dishes containing 10 mL of DMEM. In **step 9**, use 2 mL of 15% glycerol solution for the glycerol shock. Wash plate with 4 mL of media, aspirate, and replace with 10 mL fresh media.
2. Incubate 72 h in 37°C 5% CO_2 before RNA isolation.

3.2.2. Cell Lysis for RNA Analysis

1. Remove media from 72-h post-transfection cell cultures (remember to treat as a **biohazard**). Wash plate with 3 mL PBS. Repeat. Remove all residual PBS.
2. Lyse cells in tissue-culture dish in 1.8 mL GTC solution (*see* **Note 11**). Transfer lysate to a 17 × 100 mm (B-D Falcon cat. no. 2059) polypropylene tube.
3. Add 0.18 mL (0.1 vol) 2 *M* NaOAc, pH 4.0. Mix.
4. Extract RNA by adding 1.8 mL (1 vol) saturated phenol, pH 6.6, and 0.36 mL (0.2 vol.) chloroform/isoamyl alcohol (49:1).
5. Shake well to mix thoroughly. Incubate on ice for 15 min.
6. Centrifuge for 30 min at 3,000 rpm in a tabletop Sorvall RT6000 or similar centrifuge (*see* **Note 12**).
7. Transfer aqueous phase to a new 2059 tube.
8. Add 1.8 mL (1 vol) isopropanol and precipitate 1 h at –20°C or 15 min at –70°C.
9. Centrifuge for 30 min at 3,000 rpm in a tabletop Sorvall RT6000 or similar centrifuge (*see* **Note 12**). Pour off supernatant and let drain to remove residual volume.
10. Resuspend in 0.3 mL GTC solution. Transfer to RNase-free microcentrifuge tube.
11. Add 0.6 mL (2 vol) 100% ethanol and precipitate 1 h at –70°C or overnight at –20°C.
12. Centrifuge for 20 min at 20,000*g* in microcentrifuge. Pour off supernatant and wash with 70% ethanol. Carefully remove supernatant from pellet.
13. Resuspend completely in 300 μL 10 m*M* Tris-HCl, pH 8.0, 5 m*M* EDTA, 1 % SDS.
14. Precipitate with 45 μL 2 *M* NaOAc, pH 4.0, and 0.7 mL ethanol. Store at –20°C.
15. To determine concentration, spin a 50-μL aliquot at full speed in a microcentrifuge for 20 min, resuspend in water, and measure optical density at A_{260}.

3.2.3. Ribonuclease Protection Analysis

The method described here is essentially the protocol adapted from the B-D Pharmingen Riboquant™ system. The RNA probe is produced using the Ambion Maxiscript Kit. I use the reagents that are included in both kits.

1. Prepare a stock solution of linearized template DNA (or a gel-purified fragment) at a concentration of 0.5 μg/μL (*see* **Note 13**). Digest 10 μg of plasmid DNA so that the end of the template DNA is 200–400 nucleotides from the T3 or T7 polymerase start site. Following the restriction endonuclease reaction, digest the mixture with 200 μg/mL proteinase K for 30 min at 50°C. Extract with phenol/chloroform/isoamyl alcohol, followed by a chloroform/isoamyl alcohol extraction. Precipitate the DNA with 0.3 *M* NaOAc and ethanol. Dissolve the DNA in RNase-free TE at a concentration of 0.5 μg/μL.

2. Using Ambion Maxiscript Kit reagents, prepare the radiolabeled RNA probe. Mix and incubate at 37°C for 1 h: 3 µL 50 µ*M* UTP; 2 µL 3.3 m*M* each G, A, CTP mix; 10 µL α-^{32}P-UTP (100 µCi at 3000 Ci/mmol, 10 mCi/mL); 2 µL DTT (0.1 *M*); 2 µL 10X transcription buffer; 2 µL T7 or T3 RNA polymerase/RNasin mix; and 0.5 µL Template DNA (≥100 ng). Prepare markers at this time (*see* **Note 14**). Add 1 µL DNase to stop reaction, vortex, spin for a few seconds in a microcentrifuge, and incubate 30 min at 37°C. Stop DNase reaction with 1.5 µL 0.5 *M* EDTA. Add 26 µL diethyl pyrocarbonate-treated (DEPC) water, 1 µL yeast tRNA (5 mg/mL), and 50 µL Tris-saturated phenol/chloroform/isoamyl alcohol. Extract and transfer aqueous phase to new tube, discarding phenol in radioactive chemical waste. Extract one time with chloroform/isoamyl alcohol. Precipitate probe with the addition of 50 µL 4 *M* NH_4OAc and 250 µL cold 100% ethanol. After ≥ 15 min at –80°C, centrifuge 10–15 min in microcentrifuge at 4°C. Wash pellet with 70% ethanol and allow to dry. Take care not to lose the pellet. Discard all ethanol in radioactive waste. Dissolve radiolabeled RNA probe in 25 µL hybridization buffer (from B-D Pharmingen Riboquant system). Vortex well. Measure 1 µL on scintillation counter. Expect 2.5×10^5–3×10^6 counts/µL. Store probe at –20°C.
3. Follow the protocol below or the manufacturer's instruction manual for the RNase protection reaction. Prepare RNA samples by pelleting 20 µg from the ethanol precipitate and dissolving in 8 µL hybridization buffer. Prepare two 20 µg tRNA samples in 8 µL hybridization buffer as controls. One of these samples will receive RNase treatment; one will not. Dilute the riboprobes in hybridization buffer to 800 cpm/U (*see* **Note 15**).
4. Add 1 µL of each diluted riboprobe, the experimental and control, to each sample. Vortex, spin 1–2 s, add a drop of mineral oil to each tube, and quick spin again. Boil for 2–3 min, quickly transfer to 90°C, and immediately turn heat block/bath down to 56°C. Incubate samples to anneal while cooling and hybridize overnight at 56°C.
5. Prepare RNase cocktail of RNase buffer and RNAse A + T1 mix according to B-D Pharmingen Riboquant protocol (for 20 samples, mix 2.5 mL buffer and 6 µL RNase A + T1 mix). Remove RNA samples from 56°C. Pipet 100 µL RNase cocktail underneath oil into aqueous layer. Use RNase buffer alone for one tRNA control sample. Quick spin the tubes and incubate 45 min at 30°C (*see* **Note 16**).
6. Prepare proteinase K cocktail [for 20 samples, mix 390 µL proteinase K buffer with 30 µL proteinase K (10 mg/mL) and 30 µL yeast tRNA (2 mg/mL)]. Add 18 µL proteinase K cocktail to new microcentrifuge tubes. Carefully transfer the RNA digests, avoiding the oil, to the proteinase K cocktail tubes. Vortex, quick spin, and incubate 15 min at 37°C. Extract once with 130 µL Tris-saturated phenol/chloroform/isoamyl alcohol. Remove aqueous phase, avoiding interface, and transfer to a new tube (*see* **Note 17**). Precipitate samples with 120 µL 4 *M* NH_4OAc and 650 µL cold 100% ethanol for 30 min at –70°C. Prerun the sequencing gel in 0.5 × TBE at approximately 50 W/1500 V.
7. After precipitation, spin the samples for 15 min at 4°C. Wash pellets carefully with 70% ethanol (*see* **Note 18**). Let pellet dry completely and add 10 µL 1X gel-loading buffer. Vortex 2–3 min and quick spin. Prior to loading on 6% acrylamide-7 *M* urea-sequencing gel, boil 3 min, quick spin, and place on ice. Load 3 µL (*see* **Note 19**).
8. Resolve protected fragments on a sequencing gel by running at approx 50 W/1500 V in 0.5X TBE until dye front is at the bottom of the gel. Disassemble the gel and adsorb gel to Whatman 3MM filter paper. Cover with plastic wrap and dry with vacuum for ≥ 1 h at 80°C. Expose to film or a phosphorimager screen. Quantitate the ribonuclease-protected fragments using any of the phosphorimaging systems (*see* **Note 20**).

4. Notes

4.1. Reporter Molecule Analysis

4.1.1. Luciferase Transfections

1. All plasmids used for transfections should be purified by cesium-chloride density gradient. If another method of purification, such as Qiagen Maxi Preps, is used, it is recommended that the manufacturer's protocol be followed by phenol/chloroform extractions and ethanol precipitation.
2. Using a clone containing the ayw sequence, full-length genome constructs were made by linearizing the HBV DNA with restriction endonucleases at sites just upstream of the ATG of the large surface antigen, middle surface antigen, and X- and nucleocapsid genes *(2)*. These linear fragments were ligated to a promoterless luciferase vector such that the expression of LUC was under the control of the HBV promoters.
3. Promega sells the pGL3 series of luciferase plasmids, including a promoterless vector (pGL3-Basic), an SV40-promoter vector (pGL3-Promoter), and an SV40 enhancer-containing vector (pGL3-Enhancer), which are convenient for the insertion of regulatory elements. They also sell *Renilla* luciferase vectors to be used as internal controls and a dual luciferase system for the use of the firefly and sea pansy luciferases simultaneously. Tropix sells a dual-detection system for luciferase and β-galactosidase (Dual Light™). Other companies also sell various reporter-molecule vectors and detection systems.
4. The pH of the 2X HeBs buffer is very important and should be checked and adjusted if the solution is stored for a long time.
5. An alternative to the $CaPO_4$ precipitation method of transfection *(22)*, such as Lipofectamine (Invitrogen), or other commercially available lipid-mediated transfection reagents, may be used. Follow the manufacturer's recommended protocols for the appropriate cell types.

4.1.2. Luciferase and β-Galactosidase Assays

6. One should determine the linearity of the assay system being used and measure samples within this range.
7. Measuring the luminometer background with assay buffer alone helps to ensure that the equipment is functioning properly. This reading should be very low, below the level of activity in the negative control cell extract or assay background sample.

4.2. HBV RNA Analysis

4.2.1. Cell Transfection and Lysis for RNA Analysis

8. Transfection of the 1.3 genome HBV construct (**Subheading 2.2.1.**, **step 3**) into differentiated hepatoma cell lines could result in the production of HBV virions, which are potentially infectious. After transfection, the cells, culture media, and plasticware should be treated as infectious, **biohazardous** materials and handled accordingly.
9. All reagents, glassware, and plasticware should be RNase-free. Use chemicals set aside for RNA work and DEPC water (Sigma).
10. Add 0.36 mL 2-mercaptoethanol to 50 mL of guanidinium isothiocyanate solution at time of use.
11. RNA extraction kits are available from companies such as Ambion and Qiagen and can be used according to the manufacturer's instructions. The method presented here reliably yields high-quality RNA and is based on the method by Chomczynski and Sacchi *(23)*.

12. A large number of samples can be processed in this centrifuge. If the number of samples is small, a shorter spin of 10–15 min at 10,000 rpm in a Sorvall superspeed centrifuge can be used. An additional extraction may be necessary if the phases are not well separated.

4.2.2. Ribonuclease Protection Analysis

13. Follow the instructions of the Ambion Maxiscript Kit for the design of the RNA probes, but, in general, a probe length of 300–400 nucleotides, with a protected region of 100–300 nucleotides, will be efficiently synthesized and easily separated on a gel. For example, a probe containing HBV nucleotides 1658 to 1990 plus some vector sequence has been used to map the transcriptional start sites of the precore and pregenomic RNAs ***(10)***. Prepare an internal control riboprobe template by using plasmid-containing sequences from an internal reporter molecule, such as β-galactosidase, or from a cellular gene such as the mouse ribosomal protein L32 (for cell lines of mouse origin or for RNA made from mouse tissue). Design the control templates so that the length of the protected fragment will be distinct from the expected lengths of fragments in the experimental samples. Keep in mind that the riboprobe must be complementary to the mRNA sequence to hybridize and protect the mRNA.
14. Prepare radiolabeled markers for RPA. Combine and incubate at 30°C for 15 min: 1 μL 1.kb ladder (1 μg), 1 μL dC,T,GTP mix (2.5 m*M* each), 1 μL 10X Klenow buffer, 1 μL H_2O, 1 μL Klenow (5 U), and 5 μL $\alpha^{32}P$ dATP (50 μCi at 3000 Ci/mmol). Stop reaction by the addition of 1 μL 0.5 *M* EDTA. Add 39 μL STE. Separate the probe from unincorporated nucleotides using the Pharmacia G50 Probequant™ spin column. Count 1 μL on scintillation counter.
15. As the Us in the riboprobe correspond to the minus-strand sequence, count the Ts in the minus-strand sequence used as a template for the riboprobe.
16. At this time, pour a 6% acrylamide–7 *M* urea sequencing gel, approx 40 cm in length, using a standard protocol.
17. Do not worry about recovering the whole sample; it is more important to avoid the interface and obtain a clean sample. The usual recovery is approx 120 μL. Also remember that these are radioactive samples and should be disposed of accordingly.
18. These pellets may be small and slippery, so take care not to lose them. Pipet, rather than pour, the ethanol off the pellet and leave a little residual ethanol so as not to risk disturbing the pellet.
19. Run the radiolabeled 1-kb DNA ladder as approximate size markers. The yeast tRNA sample not treated with RNase should serve as a marker for the size of the probe. The RNase-treated tRNA sample should be a negative control.
20. It is important to quantitate the protected fragments and normalize each sample to the internal control band. One can correct for transfection efficiencies or for sample handling discrepancies in this way.

References

1. Honigwachs, J., Faktor, O., Dikstein, R., Shaul, Y., and Laub, O. (1989) Liver-specific expression of hepatitis B virus is determined by the combined action of the core gene promoter and the enhancer. *J. Virol.* **63**, 919–924.
2. Raney, A. K., Milich, D. R., Easton, A. J., and McLachlan, A. (1990) Differentiation-specific transcriptional regulation of the hepatitis B virus large surface antigen gene in human hepatoma cell lines. *J. Virol.* **64**, 2360–2368.

3. Guo, W., Chen, M., Yen, T. S. B., and Ou, J.-H. (1993) Hepatocyte-specific expression of the hepatitis B virus core promoter depends on both positive and negative regulation. *Mol. Cell. Biol.* **13**, 443–448.
4. Yen, T. S. B. (1993) Regulation of hepatitis B virus gene expression. *Semin. Virol.* **4**, 33–42.
5. Raney, A. K., Johnson, J. L., Palmer, C. N. A., and McLachlan, A. (1997) Members of the nuclear receptor superfamily regulate transcription from the hepatitis B virus nucleocapsid promoter. *J. Virol.* **71**, 1058–1071.
6. Tang, H., Raney, A. K., and McLachlan, A. (2001) Replication of the wild type and a natural hepatitis B virus nucleocapsid promoter variant is differentially regulated by nuclear hormone receptors in cell culture. *J. Virol.* **75**, 8937–8948.
7. Yu, X. and Mertz, J. E. (2001) Critical roles of nuclear receptor response elements in replication of hepatitis B virus. *J. Virol.* **75**, 11,354–11,364.
8. Guidotti, L. G., Matzke, B., Schaller, H., and Chisari, F. V. (1995) High-level hepatitis B virus replication in transgenic mice. *J. Virol.* **69**, 6158–6169.
9. Guidotti, L. G., Eggers, C. M., Raney, A. K., et al. (1999) In vivo regulation of hepatitis B virus replication by peroxisome proliferators. *J. Virol.* **73**, 10,377–10,386.
10. Raney, A. K., Eggers, C. M., Kline, E. F., et al. (2001) Nuclear covalently closed circular viral genomic DNA in the liver of hepatocyte nuclear factor 1α-null hepatitis B virus transgenic mice. *J. Virol.* **75**, 2900–2911.
11. Schaller, H. and Fischer, M. (1991) Transcriptional control of hepadnavirus gene expression. *Curr. Top. Microbiol. Immunol.* **168**, 21–39.
12. Aden, D. P., Fogel, A., Plotkin, S., Damjanov, I., and Knowles, B. B. (1979) Controlled synthesis of HBsAg in a differentiated human liver carcinoma-derived cell line. *Nature* **282**, 615–616.
13. Nakabayashi, H., Taketa, K., Miyano, K., Yamane, T., and Sato, J. (1982) Growth of human hepatoma cell lines with differentiated functions in chemically defined medium. ***Cancer Res.*** **42**, 3858–3863.
14. Puck, T. T., Marcus, P. I., and Cieciura, S. J. (1956) Clonal growth of mammalian cells in vitro: growth characteristics of colonies from single HeLa cells with and without a "feeder" layer. *J. Exp. Med.* **103**, 273–284.
15. Liu, C., Condreay, L. D., Burch, J. B. E., and Mason, W. (1991) Characterization of the core promoter and enhancer of duck hepatitis B virus. *Virology* **184**, 242–252.
16. Lilienbaum, A., Crescenzo-Chaigne, B., Sall, A. A., Pillot, J., and Elfassi, E. (1993) Binding of nuclear factors to functional domains of the duck hepatitis B virus enhancer. *J. Virol.* **67**, 6192–6200.
17. Crescenzo-Chaigne, B., Pillot, J., and Lilienbaum, A. (1995) Interplay between a new HNF3 and the HNF1 transcriptional factors in the duck hepatitis B virus enhancer. *Virology* **213**, 231–240.
18. Welsheimer, T. and Newbold, J. E. (1996) A functional hepatocyte nuclear factor 3 binding site is a critical component of the duck hepatitis B virus major surface antigen promoter. *J. Virol.* **70**, 8813–8820.
19. Fourel, G., Ringeisen, F., Flajolet, M., et al. (1996) The HNF1/HNF4-dependent We2 element of woodchuck hepatitis virus controls the viral replication and can activate the N-*myc2* promoter. *J. Virol.* **70**, 8571–8583.
20. Ueda, K., Wei, Y., and Ganem, D. (1996) Cellular factors controlling the activity of woodchuck hepatitis virus enhancer II. *J. Virol.* **70**, 4714–4723.

21. Sambrook. J. and Russell, D.W. (2001) *Molecular Cloning: A Laboratory Manual*, 3rd ed. Cold Spring Harbor Laboratory Press, Cold Spring Harbor, NY.
22. Graham, F. L. and Van Der Eb, A. J. (1973) A new technique for the assay of infectivity of human adenovirus 5 DNA. *Virology* **52**, 456–467.
23. Chomczynski, P. and Sacchi, N. (1987) Single-step method of RNA isolation by acid guanidinium thiocyanate-phenol-chloroform extraction. *Anal. Biochem.* **162**, 156–159.

30

In Vitro Reconstitution of ϵ-Dependent Duck Hepatitis B Virus Replication Initiation

Jürgen Beck and Michael Nassal

1. Introduction

In vitro systems, providing a defined and controllable chemical environment, have been instrumental in understanding the replication properties of many viruses. A classic example is simian virus 40 (SV40), which, in conjunction with its T antigen, uses host-encoded DNA polymerase for copying its DNA genome *(1)*. At the other end, many virus-encoded DNA and RNA polymerases, including retroviral reverse transcriptases (RTs), have been expressed in heterologous systems; when provided with a template nucleic acid and dNTPs or rNTPs, respectively, most exert easily detectable polymerase activity. Achieving the same for the RT (P protein) of hepatitis B virus (HBV) has turned out to be a very difficult, though highly desirable, goal, given the importance of P protein as the only viral enzyme and hence only enzymatic target for therapy.

Despite fundamental similarities to conventional RTs *(2,3)*, a major obstacle is that the P proteins of HBV and the animal hepadnaviruses have several unique features *(4,5)*; in particular, they initiate DNA synthesis from their pregenomic RNA (pgRNA) template in an unusual, highly specific protein-primed fashion *(6)*. Important aspects of this reaction are schematically outlined in **Fig. 1.** To this end, they all contain an extra domain at the N terminus (terminal protein, TP) providing a Tyr residue to which the first nt of the DNA is covalently attached *(7–9)*. This priming reaction requires formation of a ribonucleoprotein (RNP) complex between the RT and an RNA stem-loop structure of about 60 nt, ϵ, close to the 5' end of the pgRNA *(10–12)*; this interaction, which is also essential for encapsidation of the pgRNA *(13)* is dependent on cellular factors (sec below). After addition of two or three further nt, templated by ϵ, synthesis is arrested; the covalent P protein–oligonucleotide complex is translocated to the 3' proximal DR1* and extended from there to generate full-length minus-strand DNA *(14–17)*. This translocation as well as plus-strand DNA synthesis and circularization are probably aided by the fact that they naturally occur inside the viral nucleocapsid.

From: *Methods in Molecular Medicine, vol. 95: Hepatitis B and D Protocols, volume 1*
Edited by: R. K. Hamatake and J. Y. N. Lau © Humana Press Inc., Totowa, NJ

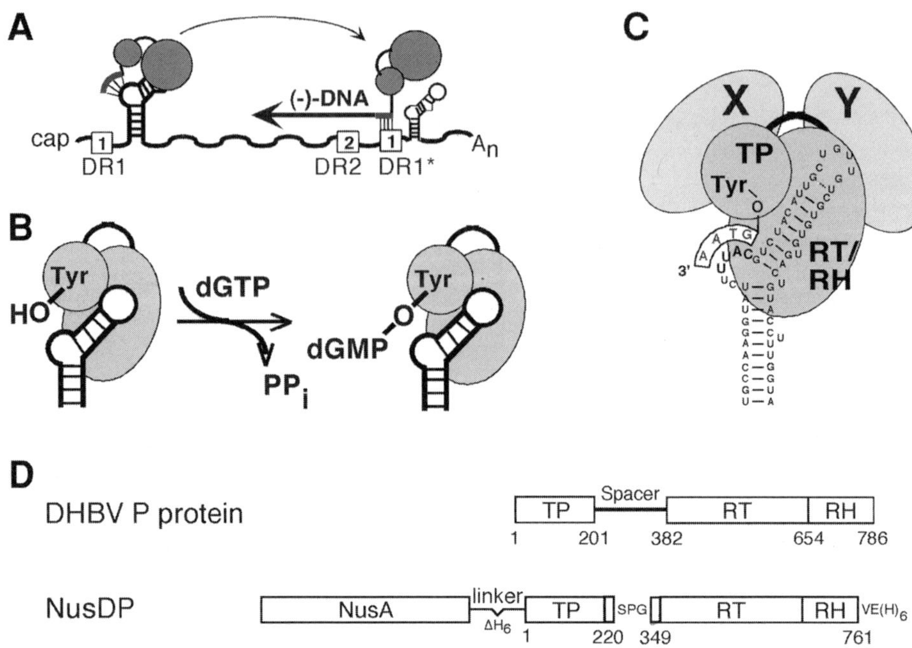

Fig. 1. Hepadnaviral replication initiation. **(A)** Outline of authentic first-strand DNA synthesis. P protein binds to the 5' proximal ϵ RNA stem loop and copies four nt from the bulged region; the first nt is covalently attached to a Tyr residue in the TP domain (small sphere). After translocation to DR1*, the primer is extended to the 5' end of the RNA template; the following steps of (+)-DNA synthesis and circularization, leading to the characteristic partially double-stranded, circular HBV genome, are not shown. **(B)** Schematic view of the priming reaction. Reaction of the phenolic Tyr OH group with dGTP leads to phosphodiester formation and release of pyrophosphate. **(C)** Model of the replication initiation complex. The sequence of the De signal is shown, along with the TP and RT/RH domains of P protein and the short oligonucleotide primer copied from the Dϵ bulge. X and Y denote cellular factors, present in RRL, that are required for P activity. Additional amino acids connecting the TP and RT/RH domains, and the C terminal His6 tag are given in single-letter code. **(D)** Comparison of the primary sequences of wild-type DHBV P protein and recombinant NusDP protein. Approximate borders of the individual P-protein domains are indicated by aa positions.

Apart from these functional complexities, a more technical problem has been that the mere generation of full-length recombinant P protein polypeptides has failed in many heterologous systems. Where it did not, such as in baculovirus-mediated expression of HBV P in insect cells, the protein is very unstable and apparently does not display the genuine ϵ RNA-dependent replication initiation activity ***(9,18,19)***.

A major breakthrough was the finding that the RT of duck hepatitis B virus (DHBV), but for unknown reasons not that of HBV, in vitro translated in rabbit reticulocyte lysate (RRL) from a DHBV ϵ (Dϵ)–containing RNA, is capable of template–directed priming and limited DNA synthesis *(6)*. Meanwhile, it is known that the ϵ stem loop does not have to be part of the RT mRNA but can also be provided as a separate small RNA molecule (*trans*-priming) *(20,21)*. Using this system, it was also discovered that factors contained in the RRL are essential contributors to RT activity.

Several lines of evidence, for instance, depletion of certain factors by antibodies, suggest that chaperones of the Hsp70 and Hsp90 class plus various co-chaperones are important *(22,23)*. It has been implied that activation of the RT proceeds similarly to activation of steroid-hormone receptors. These receptors require the sequential action of the Hsp70/Hsp40 (DnaK/DnaJ in *Escherichia coli*) system with subsequent transfer to the Hsp90/p23 co-chaperone system, facilitated by the Hip and Hop proteins *(24)* to gain binding competence to their hormone ligands. If this analogy holds, additional factors, e.g., an immunophilin, would be expected to be part of the active RT complex. This issue is not finally settled, but it should be noted that a similar model has been postulated for telomerase, a cellular RT that likewise shows no activity without additional factors *(25)*.

The in vitro translation system has been widely used to analyze the effects on replication initiation of mutations in the DHBV RT as well as in ϵ *(10,26–28)*, and detailed protocols are available *(29)*. However, a major bottleneck is the small amount of P protein that can be produced by in vitro translation (on the order of 1 ng per μL). Hence, it would be highly desirable to have an efficient heterologous source for the protein. This could then be reconstituted into functional complexes by the addition of RRL, in which all of the suspected chaperones and co-chaperones are abundant; eventually, purified factors might be used instead.

E. coli continues to be the most convenient expression system for many proteins. Recent advances in the design of vectors and *E. coli* strains have also allowed the expression of proteins that were previously difficult, or impossible, to obtain in reasonable amounts *(30,31)*. On this basis, we have reinvestigated the use of *E. coli* for expression of hepadnaviral P proteins. A systematic study of different vectors, strains, and modifications in the primary sequence of DHBV P protein revealed that the TP domain and, after removal of 25 nonessential C terminal aa the RT/RH domain, could also be efficiently expressed. Moreover, the separately generated fragments could be complemented into an active priming complex *(32)*. However, the requirement for interaction between the two domains, which in the authentic RT are part of a single polypeptide chain, seemed to limit the efficiency of complex formation.

Therefore, we recently developed a single-chain TP–RT/RH fusion protein **(Fig. 1D)**, NusDP, that is expressed at high levels in bacteria; soluble at substantial concentrations; easily purified; and able to form a priming competent complex when supplemented with RRL and, possibly, purified co-factors. Important modifications of the P-protein sequence are a short C-terminal deletion that enhances expressibility; N-terminal fusion to the *E. coli* NusA protein, which can substantially increase the solubility of many proteins that otherwise aggregate and/or precipitate; the incorporation of a His-tag to allow for affinity purification by immobilized metal affinity chromatography; and, finally, we found that the use of an *E. coli* expression strain that provides tRNAs, which are rare in *E. coli* (such as BL21 CodonPlus), greatly increases the expression level. In this way, several hundred micrograms of purified P protein can be prepared from 1 L of *E. coli* culture (*see* **Fig. 2A, B**). We also provide a protocol of a standard priming assay using RRL and in vitro transcribed wild-type Dε RNA (**Fig. 2C**). However, the system should easily be adaptable to different inputs, e.g., variants of P protein or Dε, full or partially depleted RRL, purified chaperones, as well as alterations in the general buffer, salt, pH, or temperature conditions.

2. Materials

General materials for recombinant DNA work and propagation of plasmids such as restriction enzymes, media, and antibiotics are available from various suppliers and are not separately listed below. It is also expected that users are familiar with standard biochemical techniques, such as sodium dodecyl sulfate–polyacrylamide gel electrophoresis (SDS-PAGE), and with appropriate handling of radioactive material.

2.1. Cloning of the NusDP Expression Vector

1. pET43a(+) vector (Novagen). This plasmid contains a colE1 origin of replication, an ampicillin resistance gene, and the T7 RNA polymerase promoter followed by the *E. coli* nusA gene (encoding aa 1–495) and a multiple cloning site allowing for the generation of N-terminal fusions with the NusA protein. In addition, it provides an S tag, His tag, and cleavage sites for enterokinase and thrombin. Further information can be found on the homepage of Novagen (http://www.novagen.com).
2. pET-NusDP vector. A pET43a(+)–derived vector encoding a fusion of the NusA protein with the modified DHBV P protein is shown in **Fig. 1D**.; the original His tag of the vector is removed, and instead a His tag is present at the C terminus of the fusion protein. Fragments for generating the modified NusDP protein gene were obtained by conventional techniques using plasmid pCD16 as starting plasmid; it contains the complete genome of DHBV16 *(33)* under control of the cytomegalovirus (CMV) promoter *(34)*. A detailed cloning scheme as well as the pET-NusDP vector are available from the authors upon request. The plasmid can be propagated in common laboratory strains of *E. coli*, e.g., DH5α or Top10. It is, however, highly recommended to use carbenicillin (25 μg/mL) instead of ampicillin as selection marker (*see* **Note 1**).

2.2. Bacterial Expression and Purification of NusDP Protein

1. *E. coli* BL21 CodonPlus RIL cells (Stratagene). This strain is a derivative of the commonly used BL21(DE3) cells, which carries an additional plasmid-encoding rare *E. coli* tRNAs for Arg, Ile, and Leu. Its p15A replication origin is compatible with the colE1–derived origin present on most commonly used plasmids. The vector encodes resistance toward chloramphenicol (recommended working concentration 34 μg/mL). Competent cells are commercially available from Stratagene or may be produced in-house by any standard procedure. Carbenicillin, chloramphenicol, and isopropyl-thiogalactoside (IPTG) may be purchased from any major supplier of laboratory reagents.
2. Lysis buffer: 20 m*M* Tris-HCl, pH 7.5, 500 m*M* NaCl, 5 m*M* $MgCl_2$, 1% Triton X-100, 10 m*M* imidazole, 10 m*M* β-mercaptoethanol, 1 mg/mL lysozyme.
3. Complete ethylenediaminetetraacetic acid (EDTA)-free protease inhibitor cocktail (Roche); 1 tablet dissolved in 2 mL H_2O.
4. Branson Sonifier 450 equipped with Cup Horn resonator (*see* **Note 3**).

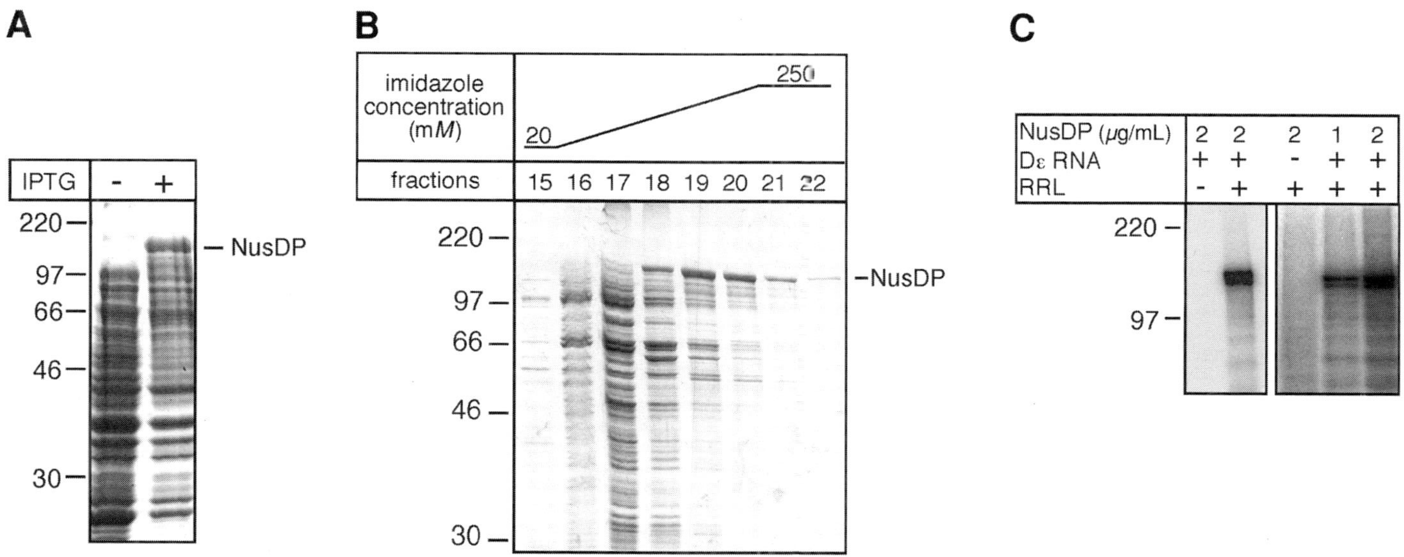

Fig. 2. Expression, purification, and activity assays of NusDP. **(A)** Control for induction. Crude SDS-lysates, obtained with or without IPTG induction, were resolved by SDS-PAGE and stained with Coomassie blue. **(B)** Affinity purification of NusDP. Cleared lysate from induced bacteria was subjected to Ni^{2+}, affinity chromatography as described in the text; aliquots from the indicated fractions were analyzed by SDS-PAGE and Coomassie blue staining. **(C)** Detection of priming activity. Reactions were performed with the indicated components and the products analyzed by SDS-PAGE and autoradiography as described in the text. Note that no signals are visible without RRL or Dε RNA. Larger amounts of NusDP yield stronger signals.

5. FPLC apparatus (*see* **Note 5**) equipped with a HiTrap Chelating HP column (both Amersham Pharmacia Biotech).
6. Column buffer: 20 m*M* Tris-HCl, pH 7.5, 500 m*M* NaCl, 5 m*M* $MgCl_2$, 0.1% Triton X-100, 10 m*M* imidazole, 10 m*M* β-mercaptoethanol.
7. Dialysis frames: Slide-a-lyzer, molecular weight cutoff 10,000 daltons (Pierce) or equivalent.
8. Protein storage buffer: 20 m*M* Tris-HCl, pH 7.5, 500 m*M* NaCl, 5 m*M* $MgCl_2$, 1 m*M* dithiothreitol (DTT), 10% glycerol.

2.3. In Vitro Transcription of Dε RNA

1. Plasmid pDε1 *(21)* harboring DHBV16 nt 2557 to 2624 under control of the T7 promoter. Other plasmids containing Dε signal under control of a phage T7 or SP6 RNA polymerase promoter are also suitable.
2. T7 MEGAshortscript in vitro transcription kit (Ambion).
3. Diethyl pyrocarbonate (DEPC)-treated water.
4. DNase I (RNase free).
5. Stop solution: 5 *M* ammonium acetate, 100 m*M* EDTA.
6. RNA gel-loading buffer: 95% formamide, 0.025% xylene cyanol, 0.025% bromophenol blue, 18 m*M* EDTA, 0.025% SDS.

2.4. In Vitro Priming Assays

1. Purified NusDP protein (*see* **Subheading 3.2.5.**).
2. In vitro transcribed Dε RNA (*see* **Subheading 3.3.**).
3. Rabbit reticulocyte lysate (RRL), micrococcal nuclease treated (Promega).
4. Two-fold priming mix: 20 m*M* Tris-HCl, pH 8.0, 20 m*M* NH_4Cl, 12 m*M* $MgCl_2$, 4 m*M* $MnCl_2$, 0.4% NP40, 20 m*M* β-mercaptoethanol, 1 m*M* spermidine, 50 μ*M* dGTP, 50 μ*M* dTTP, 0.3 μCi/μL [α-^{32}P]dATP (3000 Ci/mmol; Amersham Pharmacia Biotech).
5. Gel-drying apparatus.
6. Phosphorimager or X-ray film.

3. Methods

3.1. Cloning of a Modified NusA-DHBV P (NusDP) Protein Gene

The cloning scheme is available from the authors upon request.

3.2. Bacterial Expression and Purification of NusDP Protein

3.2.1. Transformation of pET-NusDP into E. coli Expression Strain

1. Transform 100 ng of the pET-NusDP plasmid into competent BL21 CodonPlus RIL cells; the protocol provided by the manufacturer works well but may be substituted with home-made competent cells and any of various standard transformation procedures.
2. Plate cells onto LB agar plates containing 34 μg/mL of chloramphenicol and 25 μg/mL of carbenicillin (*see* **Note 1**), and incubate at 37°C. After 16 to 20 h, easily visible colonies should have formed.

3.2.2. Selection of a Well-Inducible-Bacterial Colony

1. Pick two or more colonies from the transformation plate into 2 mL of Luria–Bertani (LB) medium containing carbenicillin (25 μg/mL) and chloramphenicol (34 μg/mL) and grow at 37°C for 8–10 h.
2. Store the bacterial cultures at 4°C.

3. Take 100 μL of each of the cultures to inoculate 2 mL LB medium containing the same antibiotics and grow at 37°C until the solution becomes visibly turbid. Keep the initial culture at 4°C as inoculum for later large-scale induction.
4. Divide each culture into two aliquots, and to one of them, add IPTG to a final concentration of 1 m*M*. Shake cells for 3–4 h at room temperature.
5. Spin down the cultures and resuspend the bacterial pellet in 100 μL of SDS-PAGE sample buffer; boil for several minutes to generate crude SDS lysates.
6. Resolve 10-μL aliquots of the SDS lysates by SDS-PAGE (7.5% acrylamide) and stain with Coomassie blue. Well-inducible clones should give an easily visible band at an apparent molecular weight of about 140 kDa if grown in the presence of IPTG (*see* **Fig. 2A**).

3.2.3. Large-Scale Induction

1. Use the total amount of the initial 2-mL culture (**Subheading 3.2.2.**) of the best expressing clone to inoculate 200 mL of LB medium with antibiotics and shake in an appropriately sized Erlenmeyer flask at 37°C until an optical density (OD) of about 0.4 at 600 nm is reached.
2. Transfer the flask to room temperature (23°C) and continue shaking.
3. Induce protein expression at an OD at 600 nm of about 0.6 by adding IPTG to a final concentration of 1 m*M* and shake the cells for 3–4 h.
4. Harvest the bacteria by centrifugation in a GSA rotor at 6000 rpm for 10 min at 4°C, discard the medium, and store the pellet at –80°C.

3.2.4. Lysate Preparation

1. Thaw the pellet on ice and resuspend the bacteria in 5 mL ice-cold lysis buffer supplemented with 100 μL protease-inhibitor cocktail. Immediately aliquot into three 2-mL tubes and incubate on ice for 30 min.
2. Add Benzonase (Novagen) to a final concentration of 50 U/mL to digest nucleic acids. Mix the lysate intensively and incubate on ice for 30 min.
3. Sonicate the lysate at 4°C in a Branson sonifier (Cup Horn) with six pulses of 10 s each interrupted by a 10-s pause (at an output level of 8); clear the lysate by centrifugation at 10,000 g for 15 min at 4°C (*see* **Notes 2** and **3**).
4. Pool the cleared lysates and filter through a 0.45-μm sterile-filter device to remove particulate material before applying the lysate to the column (*see* **Note 4**).

3.2.5. Protein Purification by Ni^{2+}-Affinity Chromatography

Perform all steps at 10°C or below.

1. Wash the HiTrap Chelating HP column (*see* **Note 5**) with 10 mL H_2O.
2. Charge the column with 1 mL of 0.1 *M* $NiSO_4$ and subsequently wash with 10 mL H_2O.
3. Equilibrate the column with at least 5-mL column buffer.
4. Load the lysate onto the column at a flow rate of 0.2 mL/min and start collecting fractions of 1-mL volume.
5. Wash the column with 10 mL wash buffer (column buffer containing 20 m*M* imidazole) at a flow rate of 0.2 mL/min.
6. Elute the fusion protein with a linear imidazole gradient ranging from 20 to 250 m*M* in 5-mL column buffer plus additional 5 mL of column buffer containing 250 m*M* imidazole at a flow rate of 0.2 mL/min.
7. Analyze 5 μL of each fraction by SDS-PAGE (7.5% acrylamide). The NusDP protein elutes at about 150 to 200 m*M* imidazole and appears in one to two peak fractions in a concentration of approx 100 μg/mL (*see* **Fig. 2B**).

8. Pool the peak fractions and dialyze for 2 h at 4°C against storage buffer in Slide-a-lyzer dialysis frames.
9. Centrifuge the dialysate at 10,000*g* for 5 min at 4°C and store the purified protein in small aliquots at –80°C.

3.3. Synthesis of Dε RNA by In Vitro Transcription

As with all RNA work, care must be taken to avoid RNase contamination. Useful hints are found in the manual supplied with the Ambion in vitro transcription kit.

1. Digest 5 μg of plasmid pDε1 with *Cla*I to obtain a 76 nt Dε RNA transcript.
2. Confirm complete digestion by analyzing 10% of the digestion sample on a 1% agarose gel.
3. Adjust the volume of the sample to 100 μL with H_2O. Purify the linearized DNA by extraction with 100 μL of TE buffer saturated phenol.
4. Add 10 μL of 3 *M* sodium acetate pH 5 to the aqueous phase and precipitate the DNA with 250 μL of ethanol.
5. Wash the DNA pellet with 70% ethanol, let air-dry, and dissolve the pellet in 10 μL of DEPC–treated H_2O.
6. In vitro transcribe 1 μg of the linearized pDε1 according to the kit manufacturer's protocol; the T7 MEGAshortscript Kit usually yields up to 100 μg RNA per 20-μL reaction (*see* **Note 6**).
7. Digest the DNA template with 2 U of DNAse I for 15 min at 37°C.
8. Add DEPC-treated water to a final volume of 135 μL and 15 μL of stop solution.
9. Extract the RNA with 150 μL of TE buffer saturated phenol.
10. Precipitate the RNA from the aqueous phase by adding 1 volume of isopropanol. Mix well, chill for at least 30 min at –20°C, and centrifuge at 4°C for 15 min at 10,000*g*.
11. Carefully remove the supernatant and wash the pellet with 200 μL of 70% ethanol.
12. Resuspend the dry pellet in 50 μL of DEPC-treated water; this typically results in a 20 μ*M* or higher concentration (*see* **Note 6**).
13. Determine the RNA concentration by measuring the ultraviolet light absorbance at 260 nm of a 1:300 dilution in H_2O. For single-stranded RNA, 1 OD at 260 nm corresponds to 40 μg/mL (*see* **Note 7**).
14. Confirm RNA integrity and concentration by native agarose gel electrophoresis: Dilute 1 μg of RNA in gel-loading buffer to a total volume of 10 μL. Denature the RNA for 2 min at 80°C, and chill on ice. Run the sample on a native 2% agarose gel alongside serial dilutions of an RNA of known concentration. Stain with ethidium bromide and estimate the concentration by visual comparison of the band intensities (*see* **Note 7**).
15. Adjust the RNA concentration to 20 μ*M* (0.5 μg/mL for the 76 nt Dε1 transcript) with DEPC-treated water and store the RNA at –80°C.

3.4. Reconstitution of the Replication Initiation Complex and Priming Assay

1. Dilute 5 μL RRL with 3.5 μL of DEPC-treated H_2O.
2. Add in vitro transcribed Dε RNA to a final concentration of 1 μ*M* (e.g., 0.5 μL of a 20-μ*M* stock solution).
3. Add 1 μL (about 100 ng) of purified NusDP protein and mix well (*see* **Note 8**).
4. Incubate the sample for 2 h at 30°C in a closed incubator (*see* **Note 9**).
5. Add 10 μL of twofold priming mix and incubate for 1 h at 37°C in a closed incubator.
6. Stop the reaction by adding 40 μL of SDS PAGE sample buffer. Analyze by SDS-PAGE or store at –20°C until further analysis.

7. Denature the samples for 5 min at 100°C and load 20 μL of each sample onto a 7.5% SDS polyacrylamide gel (20 × 20 cm, 1.5-mm spacer).
8. After running the gel for about 3 h at 40 mA, transfer the gel to Whatman paper and dry for 1 h at 75°C in a vacuum dryer.
9. Detect ^{32}P-containing bands by phosphorimaging or by autoradiography using X-ray film (*see* **Fig. 2C**).

4. Notes

1. The pET43a(+) plasmid contains the same β-lactamase gene as many other vectors; however, for unknown reasons, few (if any) colonies will be generated when the transformed bacteria are plated on ampicillin-containing plates. This problem is easily solved by using carbenicillin instead (*see also* Novagen homepage).
2. If the bacterial DNA is not completely digested and some turbid material remains in the supernatant, add a minute amount of lyophilized DNase I to the lysate, mix, and incubate for another 30 min at 4°C; centrifuge again at 10,000*g* for 15 min at 4°C.
3. The Cup Horn resonator allows for indirect sonication of samples contained in a closed tube. Depending on the induction scale, conventional Microtip or Macrotip resonators for direct sonication may be used instead; however, great care should be taken to avoid foaming, which could easily happen as a result of the content of Triton detergent in the lysis buffer.
4. Continue immediately with protein purification. Do not store the lysate for longer times.
5. The continuous imidazole gradient provided by using an FPLC apparatus will result in a sharper separation of the desired full-length Nus-DP protein from degradation products and contaminating *E. coli* proteins. Using batch procedures and other Ni^{2+} matrices should also be possible, but various imidazole concentrations for protein elution should be tested to optimize the yield of pure NusDP protein.
6. We found that the Ambion T7 MEGAshortscript Kit routinely yields the expected amounts of RNA; however, kits from other suppliers as well as homemade protocols should also work. If the RNA yield is lower, the volume of DEPC water to dissolve the RNA has to be adjusted to make up a solution of at least 20 μ*M* concentration.
7. Any residual template DNA and unincorporated nucleotides will contribute to the absorbance at 260 nm and may lead to overestimation of the actual RNA amount; running an aliquot on agarose gel as described will give a semiquantitative control for the amount of full-length RNA.
8. Do not use more than 1 μL per 10-μL reaction; higher volumes will inhibit complex formation as a result of the high salt concentration.
9. Do not use heating blocks. The vertical temperature gradient in the tube leads to reduction of the sample volume because of lid condensation. The resulting increase in salt concentration may negatively affect complex formation.

References

1. Bullock, P. A. (1997) The initiation of simian virus 40 DNA replication in vitro. *Crit. Rev. Biochem. Mol. Biol.* **32**, 503–568.
2. Das, K., Xiong, X., Yang, H., et al. (2001) Molecular modeling and biochemical characterization reveal the mechanism of hepatitis B virus polymerase resistance to lamivudine (3TC) and emtricitabine (FTC). *J. Virol.* **75**, 4771–4779.
3. Beck, J., Vogel, M., and Nassal, M. (2002) dNTP versus NTP discrimination by phenylalanine 451 in duck hepatitis B virus P protein indicates a common structure of the dNTP-binding pocket with other reverse transcriptases. *Nucl. Acids Res.* **30**, 1679–1687.

4. Nassal, M. (1999) Hepatitis B virus replication: novel roles for virus-host interactions. *Intervirology* **42**, 100–116.
5. Nassal, M. (2000) Macromolecular interactions in hepatitis B virus replication and particle assembly. In: Cann, A. J. (ed.), *DNA Virus Replication,* vol. 26. Oxford University Press, Oxford, UK, 1–40.
6. Wang, G. H. and Seeger, C. (1992) The reverse transcriptase of hepatitis B virus acts as a protein primer for viral DNA synthesis. *Cell* **71**, 663–670.
7. Zoulim, F. and Seeger, C. (1994) Reverse transcription in hepatitis B viruses is primed by a tyrosine residue of the polymerase. *J. Virol.* **68**, 6–13.
8. Weber, M., Bronsema, V., Bartos, H., Bosserhoff, A., Bartenschlager, R., and Schaller, H. (1994) Hepadnavirus P protein utilizes a tyrosine residue in the TP domain to prime reverse transcription. *J. Virol.* **68**, 2994–2999.
9. Lanford, R. E., Notvall, L., Lee, H., and Beames, B. (1997) Transcomplementation of nucleotide priming and reverse transcription between independently expressed TP and RT domains of the hepatitis B virus reverse transcriptase. *J. Virol.* **71**, 2996–3004.
10. Beck, J. and Nassal, M. (1997) Sequence- and structure-specific determinants in the interaction between the RNA encapsidation signal and reverse transcriptase of avian hepatitis B viruses. *J. Virol.* **71**, 4971–4980.
11. Knaus, T. and Nassal, M. (1993) The encapsidation signal on the hepatitis B virus RNA pregenome forms a stem-loop structure that is critical for its function. *Nucl. Acids Res.* **21**, 3967–3975.
12. Pollack, J. R. and Ganem, D. (1994) Site-specific RNA binding by a hepatitis B virus reverse transcriptase initiates two distinct reactions: RNA packaging and DNA synthesis. *J. Virol.* **68**, 5579–5587.
13. Bartenschlager, R. and Schaller, H. (1992) Hepadnaviral assembly is initiated by polymerase binding to the encapsidation signal in the viral RNA genome. *EMBO J.* **11**, 3413–3420.
14. Nassal, M. and Rieger, A. (1996) A bulged region of the hepatitis B virus RNA encapsidation signal contains the replication origin for discontinuous first-strand DNA synthesis. *J. Virol.* **70**, 2764–2773.
15. Tavis, J. E., Perri, S., and Ganem, D. (1994) Hepadnavirus reverse transcription initiates within the stem loop of the RNA packaging signal and employs a novel strand transfer. *J. Virol.* **68**, 3536–3543.
16. Wang, G. H. and Seeger, C. (1993) Novel mechanism for reverse transcription in hepatitis B viruses. *J. Virol.* **67**, 6507–6512.
17. Loeb, D. D. and Tian, R. (1995) Transfer of the minus strand of DNA during hepadnavirus replication is not invariable but prefers a specific location. *J. Virol.* **69**, 6886–6891.
18. Lanford, R. E., Notvall, L., and Beames, B. (1995) Nucleotide priming and reverse transcriptase activity of hepatitis B virus polymerase expressed in insect cells. *J. Virol.* **69**, 4431–4439.
19. Lanford, R. E., Kim, Y. H., Lee, H., Notvall, L., and Beames, B. (1999) Mapping of the hepatitis B virus reverse transcriptase TP and RT domains by transcomplementation for nucleotide priming and by protein protein interaction. *J. Virol.* **73**, 1885–1893.
20. Wang, G. H., Zoulim, F., Leber, E. H., Kitson, J., and Seeger, C. (1994) Role of RNA in enzymatic activity of the reverse transcriptase of hepatitis B viruses. *J. Virol.* **68**, 8437–8442.
21. Beck, J., Bartos, H., and Nassal, M. (1997) Experimental confirmation of a hepatitis B virus (HBV) epsilon-like bulge-and-loop structure in avian HBV RNA encapsidation signals. *Virology* **227**, 500–504.

22. Hu, J. and Seeger, C. (1996) Hsp90 is required for the activity of a hepatitis B virus reverse transcriptase. *Proc. Natl. Acad. Sci. USA* **93**, 1060–1064.
23. Hu, J., Toft, D. O., and Seeger, C. (1997) Hepadnavirus assembly and reverse transcription require a multi-component chaperone complex which is incorporated into nucleocapsids. *EMBO J.* **16**, 59–68.
24. Buchner, J. (1999) Hsp90 & Co. a holding for folding. *Trends Biochem. Sci.* **24**, 136–141.
25. Holt, S. E., Aisner, D. L., Baur, J., et al. (1999) Functional requirement of p23 and Hsp90 in telomerase complexes. *Genes Dev.* **13**, 817–826.
26. Beck, J. and Nassal, M. (1998) Formation of a functional hepatitis B virus replication initiation complex involves a major structural alteration in the RNA template. *Mol. Cell. Biol.* **18**, 6265–6272.
27. Schaaf, S. G., Beck, J., and Nassal, M. (1999) A small 2'-OH- and base-dependent recognition element downstream of the initiation site in the RNA encapsidation signal is essential for hepatitis B virus replication initiation. *J. Biol. Chem.* **274**, 37,787–37,794.
28. Tavis, J. E., Massey, B., and Gong, Y. (1998) The duck hepatitis B virus polymerase is activated by its RNA packaging signal, epsilon. *J. Virol.* **72**, 5789–5796.
29. Hu, J. and Seeger, C. (1996) Expression and characterization of hepadnavirus reverse transcriptases. *Methods Enzymol.* **275**, 195–208.
30. Hannig, G. and Makrides, S. C. (1998) Strategies for optimizing heterologous protein expression in *Escherichia coli. Trends Biotechnol.* **16**, 54–60.
31. Baneyx, F. (1999) Recombinant protein expression in *Escherichia coli. Curr. Opin. Biotechnol.* **10**, 411–421.
32. Beck, J. and Nassal, M. (2001) Reconstitution of a functional duck hepatitis B virus replication initiation complex from separate reverse transcriptase domains expressed in *Escherichia coli. J. Virol.* **75**, 7410–7419.
33. Mandart, E., Kay, A., and Galibert, F. (1984) Nucleotide sequence of a cloned duck hepatitis B virus genome: comparison with woodchuck and human hepatitis B virus sequences. *J. Virol.* **49**, 782–792.
34. Obert, S., Zachmann-Brand, B., Deindl, E., Tucker, W., Bartenschlager, R., and Schaller, H. (1996) A spliced hepadnavirus RNA that is essential for virus replication. *EMBO J.* **15**, 2565–2574.

31

Hepatitis B Viruses

A Triple Threat for Malignant Transformation of Hepatocytes

Charles E. Rogler

1. Introduction

1.1. General Description of Different Groups of Hepadnaviruses

The aim of this chapter is to provide a succinct and integrated view of hepadnaviral infections and the broad roles of these viruses in malignant transformation in the liver. This is not an exhaustive review of hepatitis B virus (HBV) molecular biology or the literature, and as such, only selected references are included. Extensive reviews of the subject can be found elsewhere and are referred to in this text *(1–4)*.

The hepadnaviruses (*Hepadnaviridae*) are DNA viruses with small DNA genomes of about 3 kbp. Following the identification of human HBV by Blumberg and colleagues in 1967 *(5)*, related viruses were soon found in woodchucks, ground squirrels, and ducks *(6)*. A major feature of hepadnaviruses is their very narrow host range and marked tissue specificity. Although the liver is the major site of viral replication, low levels of viral production have been reported in the pancreas, spleen, and peripheral blood leukocytes. The woodchuck hepatitis virus (WHV) is the mammalian virus that most closely resembles HBV in its ability to cause liver disease and, in particular, hepatocellular carcinoma (HCC; *7*).

1.2. General Description of the Viral Replication Cycle

Hepadnaviruses have partially double-stranded DNA genomes of approx 3.3 kbp that are held in a relaxed circular (RC) conformation by cohesive overlaps at their 5' ends. Following infection, the genome is converted into a covalently closed circular DNA molecule, which is localized in the nucleus, where it acts as a template for the transcription of four viral RNA species. They include pregenomic RNA (encoding the nucleocapsid protein), preS mRNA, small S mRNA, and X mRNA. Pregenomic RNA, which spans the entire genome and is terminally redundant, is packaged together with

From: *Methods in Molecular Medicine, vol. 95: Hepatitis B and D Protocols, volume 1*
Edited by: R. K. Hamatake and J. Y. N. Lau © Humana Press Inc., Totowa, NJ

the viral reverse transcriptase into subviral particles composed of 180 or 240 core subunits *(1,4)*. Following the packaging reaction, pregenomic RNA is reverse transcribed into DNA by the viral reverse transcriptase *(8)*. DNA-containing cores then interact with the viral-envelope components in the endoplasmic reticulum and, following their transport through the secretory pathway, exit the cell as enveloped virions *(1,4)*.

Although more than 90–95% of infectious Dane particles contain RC DNA genomes, approx 5% of the infectious particles contain double-strand linear (DSL) viral DNA molecules. These molecules can be circularized in hepatocytes and replicate by a mechanism that Yang and Summers have designated "illegitimate replication," because their replication leads to the formation of a spectrum of mutant viruses *(9)*. The existence of these DSL viral DNA molecules in hepatocytes may be important in hepatocarcinogenesis associated with persistent infections. Recent studies from the Rogler laboratory have shown that viruses containing only DSL DNA genomes integrate into host chromosomal DNA with a fourfold increased frequency compared with wild-type RC DNA molecules *(10)*. Newly acquired viral DNA integrations closely resemble these linear molecules in structure, whereas integrations present in HCCs from long-term carriers are generally highly rearranged, suggesting that rearrangement of integrations occurs during long-term infections *(11)*. Possible carcinogenic consequences of such rearrangements will be discussed later in this review.

2. Characteristics of Transient and Persistent Infections

2.1. Establishment and Clearance of Transient Infections

HBV generally causes transient infections in adults; however, chronic infections are common because of perinatal exposure. Transient infections are characterized by an asymptomatic incubation period that can be followed by a viremic phase, typically running a course of 1–6 mo. Although the entire hepatocyte population of the liver can be infected, virus is rapidly cleared from the serum with either coincident or delayed clearance of infected hepatocytes from the liver *(1,4)*. One scenario is that infected hepatocytes are killed by cytotoxic T lymphocytes and that regenerated hepatocytes are protected from reinfection by antibodies against the virus or by a cellular antiviral response induced by cytokines secreted by infiltrating lymphocytes *(12–14)*. An alternative possibility, initially proposed by the Chisari laboratory, is that cytokines induce an antiviral response in hepatocytes that leads to the elimination of virus and cure of the infected hepatocytes in the absence of hepatocyte killing *(12,15)*. These hypotheses are not mutually exclusive, and both mechanisms appear to play a role in natural infections, as is described below.

The second hypothesis is supported by a growing body of evidence that includes elegant studies with HBV transgenic mice. These studies demonstrate rapid clearance of viral RNA and DNA replication forms that is dependent upon the secretion of interferon γ and tumor necrosis factor α by lymphocytes that migrate to the liver *(16)*. Furthermore, infection studies with chimpanzees have shown that there is a period of viral clearance during acute infection when interferon γ and TNFα are produced and hepatocyte death is not apparent *(15)*. This is followed by a later phase of hepatocyte death, when neutralizing antibodies are produced. These data suggest that viral clearance in chimpanzees may have a previously unappreciated biphasic nature. During the first phase, virus titer is dramatically reduced via a noncytopathic cytokine–mediated mechanism; this phase is followed by a second phase in which the immune system may clear the remaining infected hepatocytes via cytopathic, CTL-mediated clearance mechanism *(15)*.

2.2. Establishment of Persistent Infections

When envelope protein particles (hepatitis B surface antigen [HBsAg]) persist in the serum of an individual for 6 mo or longer, the infection is considered chronic. The basis for chronic infection lies in the failure of the immune response to clear the infection. Consequently, infections are almost always chronic following exposure of newborn children or of immunocompromised individuals. Chronic infections in adults are often associated with severe and progressive liver disease, leading to cirrhosis and liver cancer *(2,3)*.

Interferon alpha, lamivudine, and adefovir are currently approved therapeutic agents for chronic HBV infection. The mechanism by which interferon alpha suppresses viral replication is not yet known. One possibility is that it suppresses viral replication in hepatocytes; another is that it indirectly stimulates the immune system. The latter possibility is supported by evidence indicating that patients with liver disease as a result of a strong immune response to infected hepatocytes have the best chance for recovery during therapy with the drug. The mechanism by which lamivudine inhibits viral replication is inhibition of viral DNA synthesis by the HBV reverse transcriptase *(17)*. As a consequence of monotherapy, lamivudine-resistant variants replace wild-type virus after about 1 yr of therapy. However, lamivudine-resistant variants appear to replicate at an attenuated level, compared with wild-type virus, and, perhaps as a consequence, lamivudine therapy is generally associated with noticeable amelioration of liver disease *(17)*.

3. Persistent Infections: A Triple Threat for the Malignant Transformation of Hepatocytes

3.1. The First Threat: A Cycle of Cell Death and Regeneration

Persistent infections are established in the liver when the host mounts an incomplete immune response to viral infection of the liver, as discussed above. The limited immune responses are generally responsible for a spectrum of pathophysiological reactions in the liver that vary from mild portal hepatitis to chronic active hepatitis. In humans, cirrhosis is a common sequela of persistent HBV infection, whereas in WHV-carrier woodchucks cirrhosis does not occur *(2,3)*. However, in both humans and woodchucks, a central ingredient provided by the immune response is the initiation and maintenance of a continuous cycle of cell death and regeneration in the liver. This cycle ensures that mutations that occur in regenerating hepatocytes will be fixed into cells of the next generation, and the cycle also provides an environment in which cells with a selective advantage will have the opportunity to be selectively amplified because of the need for hepatocyte replacement *(2,3)*. During long-term persistent infections, stress is placed on the regenerative capacity of the liver, and the liver begins to call upon its stem-cell compartment for replacement of lost hepatocytes.

The growth and accumulation of liver stem cells, called "oval cells," during chronic infection were first observed in WHV-carrier woodchucks *(18)*. A monoclonal antibody marker provided evidence that woodchuck oval cells proliferate near the portal tracts and then differentiate into hepatocytes as they expand out into the liver parenchyma. Interestingly, the monoclonal antibody identified some of these hepatocytes in precancerous lesions, called altered hepatic foci (AHF, ***19***). Since HCCs develop from progression of cells in AHFs, these data, plus extensive literature from rat hepatocarcinogenesis, support the notion that woodchuck oval cells are precursors of at least a subset of HCCs *(18)*. The amplification of oval cells has broad significance since it has also been confirmed to occur in HBV carrier livers *(3)*.

Under certain circumstances, HBV replication causes the production of ground-glass hepatocytes that accumulate large amounts of HBV envelope protein. A transgenic mouse model in which the large HBV envelope protein was highly overexpressed led to the production of hepatocytes in the mouse liver that resemble ground-glass cells. This pattern of large envelope overexpression caused hepatocyte injury and death and induced liver regeneration and eventually HCC in virtually all the mice *(20)*. It is interesting to note that only those hepatocytes that deleted or inactivated the transgene and eliminated envelope-protein expression survived to progress to malignancy *(20)*. Within this chronic nonimmune-mediated environment of liver damage, in which toxic oxygen radicals are overproduced and random mutagenesis is greatly increased, hepatocarcinogenesis ensues via a typical multistage mechanism. HBV DNA integration does not occur in this model because only the HBV envelope gene is present as a transgene in the mice.

These data demonstrate that overexpression of viral protein can act as a carcinogenic agent, but that the agent can be eliminated from the cells and the cells can continue to progress toward cancer. We will see later that a similar situation may exist with the HBV X protein, which is expressed during persistent infection but is absent from many HCCs. The multistage nature of hepatocarcinogenesis in mice, with the production of precancerous foci that are negative for HBV envelope proteins, clearly demonstrates the need for additional mutagenic events for carcinogenesis to proceed *(20)*. In WHV and HBV carriers, these events may be mediated by viral DNA integrations.

3.2. The Second Threat: Oncogene Activation and "Hit-and-Run" Mutagenesis via Viral DNA Integration

3.2.1. Oncogene and Growth-Factor Activation

Hepadnavirus DNA integrations into host chromosomes were first implicated in hepatocarcinogenesis, when they were observed to occur in all of the cells in HCCs from HBV carriers and soon after in HCCs from WHV-carrier woodchucks *(2,3)*. Since clonal integrations of other retroviruses had been shown to activate a cellular proto-oncogene, c-*myc*, hepadnaviral integrations were cloned and sequenced with the aim of identifying a commonly activated cellular proto-oncogene. In the case of WHV, this search led the Buendia laboratory to the identification of a *myc* gene family member, N-*myc*2, which was commonly activated in HCCs that arise in chronic carrier woodchucks *(21)*.

Interestingly, WHV DNA integrations were observed in two cellular N-*myc* genes located at two separate locations in the woodchuck genome. They included the normal N-*myc* proto-oncogene and a second N-*myc*2 gene, which is a functional retroposon ***(21)***. The N-myc2 retroposon is not expressed in normal liver and is the most frequent WHV integration target. The predominant mechanism of activation is through integration of a fragment of the WHV genome that contains either of the two strong WHV liver-specific enhancer elements. This "enhancer-insertion" mechanism is characteristic in that integration of the enhancer element can occur immediately upstream of N-*myc*2 or in the 3' untranslated region of the gene ***(2,21)***.

In an unexpected finding, a second common long-distance integration site was identified approximately 200 kb upstream from the N-*myc*2 gene ***(22)***. This site does not contain an expressed gene, and WHV DNA integration at this site is believed to mediate N-*myc*2 expression also via a long-distance enhancer-insertion mechanism that may utilize a chromatin-matrix attachment site that is near the integration site ***(22)***. A direct role of N-*myc* in the tumorigeneic phenotype has been confirmed in N-*myc* transgenic mice and in cell cultures that lose oncogenic properties when N-*myc*2 is inactivated using antisense technology ***(23)***.

Although studies with WHV DNA integrations have been successful in linking viral DNA integration with a commonly activated oncogene ***(2,3,21,22)***, parallel studies with HBV DNA integrations have not successfully identified a commonly activated oncogene ***(2,3)***. However, HBV DNA integrations into some very provocative and potentially oncogenic genes have been identified ***(24–26)***. As the list of genes affected by HBV DNA integrations in tumors increases, multiple pathways have been implicated in hepatocarcinogenesis. Alteration of a cyclin A gene implicated HBV integration in cell-cycle regulation, integration in and near a steroid hormone receptor and a thyroid-hormone receptor-associated protein suggests HBV-mediated alteration of hormone signaling in hepatocarcinogenesis, and identification of HBV integration into a telomerase–reverse transcriptase gene suggests modification of hepatocyte immortalization ***(24–26)***.

3.2.1.1. Coexpression of Insulinlike Growth Factor 2

One general finding has been that *myc* proto-oncogene activation is a double-edged sword in that it can either lead to cell proliferation or can promote apoptosis of cells, depending on the existence of co-factors. Many studies have shown that co-expression of a growth factor along with c-*myc* drives cells into growth as opposed to apoptosis. In this regard, a key observation in liver was the coordinate overexpression of the fetal liver growth factor IGF-2 plus N-*myc*2 in precancerous lesions in persistently infected woodchuck liver ***(27)***. Furthermore, IGF-2 was directly shown to block N-*myc*2–induced apoptosis of cultured liver epithelial cells and promotes the growth of cultured hepatocytes by an autocrine mechanism ***(19)***. Overexpression of these two genes is also maintained in woodchuck HCCs ***(26)***, and IGF-2 is the most commonly overexpressed growth factor in human HCCs ***(2,3)***.

Another major breakthrough came with the discovery of mutations in the β-catenin gene in many woodchuck and human HCCs ***(28)***. The mutations occurred in regions of the β-catenin gene that stabilized the protein and enabled it to be translocated to the nucleus. In the nucleus, β-catenin activates expression of cyclin genes and *myc* genes to promote malignant transformation ***(28)***.

3.2.2. Hit-and-Run Mutagenesis

HBV DNA integrations are nearly always found in HCCs that arise in young children. These integrations generally comprise viral DNA that is collinear with the HBV genome and have viral-cell DNA junctions within or near the ends of DSL HBV DNA molecules. In contrast, integrations present in tumors from older adults are almost exclusively highly rearranged, with inverted repeats and deletions of HBV DNA ***(3,11)***. Another common feature of these integrations is that they are associated with alterations of host DNA at the site of integration. Host chromosomal abnormalities linked to HBV integrations include translocations, deletions, and direct or inverted duplications ***(3,29,30)***. These mechanisms can function to inactivate tumor-suppressor genes as well as activate proto-oncogenes.

A predicted feature of the above observations is that newly acquired hepadnaviral integrations may be unstable in the genome and may function as "hit-and-run" mutagens that mediate the rearrangement of chromosomal DNA. Recent studies of the natural history of hepadnaviral integrations in cell cultures have directly demonstrated the hit-and-run mechanism and suggested that the loss of newly acquired integrations may be an important mutagenic mechanism during hepatocarcinogenesis ***(30–32)***. For example, in cell culture, host chromosomal DNA adjacent to integrated viral DNA was deleted when a viral DNA integration was lost from the cells, and a cell clone with an altered integration profile exhibited greatly increased ability to grow on soft agar ***(30)***.

Additional studies have shown that duck hepatitis B virus (DHBV) integrates frequently during acute infections. Furthermore, DHBV and HBV DNA integration in cell cultures is dramatically increased by treatments that promote DNA nicking or that block DNA repair in hepatocytes ***(31,32)***. These data support the hypothesis that sites of DNA damage may serve as integration sites. Viral DNA integrations can also accumulate in sequential cell generations ***(31)***. However, linear accumulation may be counterbalanced by hit-and-run mechanisms that reduce the total integration load of a cell.

3.2.2.1. Integration Precursor Molecules and Topoisomerase I

Cell-culture studies have also demonstrated that DSL DHBV DNA molecules integrate at a much higher frequency than circular DHBV DNA molecules ***(10)***. Linearization of viral DNA at specific sites at the 5' ends of minus- and plus-strands must occur in order for integration to preferably occur at these sites. One cellular enzyme that may participate in the integration mechanism is topoisomerase I, because it cleaves viral and cellular DNA at or near preferred sites of integration, and this enzyme can mediate nonhomologous recombination events of foreign DNA with host chromosomes ***(33)***. In fact, WHV DNA integration events can be duplicated in vitro with purified topoisomerase I, and sequence analysis of naturally occurring HBV DNA integration junctions shows an overwhelming association with preferred topoisomerase I cleavage sites both in viral and cellular DNAs at the junctions ***(34,35)***.

3.3. The Third Threat: The Hepadnavirus X Protein

A role for the mammalian hepadnavirus X (HBx) protein in hepatocarcinogenesis has been proposed from the time it was first identified in a position in the HBV genome that is analogous to the position of other oncogenes in oncogenic retroviruses *(2,3)*. However, only recently have several lines of evidence been obtained to link X-gene expression with malignant transformation of hepatocytes. The current challenge in the field is to begin to link together the disparate lines of evidence from many variable experimental systems into coherent, testable models for liver, relevant animal, and cell-culture systems. Several laboratories have begun to identify common cellular pathways affected by HBx in relevant cell-culture and transgenic mouse systems *(36)*.

3.3.1. Expression of X Protein in Chronically Infected Liver and HCCs

The X-gene promoter is weak, and a chronic problem in the field has been the determination of when and where X protein is actually expressed in chronic infections. The clearest demonstration of the presence and quantitation of X protein comes from studies of chronically infected woodchuck liver using an excellent rabbit polyclonal antibody against the complete WHV X (WHx) protein *(37)*. These studies clearly detected WHx in persistently infected hepatocytes and estimated the steady-state level to be approx 40,000 molecules per hepatocyte. Metabolic labeling demonstrated that 80% of the rapidly labeled X was cytoplasmic, with 20% located in the nucleus *(38)*.

An important finding of the woodchuck studies was that WHx was only present in tissues that performed productive WHV replication *(37)*. This included a subset of woodchuck HCCs that continued to replicate WHV *(37)*. It is important to note that WHx was *not* observed in any poorly differentiated woodchuck HCCs that were nonpermissive for WHV replication. This finding has important implications for hepatocarcinogenesis in woodchucks because it suggests that the WHx protein associates most closely with viral replication and is not required for malignancy in poorly differentiated HCCs that are nonpermissive for WHV replication.

The expression of HBx from integrated hepadnavirus DNAs has also been a controversial topic. However, recent elegant studies from the Brechot laboratory have identified HBV DNA integrations that contain mutant HBx genes that have important antiapoptotic activities *(39)*. These studies have directly demonstrated that mutant HBx proteins can be expressed from HBV integrations and that their anti-apoptotic activities can function to promote carcinogenic progression in the liver *(40)*. Both HBV and WHV transgenic mouse data support a weak tumor-promoter role for their respective X proteins *(37)*.

3.3.2. Biological Activities of X

The first biological activity associated with mammalian X proteins was that of a transacting factor *(2,3)*. In this capacity, HBx can transactivate a wide variety of promoters upstream from many different genes in a wide variety of cell types *(2,3)*. This initial activity led investigators to search for molecular mechanisms for the action of HBx and WHx and to characterize their cellular functions.

X-gene functions have been the subject of controversy. However, an increasing body of evidence has pointed to a linked group of cellular signaling pathways affected by HBx under physiologically relevant conditions. Initially, HBx was shown to activate the Ras signal transduction pathway in a variety of hepatocellular and nonhepatocellular cell lines ***(41)***. Depending on the specific culture conditions, HBx may be pro- or antiapoptotic. An extensive series of reports in this area focused on the Src signal transduction pathway, which can lead to the transactivation of important tumorigenesis genes such as c-*myc* ***(42)***. The current challenge for researchers in the signal transduction area is to determine how these signaling pathways are altered in hepatocytes during persistent infections. Clearly, X expression alone is insufficient to fully transform hepatocytes. However, recent linkage of HBx action with calcium mobilization and viral replication appears to be a key to understanding its regulatory properties and potential to act as a tumor-promoting agent ***(36)***.

The effect of HBx on tumor-suppressor pathways has also not escaped investigation. One of the most important tumor suppressors is p53, and a series of papers have provided a link between HBx and p53 action ***(1–3)***. Normally, p53 expression is upregulated in response to cell stress, and p53 sets in motion a set of gene activities that can either lead to apoptosis or cell-cycle exit. Thus, knocking out p53 removes an important brake on the cell cycle and allows mutant cells to survive and progress to malignancy. Therefore, the finding that HBx binds to p53 and blocks some of its biological actions is significant.

The initial reports have been confirmed in several cell-culture systems and in one transgenic mouse line; however, interpretation of how these findings actually relate to hepatocarcinogenesis in carrier livers remains to be elucidated. One attractive hypothesis is that mutant or wild-type HBx proteins present in the cytoplasm bind to p53 and prevent it from translocating into the nucleus ***(1,4)***. This mechanism would require continuous expression of X proteins, which is not the case in many HCCs ***(37)***. However, a significant subset of HCCs that are nonpermissive for HBV replication continue to express mutant HBx from integrated templates ***(40)***. In fact, some of these mutant-integrated HBx genes have been shown to block p53–mediated apoptosis.

4. Summary

In light of the combination of procarcinogenic mechanisms briefly outlined above, it is understandable that in the WHV-carrier woodchucks, there is virtually a 100% lifetime incidence of HCC and that in male HBV carriers there appears to be at least a 40% lifetime risk of HCC. The current therapies that limit HBV replication may also limit viral DNA integration and reduce the rate of hepatocyte turnover in the liver. Thus, the triple threat may be significantly reduced. Prospective studies of patients on long-term treatment protocols will hopefully reveal a reduced risk of HCC.

References

1. Ganem, D. and Schneider, R.J. (2000) The molecular biology of hepatitis B viruses. In: Knipe, D. and Howley, P. (eds), *Fields Virology*, Lippincott, New York.

2. Buendia, M. A. (1998) Hepatitis B viruses and cancerogenesis. *Biomed. Pharmacother.* **52**, 34–43.
3. Rogler, C. E., Rogler, L. E., Yang, D., Breiteneder-Geleef, S., Gong, S., and Wang, H. P. (1995) Contributions of hepadnavirus research to our understanding of hepatocarcinogenesis. In: Jirtle, R. (ed), *Liver Regeneration and Carcinogenesis: Cellular and Molecular Mechanism*, Academic Press, New York, 113–140.
4. Seeger, C. and Mason, W. S. (2000) Hepatitis B virus biology. *Microbiol. Mol. Biol. Rev.* **64**, 51–68.
5. Blumberg, B. S., Gerstley, B. J. S., Hungerford, D. A., London, W. T., and Sutnik, A. I. (1967) A serum antigen (Australia antigen) in Down's syndrome, leukemia and hepatitis. *Ann. Intern. Med.* **66**, 924–931.
6. Summers, J. (1981) Three recently described animal virus models of human hepatitis B virus. *Hepatology* **1**, 179–183.
7. Summers, J., Smolec, J., and Snyder, R. (1978) A virus similar to human hepatitis B virus associated with hepatitis and hepatoma in woodchucks. Proc. Natl. Acad. Sci. USA **75**, 4533–4537.
8. Summers, J. and Mason, W. S. (1982) Replication of the genome of a hepatitis B-like virus by reverse transcription of an RNA intermediate. *Cell* **29**, 403–415.
9. Yang, W. and Summers, J. (1995) Illegitimate replication of linear hepadnaviral DNA through nonhomologous recombination. *J. Virol.* **69**, 4029–4036.
10. Gong, S., Jensen, A., and Rogler, C. E. (1999) Double-stranded linear duck hepatitis B virus (DHBV) stably integrates at a higher frequency than wild-type DHBV in LMH chicken hepatoma cells. *J. Virol.* **73**, 1492–1502.
11. Nagaya, T., Nakamua, T., Tokina, T., et al. (1987) The mode of hepatitis B virus DNA integration in chromosomes of human hepatocellular carcinoma. *Genes Dev.* **1**, 773–782.
12. Chisari, F. V. (1997) Cytotoxic T cells and viral hepatitis. *J. Clin. Invest.* **99**, 1472–1477.
13. Guo, J.-T., Zhou, H., Liu, C., et al. (2000) Apoptosis and regeneration of hepatocytes during recovery from transient hepadnavirus infection. *J. Virol.* **74**, 1495–1505.
14. Kajino, K., Jilbert, A. R., Saputelli, J., Aldrich, C. E., Cullen, J., and Mason, W. S. (1994) Woodchuck hepatitis virus infections: very rapid recovery after a prolonged viremia and infection of virtually every hepatocyte. *J. Virol.* **68**, 5792–5803.
15. Guidotti, L. G., Rochford, R., Chung, J., Shapiro, M., Purcell, R., and Chisari, F. V. (1999) Viral clearance without destruction of infected cells during acute HBV infection. *Science* **284**, 825–829.
16. Guidotti, L. G., Ishikawa, T., Hobbs, M. V., Matzke, B., Schreiber, R., and Chisari, F. V. (1996) Intracellular inactivation of the hepatitis B virus by cytotoxic T lymphocytes. *Immunity* **4**, 25–36.
17. Chayama, K., Suzuki, Y., Kobayashi, M., et al. (1998) Emergence and takeover of YMDD motif mutant hepatitis B virus during long-term lamivudine therapy and re-takeover by wild type after cessation of therapy. *Hepatology* **27**, 1711–1716.
18. Fu, X. X., Su, C. Y., Lee, Y., et al. (1988) Insulin-like growth factor II expression and oval cell proliferation associated with hepatocarcinogenesis in woodchuck hepatitis virus carriers. *J. Virol.* **62**, 3422–3430.
19. Yang, D., Hixson, D., Faris, R., Affigne, S., and Rogler, C. E. (1996) Insulin-like growth factor II blocks cell death in woodchuck liver epithelial cells which overexpress N-myc2. *J. Virol.* **70**, 6260–6268.
20. Chisari, F. C., Opchin, K. K., Moriyama, T., et al. (1989) Molecular pathogenesis of hepatocellular carcinoma in hepatitis B virus transgenic mice. *Cell* **59**, 1145–1156.

21. Fourel, G., Trepo, C., Bougueleret, L., et al. (1990) Frequent activation of N-myc genes by hepadnavirus insertion in woodchuck liver tumours. *Nature* **347**, 294–298.
22. Fourel, G., Conturier, J., Wei, Y., Apiou, F., Tiollais, P., and Buendia, M. A. (1994) Evidence for long-range oncogene activation by hepadnavirus insertion. *EMBO J.* **13**, 2526–2534.
23. Wang, H. P., Zhang, L., Dandri, M., and Rogler, C. E. (1998) Antisense downregulation of N-myc 1 in woodchuck hepatoma cells reverses the malignant phenotype. *J. Virol.* **72**, 2192–2198.
24. Wang, J., Zindy, F., Chenivesse, X., Lamas, E., Henglein, B., and Brechot, C. (1992) Modification of cyclin A gene by hepatitis B virus integration in a hepatocellular carcinoma. *Oncogene* **7**, 1653–1656.
25. Dejean, A., Bougueleret, L., Grzeschik, K. H., and Tiollais, P. (1986) Hepatitis B virus DNA integration in a sequence homologous to v-erb-A and steroid receptor genes in hepatocellular carcinoma. *Nature* **322**, 70–72.
26. Gozuacik, D., Murakami, Y., Saigo, K., et al. (2001) Identification of human cancer-related genes by naturally occurring hepatitis B virus DNA tagging. *Oncogene* **20**, 6233–6240.
27. Yang, D., Alt, E., and Rogler, C. E. (1993) Coordinate expression of N-myc 2 and IGF-II in precancerous altered hepatic foci in woodchuck hepatitis virus carriers. *Cancer Res.* **53**, 2020–2027.
28. de La Coste, A., Romagnolo, B., Billuart, P., et al. (1998) Somatic mutations of the beta-catenin gene are frequent in mouse and human hepatocellular carcinomas. *Proc. Natl. Acad. Sci. USA* **95**, 8847–8851.
29. Hino, O., Shows, T. B., and Rogler, C. E. (1986) Hepatitis B virus integration site in hepatocellular carcinoma at chromosome 17:18 translocation. *Proc. Natl. Acad. Sci. USA* **83**, 8338–8342.
30. Gong, S. S., Jensen, A. D, and Rogler, C. E. (1996) Loss and acquisition of duck hepatitis B virus integrations in lineages of LMH-D2 chicken hepatoma cells. *J. Virol.* **70**, 2000–2007.
31. Petersen, J., Buerkle, A., Zhang, L., and Rogler, C. E. (1997) Increase in the frequency of hepadnavirus DNA integrations by oxidative DNA damage or inhibition of DNA repair. *J. Virol.* **71**, 5455–5463.
32. Dandri, M., Burda, M. R., Burkle, A., et al. (2002) Increase in de novo HBV DNA integrations in response to oxidative DNA damage or inhibition of poly(ADP-ribosyl)ation. *Hepatology* **35**, 217–223.
33. Pourquier, P., Jensen, A. D., Gong, S. S., Pommier, Y., and Rogler, C. E. (1999) Human DNA topoisomerase I-mediated cleavage and recombination of duck hepatitis B virus DNA in vitro. *Nucl. Acids Res.* **27**, 1919–1925.
34. Wang, H. P. and Rogler, C. E. (1991) Topoisomerase I mediated integration of hepadnavirus DNA 'in vitro.' *J. Virol.* **65**, 2381–2392.
35. Schirmacher, P., Wang, H. P., Stahnke, G., Will, H., and Rogler, C. E. (1995) Sequences and structures at hepadnaviral integration recombination sites implicate topoisomerase I in hepadnaviral DNA rearrangements and integration. *J. Hepatol.* **22**, 21–
36. Bouchard M. J., Wang L. H., and Schneider R. J. (2001) Calcium signaling by HBx protein in hepatitis B virus DNA replication. *Science* **294**, 2376–2378.
37. Dandri, M., Schirmacher, P., and Rogler, C. E. (1996) Woodchuck hepatitis virus X protein is present in chronically infected woodchuck liver and woodchuck hepatocellular carcinomas which are permissive for viral replication. *J. Virol.* **70**, 5246–5254.
38. Dandri, M., Petersen, J., Stockert, R., Harris, T., and Rogler, C. E. (1998) Metabolic labeling of woodchuck hepatitis virus X protein in naturally infected hepatocytes reveals a bimodal half-life and associated with the nuclear framework. *J. Virol.* **72**, 9359–9364.

39. Tu, H., Bonura, C., Giannini, C., et al. (2001) Biological impact of natural COOH-terminal deletions of hepatitis B virus X protein in hepatocellular carcinoma tissues. *Can. Res.* **61**, 7803–7810.
40. Sirma, H., Giannini, C., Poussin, K., Paterlini, P., Kremsdorf, D., and Brechot, C. (1999) Hepatitis B virus X mutants present in hepatocellular carcinoma tissue abrogate both the antiproliferative and transactivation effects of HBx. *Oncogene* **18**, 4848–4859.
41. Benn, J. and Schneider, R. J. (1994) Hepatitis B virus HBx protein activates Ras-GTP complex formation and establishes a Ras, Raf, MAP kinase signaling cascade. *Proc. Natl. Acad. Sci. USA* **91**, 10,350–10,354.
42. Klein, N. P., Bouchard, M. J., Wang, L. H., Kobarg, C., and Schneider, R. J. (1999) Src kinases involved in hepatitis B virus replication. *EMBO J.* **18**, 5019–5027.

Index